Comprehensive Aesthetic Rejuvenation

Series in Cosmetic and Laser Therapy

Series Editors

David J. Goldberg, Nicholas J. Lowe, and Gary P. Lask

Published in association with the *Journal of Cosmetic and Laser Therapy*

Comprehensive Aesthetic Rejuvenation
A Regional Approach

Edited by

Jenny Kim, MD PhD

*Associate Clinical Professor of Medicine, Division of Dermatology, David Geffen School of Medicine,
University of California, Los Angeles, and Department of Dermatology,
Veteran Affairs Greater Los Angeles Healthcare System,
Los Angeles, California, USA*

Gary Lask, MD

*Clinical Professor and Director of Dermatologic Surgery and the Dermatology Laser Center,
David Geffen School of Medicine, University of California, Los Angeles, California, USA*

Andrew Nelson, MD

*Assistant Clinical Professor, Department of Dermatology, Tufts University School of Medicine,
Boston, Massachusetts, USA*

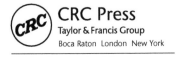

CRC Press
Taylor & Francis Group
Boca Raton London New York

CRC Press is an imprint of the
Taylor & Francis Group, an **informa** business

CRC Press
Taylor & Francis Group
6000 Broken Sound Parkway NW, Suite 3000
Boca Raton, FL 33487-2742

First issued in paperback 2019

ISBN-13: 978-0-415-45894-8 (hbk)
ISBN-13: 978-0-367-38194-3 (pbk)

Library of Congress Cataloging-in-Publication Data

Comprehensive aesthetic rejuvenation : a regional approach / edited by Jenny Kim, Gary Lask, Andrew Nelson.
    p. ; cm. -- (Series in cosmetic and laser therapy)
  Includes bibliographical references and index.
  ISBN 978-0-415-45894-8 (hardback : alk. paper)
  I. Kim, Jenny (Jenny Jiyon) II. Lask, Gary P. (Gary Philip) III. Nelson, Andrew, 1979- IV. Series: Series in cosmetic and laser therapy.
  [DNLM: 1. Reconstructive Surgical Procedures--methods. 2. Aging--physiology. 3. Esthetics. 4. Rejuvenation. 5. Surgical Procedures, Minimally Invasive--methods. WO 600]
  617.9'52--dc23

2011033579

Typeset by Exeter Premedia Services Private Ltd., Chennai, India

Visit the Taylor & Francis Web site at
http://www.taylorandfrancis.com

and the CRC Press Web site at
http://www.crcpress.com

Contents

Contributors

Gurpreet Ahluwalia
Dermatology Clinical R&D, Allergan, Inc., Irvine, California, USA

Mathew Avram
Wellman Center for Photomedicine, Department of Dermatology, Massachusetts General Hospital, Harvard Medical School, Boston, Massachusetts, USA

Frederick Beddingfield
Division of Dermatology, David Geffen School of Medicine, University of California, Los Angeles, and Dermatology Clinical R&D, Allergan, Inc., Irvine, California, USA

David Beynet
Division of Dermatology, David Geffen School of Medicine, University of California, Los Angeles, California, USA

James C. Collyer
Division of Dermatology, University of Washington and Westside Dermatology, Seattle, Washington, USA

Andrew L. DaLio
Department of Microsurgery, Division of Plastic and Reconstructive Surgery, David Geffen School of Medicine, University of California, Los Angeles, California, USA

Joseph F. Greco
Division of Dermatology, David Geffen School of Medicine, University of California, Los Angeles, California, USA

H. Ray Jalian
Wellman Center for Photomedicine, Department of Dermatology, Massachusetts General Hospital, Boston, Massachusetts, USA

Derek Jones
Skin Care and Laser Physicians of Beverly Hills, and Division of Dermatology, David Geffen School of Medicine, University of California, Los Angeles, California, USA

Jenny Kim
Division of Dermatology, David Geffen School of Medicine, University of California, Los Angeles, California, USA

Gary Lask
Division of Dermatology, David Geffen School of Medicine, University of California, Los Angeles, California, USA

Tom S. Liu
Liu Plastic Surgery, Los Altos, California, USA

Paul J. McAndrews
Paul J. McAndrews, MD, Inc., Pasadena, California, USA

Howard Murad
Division of Dermatology, David Geffen School of Medicine, University of California, Los Angeles, and Murad, Inc., El Segundo, California, USA

Diane Murphy
Global Medical Writing, Allergan Inc., Irvine, California, USA

Andrew Nelson
Department of Dermatology, Tufts University School of Medicine, Boston, Massachusetts, USA

Corey Powell
Sally Hershberger Salon, Los Angeles, California, USA

Quyn S. Rahman
Atlanta Dermatopathology and Pathology Associates, P.C., Atlanta, Georgia, USA

Cherilyn Sheets
Newport Coast Oral Facial Institute, Newport Beach, California, USA

Anastasia Soare
Anastasia Beverly Hills Salon, Beverly Hills, California, USA

Stefani Takahashi
Department of Dermatology, Keck School of Medicine, University of Southern California, Los Angeles, California, USA

Daniel I. Wasserman
Riverchase Dermatology and Cosmetic Surgery, Naples, Florida, USA

Jamie Zussman
Division of Dermatology, David Geffen School of Medicine, University of California, Los Angeles, California, USA

An approach to the aging process and rejuvenation
Andrew Nelson, Gary Lask, and Jenny Kim

KEY POINTS

- The goals of rejuvenation are to soften the signs of aging by minimizing and reversing the natural changes that are responsible for the aging process
- Aging occurs due to a complex interplay between intrinsic (natural) changes and extrinsic (external) damage
- In order to achieve the ideals of beauty, a multimodality approach combining many different techniques is necessary to address all of the changes
- It is our goal to describe these different techniques, as well as how they can be combined synergistically, to help your patients achieve a rested, rejuvenated appearance

---

Aging is a natural process of life. As we grow older, our features and appearance change. Some of these changes can be wonderful, while there are others that we wish we could avoid. For thousands of years, people have been trying to change their appearance in order to accentuate their desirable features while minimizing others; there are reports of cosmetics being used as far back as ancient Egypt. More recently, there has been an explosion in the number of minimally invasive procedures to help reduce the signs of aging. As a result, more patients are seeking out these minimal downtime procedures, and more physicians are offering these services.

In order to offer patients the ideal rejuvenation treatment option, it is necessary to understand the aging process and the underlying mechanism for these changes. For instance, it is important to understand the mechanistic difference between dynamic rhytides due to muscular activity versus static rhytides due to an overall loss of facial volume and hyaluronic acid. Dynamic rhytides are best addressed through the administration of botulinum toxins, while a loss of facial volume requires restoration with a dermal filler product. Throughout this book, we will discuss the aging process from a basic science perspective, as well as provide a strong clinical perspective, in order to understand the reasoning behind the different treatment options. With a thorough understanding of how the aging process results in undesired changes, it is then possible to understand the best options to reverse or minimize these effects.

It is also necessary to keep in mind that the best cosmetic outcomes will typically result from a multimodality approach. There is no single magic bullet that can address all of the different changes associated with aging. Instead, different options will address differing aspects of the aging process. By combining different approaches, it is possible to offer your patients the best opportunity to achieve their ideal goals of rejuvenation. The best results will typically occur from combining a holistic approach, beginning with good nutrition, including essential vitamins and minerals for healthy skin, topical medical therapies, injectable products, minimally invasive laser and light source therapies, and even invasive surgical procedures.

When patients present for cosmetic consultations, they typically do not ask for a specific procedure. Rather, most patients describe the areas of their face or body that have aged and changed; it is then up to the proceduralist to help the patient understand their options and make an informed decision regarding which therapeutic options will help to best achieve their goals. Throughout the remainder of this book, we will therefore approach rejuvenation from a regional body area perspective. Rather than discussing each therapy on its own, we will instead focus on how to rejuvenate an area of the body. This approach allows us to discuss all the therapeutic options for rejuvenating that body area, as well as discuss how to combine the therapies together to achieve the best outcome. This approach allows the proceduralist to offer the most comprehensive approach to rejuvenation to their patients, and to help the patients achieve their best cosmetic outcome.

THE FOUR RS OF REJUVENATION

The four Rs represent an easy and effective way to approach rejuvenation. These four aspects: relax, refill, resurface, and redrape, attempt to address the different aspects of the aging process.

Relax

Dynamic rhytides often represent one of the most visible aspects of the aging process. These lines develop from overactivity of the underlying muscles. While smiling and laughing are a part of life, the wrinkles that they cause no longer need to be. Botulinum toxins, including Botox® and Dysport®, can safely and effectively be used to temporarily reduce the appearance of these lines. Due to their effectiveness and positive outcomes, they are now the most common cosmetic procedure performed in the United States. Botulinum toxins are extremely effective in relaxing dynamic rhytides on the upper and lower face, including the neck. Rather than discussing botulinum toxins in a single section, we will focus on how to incorporate botulinum toxins into an approach to rejuvenation.

Throughout the rest of this book, we will discuss the potential uses of botulinum toxins in the rejuvenation of different regions of the body, particularly showing how to incorporate botulinum toxins into a multimodality treatment approach.

Refill

As we age, our body's natural stores of collagen, hyaluronic acid, fat, and bone slowly redistribute and decrease. These changes alter the shape of our face and body. Historically, few products were available to restore this lost volume, and these original products often had risks such as hypersensitivity allergic reactions or long-term granulomatous reactions. Fortunately, there are now products such as hyaluronic acids (Restylane®, Juvederm®), calcium hydroxylapatite (Radiesse®) and collagens that can safely and effectively replace our lost volume and restore the natural shape to our patients' faces. These filler products can be used in many areas, including the upper face, lower face, neckline, ears, and hands to replace lost volume. Throughout the book, we will discuss the safe and effective incorporation of these products into a regional rejuvenation approach.

Unfortunately, the aging process can also redistribute excess adipose tissue to areas we would prefer to avoid, such as the love handle and flank areas. While liposuction remains the gold standard for removing excess adipose tissue, there are now laser, radiofrequency, cryolipolysis, and other technologies to treat these changes through non-invasive means. An understanding of the uses of all of these technologies, as well as their limitations, is necessary to achieve complete rejuvenation for our patients.

Resurface

Extrinsic components of the aging process, particularly ultraviolet light, ultimately result in mottled discoloration, textural changes, and other undesired effects. These changes can often be some of the most visible effects of the aging process. Resurfacing the skin attempts to treat and remove these damaged superficial layers of the skin, in order to expose the healthy, less damaged skin below. There are many different approaches to resurfacing the skin, including medical therapies and chemical peels. More recently, many different laser technologies have been developed to achieve similar goals. These laser technologies range from non-ablative visible and infrared lasers to ablative CO_2 and erbium lasers. More recently, fractional devices have been developed, which attempt to achieve similar outcomes as fully ablative devices while minimizing the side effects associated.

Given the rapid development of novel technologies to resurface the skin, it is important for the physician to understand the mechanisms and theories behind these devices. With this background, it is possible for the physician to apply this knowledge and continue to evolve their practice as new devices are developed. While laser devices result in wonderful improvements for patients, the best outcomes typically occur when combining the technologies with botulinum toxins and/or dermal filler products. We will discuss each of these technologies, their application to regional body rejuvenation, and how to incorporate them into a multimodality approach to achieve the best cosmetic outcomes.

Redrape

Our initial goal for cosmetic patients is to achieve their rejuvenation goals with the safest, most effective, least downtime, minimally invasive procedures possible. There are, however, many cases where the cosmetic goals of the patient can be best addressed through surgical procedures. It is important for all proceduralists to be familiar with these procedures, their outcomes, and limitations. These surgical procedures may result in some of the most dramatic cosmetic improvements for your patients, but may also have associated downtime.

We discuss the incorporation of surgical procedures into the rejuvenation of the body. While the exact details of the surgical technique may be beyond the scope of this book, it is nonetheless important for physicians to understand and be aware of the benefits and limitations of these procedures. Physicians can then properly counsel patients on their cosmetic options, as well as help the patient to make an informed choice regarding the approach to cosmetic rejuvenation.

CONCLUSIONS

The field of cosmetic rejuvenation has undergone a dramatic transformation in the last two decades. The incorporation of botulinum toxins, dermal filler products, laser technologies, and minimally invasive surgeries allow nearly all patients to achieve their goals of cosmetic rejuvenation simply, safely, and effectively. The four Rs of rejuvenation are a simple and effective method to describe rejuvenation techniques. However, it is not possible to achieve the best outcome by only using one of these techniques. While we often talk about new technologies and techniques as being independent, the reality is that each has its benefits and limitations. Rather than focusing on each of the single techniques on their own, it is better to learn how to incorporate them together to achieve the best cosmetic outcome.

Many textbooks have been devoted to cosmetic rejuvenation. This textbook is unique in that we approach rejuvenation from a body region, multimodality approach. When your cosmetic patient presents and tells you that they want their eyes to look younger, your goal should be to think about how to incorporate botulinum toxins, dermal fillers, lasers, cosmetic peels, and surgery to achieve the best outcome. With that in mind, this textbook is organized into different sections and chapters, each focusing on a specific body region or patient type. The techniques relevant to that body region are then discussed together, focusing on all the options for rejuvenation and how to use them synergistically. With this approach in mind, proceduralists will be able to help their patients achieve their ideals of beauty and rejuvenation.

Skin aging and function
Howard Murad

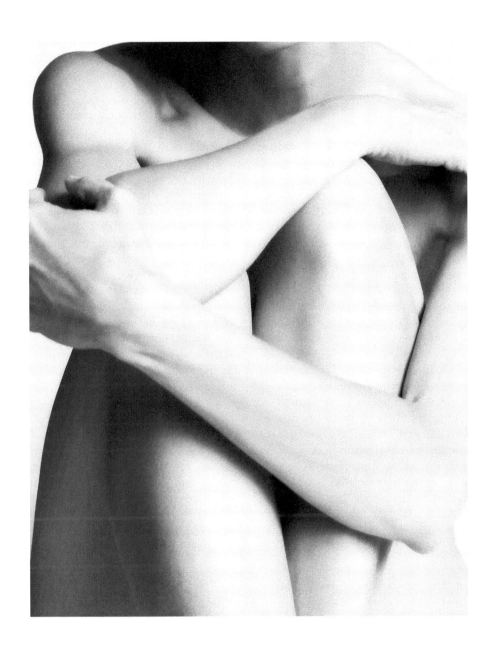

KEY POINTS

- Aging is a complex process of many interrelated changes
- Aging can be attributed to intrinsic (genetic), extrinsic (environmental), and hormonal causes
- Excessive water loss may be a prominent component of the aging process
- Dysregulation of the immune system occurs as we age, generating damaging reactive oxygen species and matrix metalloproteinases
- Hormonal changes, such as the loss of estrogen and androgen imbalance, also contribute to the aging process
- The ideal skin care protocol should attempt to maintain water in the skin, reduce the effects of free-radicals, and restore the skin's normal immune function

As long as humans have existed, the search for eternal youth has pressed forward. While the true fountain of youth eluded Spanish explorer Juan Ponce de Leon, cosmetic scientists have continued their enduring quest for the antidote to aging. Aging has perplexed researchers for millennia. Decades of scientific study have been dedicated to defining the exact mechanisms of cellular deterioration, aging, and apoptosis. Preventing and reversing cellular aging has been an eternal crusade among researchers, the new explorers, and the basis for many prescription and over-the-counter product claims. Fundamentally, we now know that the key to healthy skin is found at the cellular level and that a youthful epidermis is dependent on an optimal cellular condition. In short, healthy cells function properly and replicate predictably, preserving a person's health, and ultimately outward appearance, until natural aging can no longer be stalled.

There are more than 300 theories on aging. The most likely theory is that cells lose their ability to reproduce because of accumulated damage. That damage can be influenced or even caused by several forces such as intrinsic, extrinsic, or hormonal influences. In addition, systemic diseases and the state of the patient's immunity are also factors in this process. However, at the top of the list, cellular damage occurs because of free radicals or reactive oxygen species (ROS).

To devise an effective multilateral, whole-health campaign that promotes healthy skin, a keen understanding of aging must be gleaned.

TYPES OF AGING

Aging is subdivided into three areas: intrinsic (genetic), extrinsic (environmental), and hormonal aging.

Intrinsic aging is considered the natural aging process apart from sun and pollutant exposure or ingested toxins, etc., and is largely the result of genetics. Intrinsic aging can be determined through heredity; thus, a patient's parents will offer clues to his or her aging process. Intrinsic aging causes collagen and elastin reductions in addition to intracellular water loss.

Extrinsic aging is environmental aging and results because of a combination of external injury and compromised internal cellular functions. As such, it is a type of aging that can be controlled. Factors such as sun exposure, smoking, stress, poor diet, and intake of drugs or alcohol contribute to the extrinsic aging process. Extrinsic aging effects can be reduced with preventive and corrective care. With extrinsic aging, skin thins; there is also a loss of collagen and elastin as well as intracellular water. Finally, there is an increase in hyperpigmentation, redness, and dryness (Figs. 1.1.1, 1.1.2).

Hormonal aging occurs as levels of estrogen decline. Low estrogen levels result in the weakening of the collagen and elastin fibers. Skin becomes thinner and more fragile. There is an increase in facial hair and breakouts, and reduced water content within cells among other internal metamorphoses. In women, although the eventual dryness and inelasticity of skin that come with age are inevitable facts of life, the aging process is a cumulative one that occurs at varying rates from individual to individual. In addition, aging for women commences far before menopause begins. In fact, by the time a woman reaches her 20s, the hormonal aging process has already started. The reasons why this happens vary and include many factors such as stress and lifestyle; for example, smoking can accelerate hormonal aging (1).

All female patients will experience a combination of the three types of aging to certain degrees. Topical treatment can do much to assist in collagen and elastin repair, and preventive behavior and lifestyle choices will help maintain results and circumvent new damage from forming. However, female hormonal aging is the most troublesome to address effectively as it requires an inclusive approach and a great understanding of the body's systems and complex interactions. Fundamentally, however, all three types of aging can be addressed with one simple element—water.

WATER LOSS ACCOMPANIES AGING

Water is by far the most abundant substance in the body. It accounts for one-half to three-fourths of the body's weight, depending on age, sex, and body composition. Water is essential to life as all metabolic processes occur in a water medium. Life can be described as a process during which a highly hydrated state of fertilized oocytes, embryos, newborns, etc. is transformed into a gradually more and more dehydrated one (2). A newborn infant is 75–80% water, but a gradual process of water loss continues throughout life until, in old age, water accounts for only about 50–60% of a woman's body weight and 60–65% of a man's body weight. As we age, we naturally lose water inside our cells and tissues. This process is useful until an organism reaches its optimum performance requiring a given amount of enzymes, muscle fibers,

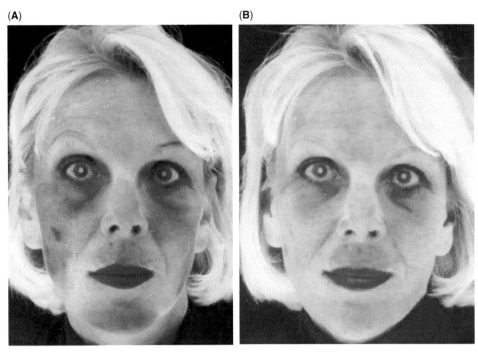

Figure 1.1.1 (**A**) Sun-damaged skin. (**B**) Appearance of the skin after 5 weeks of vitamin C, sunscreen, and internal supplementation.

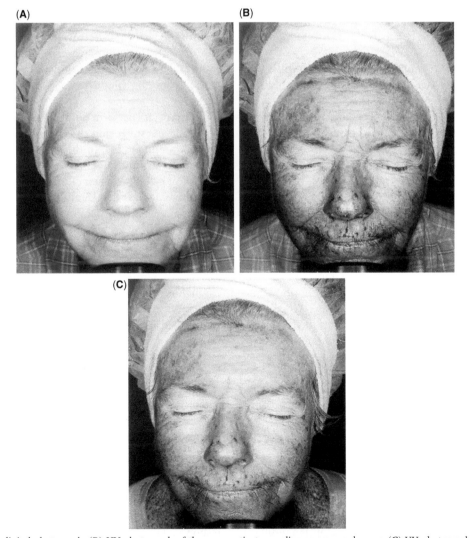

Figure 1.1.2 (**A**) Plain clinical photograph. (**B**) UV photograph of the same patient, revealing severe sun damage. (**C**) UV photograph after a treatment with vitamin C, revealing a significant reduction in pigmentation.

collagen, neurofilaments, etc. Unfortunately, the tendency for cellular dehydration continues with age progression. This dehydration helps accumulate intracellular dry mass, which has serious consequences. First, dehydration slows down and stops an organism's growth. Second, further increases in the physical density of cell colloids compromise basic cellular functions and this increases the free-radical efficiency and damage of cells. Lastly, the in situ enzyme catalytic rate constants are all strongly dependent on the density of their microenvironment (3,4).

Nagy's Membrane Hypothesis of Aging elaborates on the role of the plasma membrane in differentiation and aging. Structural and functional alterations occur throughout life to every cell's plasma membrane because of free radical–induced cross-linking of proteins and lipids, molecular damage, and residual heat formed during each discharge of the resting potential. Damaged plasma membrane is continually renewed through de novo synthesis, but certain accumulations of residual damage are inevitable. The implication is that there are functional changes within the cells, such as a gradual decrease in potassium permeability, with an increase in the intracellular potassium content and a consequent colloid condensation. It also implies there is a loss of intracellular water and an increase of dry mass content, which inhibits enzyme activity, decreases RNA rates, and decreases the activity of the genes for protein synthesis. In addition, it suggests that there is an accumulation of waste products in cells (lipofuscin) (2–4). Interestingly, studies show that the elderly, especially if diseased, display reduced intracellular water (5).

Drinking water alone is not the solution to replenish this decline in intracellular water during aging. The body produces some of the structural elements necessary for cells, but not all of them (e.g., essential amino acids). Another problem is that as the body ages, its production of cell membrane and of connective tissue–building substances slows down. To make cell membranes stronger (with increased intracellular water), encourage connective tissue regeneration (and hydration), mitigate free-radical damage to neuropeptides, and decrease inflammation, the body must be flooded with appropriate dietary nutrients.

Through the use of appropriate nutrients and the avoidance of deleterious lifestyle habits, the body is able to build the healthy cells needed to repair its tissues and improve total well being. Dehydrated cells are not resilient and do not function properly and this affects the immune response. When cells deteriorate, disorders, diseases, and death occur; therefore, it is important to regulate cellular hydration and volume in order to maintain regular cell functions (6). Plainly, when the delicate balance between free-radical generation and the body's defense mechanisms with antioxidants is disturbed, the consequences can range from natural aging to a variety of benign and precancerous lesions to ultimately neoplastic transformations (7).

INTRINSIC AND EXTRINSIC AGING AND IMMUNITY

On the outermost cutaneous layers, the major change that occurs with both intrinsic and extrinsic aging is that the skin becomes wrinkled, yellow, lax, dry, and leathery. In addition, precancerous and even cancerous lesions develop as a result of repeated sun exposure (8).

As skin ages and experiences environmental damages, cutaneous functions such as protection, secretion, absorption, and thermoregulation are detrimentally affected by as much as 60%. In addition, skin barrier function is impaired, skin cell turnover slows down, and fibroblasts and keratinocytes reduce in number (9). Skin that is chronically photodamaged is metabolically hyperactive with epidermal hyperplasia (sometimes neoplasia) and an increased deposition of abnormal elastic fibers, collagen, and glycosaminoglycans (GAGs) (10). Intrinsic aging exhibits epidermal atrophy, retraction of the rete pegs, flattening of the dermo–epidermal interface, and deposition of pseudoxanthoma-elasticum–like papillary dermal elastolysis (11–13).

Specifically, when the sun burns the skin, the Langerhans cells become less effective and diminished. In fact, Langerhans cells are nearly completely depleted within 24 hours after a sunburn. Exposure to ultraviolet radiation triggers a panoply of cellular defenses under the skin. UVB rays attack the living cells of the epidermis. The UVA rays, which are longer and penetrate deeper, attack the structures within the dermis and the epidermis. The side effect of this biological strategy is that the cells of the blood vessels become larger and the walls become thinner. Water leaks from the bloodstream through these vessels into the surrounding tissue, causing swelling within an hour. The cells of the blood vessel walls release cytokines, but despite the efforts, cell damage and apoptosis occur while lipids of the keratinocyte cell membrane walls are destroyed. Sun-induced inflammatory cascades are hazardous to the entire body because they increase free-radical formation and cause ripple effects that travel from the bloodstream through every system and organ.

Keratinocytes perform numerous immunologic tasks, many of which are still being discovered. Keratinocytes represent innate immunity (14). In the last decade, it has been discovered that keratinocytes express toll-like receptors, potent sources of cytokines, chemokines, and antimicrobial peptides. It has become clear that keratinocytes may be more than active participants in epidermal immune responses; they may actually play a key, initiating role. They may be involved in encouraging epidermal growth factors and fibroblast growth factors as well.

Adaptive immunity is a second line of protection that builds throughout our lives. Also known as active immunity, it involves the lymphocytes, and develops as we are exposed to diseases or immunized against diseases through vaccination. The adaptive immune response is characterized by its specificity, and by the fact that it becomes more effective with each successive encounter with the same antigen (15). Crucial components of an adaptive immune response are antigen-presenting cells. In the epidermis, Langerhans cells present antigens. Langerhans cells are abundant in the epidermis. These dendritic cells break up the invading microorganisms and antigens and present the material to other immune system cells such as T-cells, which secrete cytokines.

At the cellular level, the skin's Langerhans cells and keratinocytes attack immediately when skin is assaulted. This initiates an inflammatory cascade, which triggers a two-stage immune response. First, inflammatory mediators (e.g., interleukins, prostaglandins, etc.) are produced in the area surrounding the damaged cells. Second, macrophages and neutrophils migrate to the site of inflammation, where they release two classes of beneficial molecules—ROS as well as proteolytic enzymes (neutrophil elastase and collagenase). Together, these compounds provide protection from infections while promoting removal and repair of damaged cells and connective tissue.

With the aging process, the skin develops an ability to create a disproportionate immune response, one that goes beyond what is needed to repair the environmental insult or stress-induced damage. More specifically, the immune response produces an overaccumulation of ROS and matrix metalloproteinases (MMPs), enzymes that degrade the skin matrix (16). The results are damage to uninjured tissue and the edema and redness that are often associated with inflammation.

One way to quell these reactions is to use durian extract. By acting at both stages of the immune response, the antioxidants and omega-3 fatty acids present in durian extracts can serve as potent anti-inflammatory agents, reducing the exaggerated immune response in adult tissue.

Moreover, omega-3 essential fatty acids (EFAs), in particular eicosapentaenoic acid and docosahexaenoic acid, have been shown to inhibit the production of inflammatory mediators that begin the inflammation cascade. The scientific literature reports that omega-3 EFAs reduce inflammation caused by prostaglandins and exposure to ultraviolet radiation (17,18).

Antioxidants, in general, are well known for their health benefits as protectants against the deleterious effects of aging and inflammation (19). The antioxidant constituents of durian have been associated with numerous health benefits (20). In particular, quercetin helps to reduce inflammation by quenching excessive ROS and inhibiting MMP activity (21–25).

Together, the omega-3 EFAs and antioxidants in durian act synergistically by moderating the induction of inflammatory mediators, decreasing cellular and tissue damage caused by excessive levels of ROS, and inhibiting the breakdown of collagen and elastin by MMPs.

However, the fact remains that as the human body ages, its epidermal immune response diminishes. Langerhans cells are diminished; keratinocytes lose their ability to release cytokines and growth factors; cellular proliferation declines; and the dermal layer atrophies, causing a loss in resiliency. It is important to note that inflammation in a healthy body, when not an overreaction, chronic or irreparable, results in increased general health and skin health because of the repair process happening at the cellular level. As such, controlling the immune system's inflammation response for rejuvenation purposes has been the subject of recent research.

HORMONAL AGING

While there have been great advances in hormone research, a predictable hormone sequence from female to female is non-existent, which increases the difficulty in treatment for imbalances. In women, estrogen levels will determine the extent of hormonal aging.

The overall ratio between hormones is important. In all cases, saliva or blood tests can be used to determine hormone imbalances. Based on saliva and blood test results, proactive measures can be incorporated into a patient's protocol.

The primary issue found in those experiencing hormonal aging is estrogen loss. Estrogen is skin's best ally, therefore, the goal is to prolong menopause from occurring for as long as possible and this can be done at any time from age 20 upward, not just the "perimenopausal" years. Estrogen helps prevent aging in many ways. It prevents a decrease in skin collagen in postmenopausal women, and increases the skin's collagen content thereby maintaining skin thickness. In addition, estrogen helps skin maintain moisture as it increases the levels of acid mucopolysaccharides and hyaluronic acid in the skin, which could play a role in maintaining the stratum corneum barrier function. It has been suggested that estrogen increases cutaneous wound healing because of its cytokine-regulating role. In fact, topical estrogen has been found to accelerate and improve wound healing in elderly men and women. Preliminary studies have suggested that estrogen may actually improve the quality of scarring (26).

To combat hormonal aging, a comprehensive program must be initiated. This is a partnership between the patient, physician, aesthetician, and lifestyle practitioner, and its goal is to promote whole-body health. Working together, anti-aging facials, maintenance home care, medical treatments, prescription medication (if needed), nutrition and supplement recommendations, exercise, and adjunct therapies such as acupuncture and massage may be used to inclusively address all avenues of hormonal aging. To begin with, a skin care regimen for hormonally aging skin should consist of the following:

- Antioxidants to disarm free radicals, which ultimately damage the cell membrane and cause it to lose water
- Anti-inflammatory agents to reduce inflammation, which releases free radicals that damage cellular structures and cause water loss
- Natural moisture factors to absorb water from the environment and act as a reservoir for water in the skin
- Hydrophobic agents such as ceramides, which prevent water loss from all cells and maintain the skin's barrier function. These can also be essential in repairing and maintaining cell membranes
- Fatty acid and glucosamine supplements to encourage the body to make its own water-holding molecules
- Lecithin and its building blocks, phosphatidylcholine and choline, to maintain cell walls

Beyond the aforementioned recommendations, an option for some women is hormone replacement therapy (HRT), sometimes called postmenopausal hormone therapy. HRT should only be used as a last resort. Alternative methods to HRT are also being used to relieve menopausal symptoms. Called bioidentical hormones, these alternative products come from botanical, herbal, and animal sources and they mirror the effects that estrogen may provide, thus they offer some relief in alleviating menopausal symptoms. The popularity of bioidentical hormones has grown considerably in direct relation to the growth of the natural and organic market. Some literature speculates that these "natural" hormones are safer than synthetic ones, but there are no conclusive studies that indicate this to be a fact. Bioidentical hormones are found in plants and animals, extracted and processed into a form that can be readily used such as cream, patch, or supplement. Examples of sources for these hormones are evening primrose, black cohosh, red clover, chasteberry tree, soy, wild yams, pigs, and horses. They are available as FDA-approved prescriptions (Estrace®, Warner Chilcott, Dublin, Ireland; Climara®, Bayer HealthCare Pharmaceuticals Inc., Wayne, New Jersey; Vivelle-Dot®, Novartis Pharmaceuticals Corporation, East Hanover, New Jersey; Prometrium®, Abbott Laboratories, North Chicago, Illinois; Vaniqa®, SkinMedica Inc., Carlsbad, California). Bioidentical hormone ingredients used in over-the-counter products are usually plant-derived; hence, labels may promote them as "phytoestrogens" (phyto meaning "plant").

There are many effective topical and internal ingredients available, but with regard to hormonally aging skin, some are better than others. Many ingredients can be delivered through in-spa services as well as in home care products. Others can be found in supplement form and in the foods consumed. Because education is part of every treatment protocol, patients should be provided with as much information as possible so they may augment their home care. Specifically, the following list includes a few simple and effective recommendations:

- Apricot, evening primrose and borage seed oils protect the skin's natural barrier, increasing moisture retention.
- Papaya enzymes gently exfoliate to reveal a brighter, softer skin.
- Soy and wild yam extracts are natural, plant-based estrogens.
- Clove flower and iris extracts tone and firm skin.
- GAGs inhibit collagen breakdown.
- Shiitake mushroom extract conditions and firms skin.
- Shea butter superhydrates and restores skin's vibrancy.
- Chaparral extract inhibits facial hair growth and is clinically proven to reduce facial hair growth by 22% in 12 weeks.
- Melatonin induces calm and encourages restful sleep.
- Glucosamine boosts collagen production and eases joint pain.
- Biotin strengthens hair, skin, and nails.
- EFAs hydrate from the inside out and reduce inflammation.
- B-complex vitamins offer overall health benefits.

With estrogen loss, the skin and body are affected in many ways. Although there are no established rules for managing menopausal skin, proper skin care and long-term preventive techniques can help lessen its visible influence. Without treatment, skin will continue to degenerate after menopause. Estimates have indicated that skin loses up to 30% of its collagen in the first five years after menopause. Moreover, as skin thins by approximately a percentage point a year, the decelerated cell renewal rate leaves increasing numbers of dead skin cells on the surface (27,28).

In the years before menopause, skin becomes progressively sensitive and dry. Apricot, evening primrose, and borage seed oils can be used to strengthen the skin's barrier function and help it stay hydrated. Exceptionally dry skin conditions will benefit from shea butter. Conversely, because estrogen suppresses the sebaceous glands, a decline in estrogen stimulates the sebaceous glands to overproduce. In this circumstance,

soy and wild yam extracts are beneficial because as natural plant-based estrogens, they help keep the sebaceous gland production balanced. These phytoestrogens are also useful because they help normalize cell turnover, which slows down during hormonal aging. Using papaya enzymes and other gentle exfoliators, dead skin cell removal is essential in hormonally aging skin as an accumulation of dead cells and excessive oils will combine to create acne. Topical exfoliators like papaya enzyme will help control skin discoloration as well and will help skin in preparing firming and toning ingredients like clove flower and iris extracts. Hair, skin, and nails all become weaker with estrogen loss, so adding biotin is essential as it is necessary for cell growth. Specifically, skin loses its firmness; so, in addition to biotin, there is a need to increase ingredients like shiitake mushroom extract and GAGs, which will make skin more resilient as they inhibit collagen breakdown.

Hormonal aging disrupts sleep, which can cause health and cosmetic consequences. Sleeplessness promotes edema and darkness in the ocular region. Without sleep, cortisol cannot return to baseline values and this can lead to adrenal fatigue, weight gain, and impaired immunity. Studies have shown that cortisol levels the day after a sleepless night are reduced, which makes a patient less able to handle normal stress. Hypertension is a side effect of lack of sleep as well as confusion, memory loss, and depression. Sleep is also important to sex drive and digestion. The body requires sleep to metabolize glucose, and as such, sleep loss may promote diabetes. In addition, wound healing is decreased with sleeplessness. To combat sleeplessness, melatonin can be used, as well as B vitamins, which support and increase the rate of metabolism; maintain healthy skin and muscle tone; enhance immune and nervous system functions; and combat the symptoms and causes of stress, depression, and cardiovascular disease (CVD).

CVD is a great concern with aging women. According to the American Heart Association, one in three female adults has some form of cardiovascular disease. With hormonally aging women, less estrogen translates to more freely circulating androgens, which can lead to androgen excess. Androgen excess is associated with insulin resistance, dyslipidemia (high cholesterol), hypertension, and vascular diseases; therefore, it is a forerunner for CVD. Symptoms of androgen excess include more hair on the face and less on the scalp as well as worsening acne. To help control excessive hair growth, chaparral extract or a cream prescription of Vaniqa® (SkinMedica Inc., Carlsbad, CA) could be used.

With estrogen loss there is also less circulation and less circulation will adversely affect skin as nutrients have a difficult time reaching the skin layers effectively. In addition, less circulation increases inflammation on skin and in the body, which can contribute to inflammatory diseases and conditions such as CVD, arthritis, acne, and rosacea. To combat inflammation, EFAs need to be introduced to the diet as they inhibit transcription factors that are linked to proinflammatory cytokine production. Coenzyme Q10 also has many cardiac benefits and is known to reduce oxidation and increase cellular energy, so supplementing the diet with it can be very beneficial to overall health.

These processes and how they are all linked highlight the importance of exercise for women as they age to enhance circulation, combat CVD, and reduce stress. Estrogen declines cause muscle loss and weight gain, which can contribute to many issues within the body like arthritis and joint pain, for which glucosamine can be used. But perhaps the biggest benefit to exercise is its effect on mood.

ANDROGENIC IMBALANCE CONTRIBUTES TO AGING

Androgen is skin's worst hormonal enemy. Acne can be aggravated or initiated by increased androgen levels (29). For this reason, any disease, condition, or concomitant hormonal issue that raises androgen levels in women must be addressed to achieve results with acne.

Researchers believe acne worsens because of increased adrenal androgens, which happens as dehydroepiandrosterone (DHEA) levels build up. It is thought that glucocorticoids, such as cortisol, also exacerbate acne (30). Both hormones are released during periods of emotional stress. These hormones stimulate the sebaceous glands and cause excess oil to build up in pores, which leads to acne formation.

DHEA that is found naturally in the body decreases with age, beginning in the fourth decade of life (31). Many people take DHEA orally as a nutritional supplement as available data suggest its influence on stimulating the immune system and its ability to improve memory. While it is often called the "youth hormone," it has a common side effect for its users—an oily, acneic skin.

Cortisol is the "stress hormone," which assists the body during stressful situations, initiating the "fight or flight" response. It is responsible for increasing blood pressure and sugar levels and it also has an immunosuppressive action.

Androgens are bound in blood to the sex hormone binding globulin (SHBG) and albumin (blood plasma protein). Androgens circulate in a bound and unbound fashion. In healthy women, 80% of testosterone is bound to SHBG, 19% is bound to albumin, and 1% circulates freely in the blood stream. In women who are hirsute, 79% is bound to SHBG, 19% is bound to albumin, and 2% circulates freely (32). Only a slight imbalance can cause a large effect.

Androgen excess occurs as a result of the production of DHEA in the adrenal gland, production of testosterone in the ovary, and in some other peripheral areas in the body. It can also occur as a result of metabolic syndromes like diabetes (hyperinsulinism), hypothyroidism, acromegaly, obesity, or because of progesterone-containing medications such as norethindrone, norgestrel, desogestrel, and norgestimate.

Polycystic ovarian syndrome (PCOS) can also increase testosterone levels in the bloodstream. Signs of PCOS include an increase in facial hair or abnormalities of hair in general such as hair thinning on the scalp as well as an increase in the male escutcheon. Abnormal periods will occur and these patients usually will have used many acne programs without success. If PCOS is suspected, blood work can be performed to confirm a diagnosis.

Oral contraceptives increase sex hormone binding globulin, which decreases the amount of testosterone circulating freely. Yasmin® and Diane®-35 are two birth control pills with low androgenic activity and these two pills are good for use with polycystic ovarian syndrome. Alternatively, flutamide or spironolactone may be useful. Pregnancy must be avoided while on these drugs because they can cause birth defects. Spironolactone has

been used to treat hypertension, so if prescribed, blood pressure readings and potassium levels must be checked regularly. Other therapies must be considered if a patient is already using hypertension medication.

Men also suffer from hormonal aging in the form of androgen imbalance. Termed "andropause," or male menopause, men face a litany of external symptoms from androgen loss, which naturally occurs as age progresses. Specifically, men will experience a reduction in the production of testosterone and DHEA. Hair disorders are commonplace such as excessive hair growth in the eyebrows and on or in the ears. In addition, men may experience the formation of deeper wrinkles and a lack of skin vitality. Physically, men may develop redundant, pendulous breast tissue, experience decreased muscle mass and strength, as well as declined sex drive. There is also increased fatigue, body fat, CVD risk, as well as emotional or psychological behavioral changes in men experiencing hormonal aging. Many of the external therapies that are used to treat hormonal imbalance in women are also beneficial for men. Moreover, a complete inclusive protocol will do much to assist men with their topical, systemic, and emotional symptoms during hormonal aging.

DESIGNING THE IDEAL SKIN CARE PROTOCOL

There are two basic principles to consider in any skin care protocol that leads to healthy skin. First, intracellular water must be enhanced to improve cell functions, which hastens healing and cutaneous immunity. Second, the skin's barrier function must be considered, and if compromised, must be strengthened and fortified.

The skin's extracellular, natural lipids must be regulated as these lipids hold water, surround the skin cells, and provide a permeable barrier. Keratinized corneocytes of the stratum corneum, lipids, and natural moisturizing factors work in synergy to provide an efficient barrier against water loss and promote hydration, which preserves the lower epidermal and dermal layers of skin to maintain skin's flexibility and function. In other words, these protective elements shield the skin from desiccation and environmental assaults. When lipids are lost, the spaces between the cells dry out and allow irritants or pathogens to enter. Missing lipids also increase trans-epidermal water loss. To address this, humectant moisturizers can be applied, but these products must also have barrier properties to prevent moisture loss.

Beyond cellular water and the skin barrier, a complete and custom skin treatment plan can be commenced based on information collected during a thorough patient consultation.

PATIENT CONSULTATION AND EVALUATION

Patient consultations must consist of examinations that consider all that is visible externally as well as the "invisible" or internal factors. Superficial, external examinations will steer topical therapies, but they do not adequately address the root cause of any condition and cannot illuminate fully what is happening at the cellular level. We now know that this mode of evaluation and treatment only produces marginal, short-term results. Old patterns of medical skin treatment only address the outermost cutaneous concerns with medication or methods that suppress symptoms. The new movement in cutaneous medical care is to encourage corporal homeostasis and health, which extends rejuvenation to the dermal and epidermal layers. The skin and its many layers are not autonomous. The epidermis is connected to every part of the body and in turn, every part of the body is connected to it. It is therefore important to devise a consultation examination that analyses external, internal, and emotional issues that may be involved with the client's skin and body health. Long-term solutions can only be achieved through a collaborative effort among medical professionals as well as aesthetics and lifestyle practitioners.

To begin the consultation, address the impact the patient's skin condition has on his/her quality of life. Practice I VOTE:

> *Inquire* about how their skin affects their social life, emotions, self-esteem, and ability to do work and enjoy leisure activities.
> *Validate* their experience by acknowledging the impact their skin's condition has on them and their quality of life.
> *Offer* to discuss ideas and find additional resources (e.g. articles, referrals, etc.).
> *Tell* patients that you are committed to helping them, improving their skin and quality of life.
> *Evaluate* their quality of life throughout the course of treatment.

The Impact of Skin Types

The skin evaluation is a narrowing process. To start with, skin type must be classified into dry, normal, or oily.

Dry Skin

Dry skin has small, fine pores, even across the nose and chin areas. There may be some cutaneous flaking. Over the cheeks, skin is thin and, in general, skin may appear transparent and delicate, as capillaries are easily visible. Skin may appear smooth, but exhibit rough texture. Patients may complain of skin tightness and that moisturizer only restores comfort for short durations. Harsh weather intensifies patients' complaints. Red, scaly patches may appear after outdoor activities. Superficial lines are etched on cheeks because normal creases in the skin are more obvious when there is not enough moisture to soften them. Moisturizing creams and lotions absorb quickly after applications.

Normal Skin

Normal skin exhibits medium-sized pores, with a proliferation of pores along the nasal and chin areas, which may be oilier than the cheeks and ocular region. There are few if any comedones present. The complexion appears bright and texture is smooth. Normal skin tolerates temperature extremes well without irritation or chapping. Skin adapts well to weather changes and may become drier in cool climates and slightly oilier in warm climates.

Oily Skin

Oily skin has many noticeable pores. Skin tone may be sallow but appear shiny at times. It will feel oily, especially along the nose and across the forehead and chin. Skin will have fewer wrinkles than the norm according to age group. While there are few if any small wrinkles, deeper lines will predominate. This skin type tolerates cold and wind well, but not hot, humid weather, which stimulates sebaceous oil production. Foundation disappears after about an hour or two, and moisturizing lotions and creams are absorbed slowly. It is generally assumed that oily skin types are more prone to acne; however, every skin type can be troubled with acne.

The Differences Between Age Groups

Beyond skin type, age group will reveal more about the client's hormonal state, stress levels, lifestyle, and concerns. Biologically, we can categorize patients by age group to determine their aging rate with regard to the norm. The categories include teens; women in their 20s; and women in their 30s and above. After age group, the consultation can focus on any skin conditions such as acne, cellulite, skin disorders, etc.

Teens

Skin is taut. There are no wrinkles. Acne may be present and is associated with hormonal fluctuations because of puberty growth spurts. When puberty is over, acne improves or even disappears. For girls, menstruation begins. Interestingly, high-stress environments have been shown to delay puberty, which usually begins between the ages of 9 and 14.

Twenties

Skin is starting to lose collagen and elastin; the beginnings of wrinkles are visible, particularly in the ocular region. Skin pigment is usually uniform. If contraceptive pills are used, some pseudomelasma or discoloration may occur. The decline in hormone levels begins for many women. Premenstrual syndrome (PMS) may be experienced soon after puberty and can last until menopause. PMS may indicate a progesterone deficiency, hypothyroidism, or chronic stress. Hormonal imbalances cause skin symptoms at both ends of the spectrum such as acne and oiliness, or dryness and dull skin. Declining hormone levels cause skin thinning. Hormonal imbalance in this age group is largely due to stress, as stress stimulates the overproduction of DHEA and cortisol.

Thirties Plus

Stress still causes hormone imbalance, but there is a steady decline in natural hormones and this decline results in an imbalance that becomes more pronounced. There is more skin thinning, dead skin cell buildup, and skin discoloration. Sometimes acne is present, but lesions are cyst-like, long lasting, and "underground." While the onset of menopause usually occurs between the ages of 45 and 55, some women in their early 30s experience menopausal sleeplessness, weight gain, irritability, temporary memory loss, hot flashes, brittle hair, and dry skin. Irregular periods, excessive hair growth in unexpected places like the chin, in addition to the presence of acne, could all possibly indicate underlying polycystic ovarian syndrome in patients. Women who are nutritionally deficient, smoke, or do not have children will approach menopause at an earlier age than they normally would have without these factors. Constant, unrelenting stress has also been shown to accelerate hormonal aging as stress hormone overproduction can cause symptoms associated with adrenal gland fatigue. Adrenal fatigue has been described in literature to be a factor in many related conditions, including fibromyalgia, hypothyroidism, chronic fatigue syndrome, arthritis, and premature menopause, and may cause many undesirable side effects such as acne, hair loss, depression, weight gain, a decline in the immune system, and insomnia.

CONCLUSIONS

Just as Ponce de Leon sought the fountain of youth, so do millions of patients every day. Unfortunately, there are literally millions of products on the market, all of which purport to have the one true cure for the aging process. As is readily apparent, there are many different causes for the aging process, and as such, patients will likely require multiple products and interventions in order to help slow down the aging process. With a keen understanding of the aging process, it is possible for physicians to help safely guide patients on their quest for eternal youth.

REFERENCES

1. Buela U. Determinants of the age at natural menopause. Przegl Lek 2002; 59: 165–9.
2. Nagy IZs. The frustrating decades of biological aging theories and the hopes for the future. Anti-Aging Bull 2003; 4: 22–31.
3. Nagy IZs. The membrane hypothesis of aging: its relevance to recent progress in genetic research. J Mol Med 1997; 75: 703–14.
4. Nagy IZs. Enzyme activities in the light of the membrane hypothesis of aging. Mech Aging Dev 2001; 122: 811–21.
5. Ritz P. Chronic cellular dehydration. J Gerontol 2001: 56A: 349–52.
6. Lang F, Waldegger S. Regulating cell volume. Am Sci 1997; 85: 456–63.
7. Murad H, Tabibian M. The effect of an oral supplement containing glucosamine, aminoacids, mineral, and antioxidants on cutaneous aging. J Dermatolog Treat 2001; 12: 47–51.
8. Kligman AM, Kligman LH. Photoaging. In: Fitzpatrick TB, Eisen AZ, Wolff K, et al., eds. Dermatology in General Medicine. McGraw-Hill: New York: 1993, p. 2972.
9. Ghersetich I, Lotti T, Campanile G, et al. Hyaluronic acid in cutaneous intrinsic aging. Int J Dermatol 1994; 33: 119–22.
10. Kligman LH. Photoaging: manifestations, prevention and treatment. Clin Geriatr Med 1989; 5: 235–51.
11. Fenske NA, Lober CW. Structural and functional changes or normal aging skin. J Am Acad Dermatol 1986; 15: 571–85.
12. Montagna W, Carlisle K. Structural changes in aging human skin. J Invest Dermatol 1979; 73: 47–53.
13. Rongioletti F, Rebora A. Firoelastolytic patterns of intrinsic skin aging: pseudoxanthoma-elasticum-like papillary dermal elastolysis and white fibrous papulosis of the neck. Dermatology 1995; 19: 19–24.
14. Pivarcsi A, Nagy I, Kemeny L. Innate Immunity in the Skin: How Keratinocytes Fight Against Pathogens. Curr Immunol Rev 2005; 1: 29–42.
15. Schwarz T. Skin immunity. Br J Dermatol 2003; 149: 2–4.
16. Ferguson MWJ, O'Kane S. Scar-free healing; from embryonic mechanisms to adult therapeutic intervention. Phil Trans R Soc Lond B 2004; 359: 839–50.
17. Danno K, Ikai K, Imamura S. Anti-inflammatory effects of eicosapentaenoic acid on experimental skin inflammation models. Arch Dermatol Res 1993; 285: 432–5.
18. Storey A, McArdle F, Friedmann PS, Jackson MJ, Rhodes LE. Eicosapentaenoic acid and docosahexaenoic acid reduce UVB- and TNF-alpha-induced IL-8 secretion in keratinocytes and UVB-induced IL-8 in fibroblasts. J Invest Dermatol 2005; 124: 248–55.
19. Hu HL, Forsey RJ, Blades TJ, et al. Antioxidants may contribute in the fight against ageing: an in vitro model. Mech Ageing Dev 2000; 121: 217–30.
20. Leontowicz H, Leontowicz M, Haruenkit R, et al. Durian (Durio zibethinus Murr.) cultivars as nutritional supplementation to rat's diets. Food Chem Toxicol 2008; 46: 581–9.
21. Haruenkit R, Poovarodom S, Leontowicz H, et al. Comparative study of health properties and nutritional value of durian, mangosteen, and snake fruit: experiments in vitro and in vivo. J Agric Food Chem 2007; 55: 5842–9.
22. Casagrande R, Georgetti SR, Verri WA Jr, et al. Protective effect of topical formulations containing quercetin against UVB-induced oxidative stress in hairless mice. J Photochem Photobiol B 2006; 84: 21–7.
23. Casagrande R, Georgetti SR, Verri WA Jr, et al. In vitro evaluation of quercetin cutaneous absorption from topical formulations and its functional stability by antioxidant activity. Int J Pharm 2007; 328: 183–90.
24. Lim H, Kim HP. Inhibition of mammalian collagenase, matrix metalloproteinase-1, by naturally-occurring flavonoids. Planta Med 2007; 73: 1267–74.
25. Sin BY, Kim HP. Inhibition of collagenase by naturally-occurring flavonoids. Arch Pharm Res 2005; 28: 1152–5.
26. Ashcroft GS, Dodsworth J, van Boxtel E, et al. Estrogen accelerates cutaneous wound healing associated with an increase in TGF-beta1 levels. Nat Med 1997; 3: 1209–15.
27. Affinito P, Palomba S, Sorrentino C, et al. Effects of postmenopausal hypoestrogenism on skin collagen. Maturitas 1999; 33: 239–47.
28. Brincat M, Moniz CJ, Studd JW, et al. Long-term effects of the menopause and sex hormones on skin thickness. Br J Obstet Gynaecol 1985; 92: 256–9.
29. ligman AM. An overview of acne. J Invest Dermatol, 1974; 62: 268–87.
30. Lee S, Tsou A, Chan H. Glucocorticoids inhibit the transcription of interleukin. Proc Natl Acad Sci USA 1998; 85: 1204–8.
31. Zdrojewicz Z, Ciszko B. Dehydroepiandrosterons (DHEA)-structure, clinical importance and the role in the human body. Postepy Hig Med Dosw 2001; 55: 835–54.
32. Sabatini Luca. Androgen Excess. eMedicine WebMD 2007; http://www.emedicine.com/med/TOPIC3489.HTM#section~References; (Epub 16 June 2008).

BIBLIOGRAPHY

Murad H. Wrinkle-Free Forever. New York: St. Martin's Griffin, 2003.
Murad H. The Cellulite Solution. New York: St. Martin's Press, 2005.

1.2 Cosmeceuticals
Gurpreet Ahluwalia

> **KEY POINTS**
> - Cosmeceuticals are a rapidly expanding frontier in aesthetic medicine
> - Cosmeceuticals possess biological activity to provide skin benefits
> - Topical retinoids and antioxidants provide photoprotection, as well as reverse and prevent photodamaged skin
> - Cosmeceuticals promote healthy skin through hydration, exfoliation, and improvement of skin texture and wrinkles

Cosmeceuticals are a rapidly expanding frontier in beauty medicine. Cosmeceuticals, a term introduced by Albert Kligman almost three decades ago at a meeting of the Society of Cosmetic Chemists, refers to products that have biological activity and provide skin benefits more than what can be achieved using a purely cosmetic product. Most cosmeceuticals are intended for facial application to treat conditions such as photodamaged skin, improve skin tone and texture, and reduce the appearance of wrinkles and skin hyperpigmentation. As our understanding of skin science, especially molecular mechanisms, behind skin aging and skin damage has grown, the field of cosmeceuticals has dramatically developed. The emergence of new active ingredients and advances in delivery technology and formulation science are also contributing factors for the rapid pace of development of beauty medicine products.

AN INTRODUCTION TO COSMECEUTICALS

Several topical drugs, whether prescription or over-the-counter (OTC), have been shown to provide significant cosmetic benefits for patients. Multiple formulations of topical retinoids improve photodamaged skin and reduce wrinkles, while minoxidil (Rogaine®, McNeil-PPC Inc, Fort Washington, Pennsylvania) and bimatoprost (Latisse®, Allergan Inc, Irvine, California) have been shown to stimulate hair growth on the scalp and eyelashes, eflornithine (Vaniqa®, SkinMedica Inc., Carlsbad, California) reduces hair growth, and generic hydroquinone reduces skin pigmentation. Interestingly, for most of these products, the cosmetic benefits were discovered serendipitously. Retinoids were initially developed for acne treatment (Retin-A®, Ortho Dermatologics, Los Angeles, CA; Accutane®, brand name Accutane® no longer available, though generic versions are produced by several manufacturers), minoxidil for the treatment of hypertension (Loniten®, brand name Loniten® no longer available, though generic versions are produced by several manufacturers), and bimatoprost for glaucoma treatment (LUMIGAN®, Allergan Inc, Irvine, CA). Eflornithine, a selective and potent ornithine decarboxylase inhibitor was being used for African sleeping sickness when it was discovered that the same enzyme is involved in the regulation of hair growth, which led to its development as a hair growth–reducing agent. These topical agents are all available by prescription. Many cosmetic companies have attempted to replicate similar effects through cosmeceuticals. Although these cosmeceuticals may not have the efficacy of the prescription products for the select indication, they do fill a meaningful needed gap for the consumers.

From the regulatory perspective, the U.S. Food and Drug Administration (FDA) legally differentiates topical cosmetic and drug products by their intended uses. Cosmetic products are defined as substances that cleanse, beautify, promote attractiveness, or alter appearance without affecting the body's structure and function. Drugs, on the other hand, are defined as products intended for diagnosing, treating, or preventing diseases, or affecting the structure or function of living tissue. In practice, it is the intended use and the product claims that dictate whether the product is classified as a cosmetic/cosmeceutical or a drug, rather than its actual components. Cosmeceuticals are also not required to undergo the regulatory marketing approval process required for drugs. Companies marketing these products may not make claims that fall under the regulatory definition of drugs, for example, a cosmeceutical product may claim to improve the appearance of wrinkles but not claim to treat the wrinkles. Even though the FDA does not review or approve the ingredients found in cosmeceuticals, it does closely monitor product claims, whether they are explicit or implied, that it may consider falling under the drug category. The FDA can then force companies to remove products from the marketplace by issuing warning letters if it believes the product or its claims to fall under the drug category. In addition, the FDA can have a product removed from the marketplace even with cosmetic claims if it believes that the active ingredient in the product can cause harm to the public.

For years, cosmeceutical marketers have been pushing the envelope in making claims that imply drug-like activity. However, they are carefully worded so as not to invite FDA scrutiny. Topical products with significant biological and biochemical activity that alter the structure and function of skin, such as tretinoin and hydroquinone, get classified as drugs. However, claims such as the ability to improve skin tone, texture or radiance, decrease the appearance of fine lines and wrinkles, provide enhanced anti-aging benefits, or improve photodamaged skin are considered cosmeceutical claims. These cosmeceutical claims are in most part made based on the defined cellular or biochemical actions of the active ingredients. The claims are generally tied to an individual active ingredient where the activity may have been demonstrated in an in vitro model.

From the science perspective, one must ask these questions related to the claimed activity of a cosmeceutical. (1) Can the claimed active ingredient be effectively delivered through the stratum corneum barrier layer to the targeted skin site in concentrations that have pharmacological activity to elicit the desired biological response? (2) How well has the mechanism of action been defined for the active ingredient as it relates to skin metabolism and the claimed activity? The skin's outermost layer, the stratum corneum, is composed of nonviable corneocytes that present an effective barrier to water loss, as well as a significant barrier to entry for exogenous materials. A variety of claimed cosmeceutical active ingredients, when incorporated in simple formulations, cannot penetrate through this barrier layer to be able to reach their target. Substances such as proteins and peptides, sugars, nucleic acids, highly charged molecules, and substances with molecular weight above 1000 kD have a very low probability to penetrate an intact skin in any significant amount. The physiochemical properties of the molecule, such as the hydrophilic/lipophilic nature, also play an important role in its skin penetration. Additional compounds known as penetration enhancers may be necessary to facilitate absorption of the active ingredient across the stratum corneum. It is important to consider these questions when attempting to determine the likely efficacy of a cosmeceutical agent.

AGING OF THE SKIN: PHOTOAGING VS. INTRINSIC AGING

With age, human skin undergoes morphological, structural, and biochemical alterations that result in the aged look characterized by fine lines and wrinkles, textural changes, uneven tone, pigmented spots, and loss of elasticity (1). These skin changes can be due to either intrinsic chronological aging resulting from metabolic changes in cells, or extrinsic aging mostly as a result of ultraviolet (UV) irradiation causing photodamage (2). Though the end results may be similar, the excessive chronic UV exposure which is the primary cause of photodamage undoubtedly accelerates the aging process (3,4).

Several theories of aging have been proposed (5), the most widely accepted being that oxidative stress caused by oxygen free radicals is the underlying cause of aging (6). UV-generated active radical oxygen species (ROS) and hydrogen peroxide are responsible for triggering a cascade of biochemical events that ultimately lead to cellular damage (7). ROS generated by UV irradiation can cause cross-linking and glycation of extracellular matrix proteins including collagen and elastin and cause lipid peroxidation (8). The result is a marked decrease in new collagen synthesis in the papillary dermis (9). The net amount of collagen in skin is further impacted by a stimulation of the expression of Matrix metalloproteinases (MMPs) by free radicals, which causes a steady degradation of the collagen network that supports skin structure. Studies show that immediately after a suberythemal dose of UV radiation, skin reacts by inducing the expression of Matrix metalloproteinases through signal transduction, transcription factors, and cytokine release mechanisms (10). The overall collagen reduction and thinning of dermis results in the loss of skin firmness and elasticity and causes wrinkles. Additional factors that affect cells' ability to neutralize or fight oxidative stress in the aging skin include telomere shortening (11) and hormonal changes (12).

Chronological aging, characterized at the subcellular level as damage caused by ROS and telomere shortening due to intrinsic metabolic processes may be difficult to prevent or reverse (13); in contrast, damage related to ROS generated by UV radiation may be completely preventable and somewhat effectively treatable by active ingredients incorporated in cosmeceuticals. Human skin contains a number of endogenous antioxidants and detoxifying enzymes including glutathione, catalase, superoxide dismutase, and various reductases that either function to prevent free-radical formation or play a role in neutralizing them under normal physiological conditions (14).

Photoaging is a result of repetitive, chronic exposure of the skin to UV radiation that causes the patient's skin to appear older than their chronological age. UVA is considered to be the most photodamaging. Some of the most effective ingredients against UVA damage include zinc oxide, titanium dioxide, benzophenone, benzophenone complexes, avobenzone, and ecamsule. In the benzophenone class, oxybenzone has weak UVA protection, and can be more effectively used in combination with an ingredient with stronger UVA protection, such as avobenzone. Because of the well-established involvement of UV radiation in causing photodamage, many cosmeceuticals incorporate sunscreens, and can then make claims such as "provides anti-aging benefits."

Damaged skin, whether due to chronological aging or photoaging, is characterized by excessive fine lines, wrinkles, rough/dry/scaly texture, uneven tone, brown spots, and an ashy appearance. In addition, the skin becomes less firm and has a significant loss of elasticity. The changes are most commonly seen on sun exposed areas such as the hands, face, and neck. Many of the cosmeceutical active agents are directed at treating and/or preventing these changes. The most commonly used active ingredients to address these changes include antioxidants to preventing oxidative damage, moisturizers to enhance skin hydration, retinoids to treat photodamaged skin and wrinkles, and lightening creams to reduce skin hyperpigmentation.

PREVENTING OR REVERSING OXIDATIVE SKIN DAMAGE

First suggested by D. Harman in 1956, the theory that free radicals are responsible for skin aging is now widely accepted. Free radicals in cells result in nucleic acid damage, lipid peroxidation, and inflammation that accumulate over time to cause skin aging (15,16). It is not surprising, therefore, that topical antioxidants are one of the largest areas of interest in cosmeceuticals. Antioxidants, such as vitamins C and E, coenzyme Q10, alpha-lipoic acid, and several botanicals such as polyphenols from green tea and flavonoids from grape seed extract are some of the common ingredients found in cosmeceuticals to prevent and reverse damage from free radicals.

At the intracellular level, vitamin C or ascorbic acid is highly effective in neutralizing reactive free radicals created by UV radiation; in addition, it has collagen stimulating properties. Vitamin C serves as a cofactor for the enzymes prolyl hydroxylase and lysyl hydroxylase. These two key enzymes are responsible for post-translational modification of type-I and type-III procollagen that give structural integrity to the collagen fibers (17,18). While the antioxidant properties of vitamin C are well established, there are topical delivery and formulation issues that must be considered for effective cosmeceutical use of this molecule. Vitamin C has poor skin penetration, undergoes rapid oxidation, and can have compatibility issues with other ingredients in a topical formulation. Some derivatives of ascorbic acid, including ascorbyl phosphate, ascorbyl palmitate, and ascorbyl glucoside, have been developed to address these issues. The form of vitamin C that is commonly used in skin care products is ascorbyl palmitate; this is a lipid form of vitamin C, which gives it a better stability in the topical formulation and allows for greater absorption into the skin.

Vitamin E, or alpha-tocopherol, is another vitamin that has established antioxidant properties and has benefits in preventing and treating photodamaged skin (19,20). In its physiological role, it is a lipid soluble vitamin which protects cell membranes from lipid peroxidation. There is substantial literature on the effects of topical vitamins C and E in preventing or reversing UV-induced skin damage (21–25).

Another natural molecule involved in providing protection against free radical damage is coenzyme Q10 (CoQ10) or ubiquinone, which is thought to protect vitamin E from UV radiation–induced depletion (26).

Alpha lipoic acid is another potent antioxidant that has a unique property of being either hydrophilic or hydrophobic so it can be used in most cosmeceutical formulations.

In addition to these physiological molecules there are a number of botanical agents that function as effective antioxidants, including lycopene, grape seed extract, and green tea polyphenols. In vitro data show that the grape seed extract, which is rich in the bioflavonoid antioxidant proanthocyanidin, has more potent free radical scavenging activity than either vitamin C or E (27). Ellagic acid found in pomegranate is thought to increase the levels of glutathione, a natural antioxidant present in cells. The polyphenols present in green tea leaves, including the potent catechin antioxidant epigallocatechin gallate, have been shown in various systems to modulate cellular metabolism, proliferation, and inflammatory pathways (28).

Increasing skin hydration is one of the most effective ways to temporarily improve the appearance of photodamaged skin, as well as improve fine lines and wrinkles. Skin hydration can be increased by attracting and holding water at the skin surface or by reducing the water loss from skin, referred to as transepidermal water loss (TEWL). There are three categories of effective ingredients to enhance skin hydration: occlusives, humectants, and hydrophilic materials (29). The occlusive agents, of which petrolatum is the gold standard, create a barrier at the skin surface and prevent water evaporation (30). Other more cosmetically elegant occlusive agents that are typically present in a formulation include dimethicone, mineral oil, waxes, and lanolin. Humectants are hygroscopic agents that attempt to absorb ambient water thereby increasing skin hydration; commonly used humectants include glycerin, urea, propylene glycol, sorbitol, pyrrolidone carboxylic acid, gelatin, hyaluronic acid (HA), and proteins (30–32). HA is the most important natural moisturizing component of skin, but unfortunately, it decreases with age (33). However, as much as HA is involved in maintaining skin health, because of its high molecular weight and anionic polysaccharide structure it is unlikely that any topically applied HA penetrates to the viable skin layers.

Although ingredients that provide moisturization and skin hydration are regulated as cosmetics, they nonetheless may affect the structure and function of skin. They are extensively and effectively utilized either as sole ingredients or with other active ingredients in cosmeceuticals to provide various skin benefits. Effective moisturizers can change both the appearance and the tactile feel of skin by changing corneocyte adhesion at the skin surface, as well as the resultant light reflectance at the surface. Depending on the ingredients, the effects can last from a few minutes to several hours. Additionally, these compounds can help maintain the skin at optimal hydration by improving the barrier properties of the skin, which in turn reduces TEWL and increases skin hydration. Many cosmeceuticals incorporate ceramides, free fatty acids, and cholesterol to help achieve these goals.

Skin texture is caused by the excessive accumulation of dead keratinized skin, resulting in peaks and valleys at the skin surface. The appearance and tactile feel of skin surface roughness, scaliness, and dryness can be partially explained by abnormalities in corneocyte production, maturation, adhesion, and separation. By exfoliating the superficial, loosely coherent corneocytes, a significant improvement in the skin texture can be achieved. Further skin benefits can occur when dermal cell proliferation, differentiation, and collagen production are simultaneously stimulated to reduce the appearance of wrinkles.

Exfoliation

The most common exfoliating agents are alpha-hydroxy acids (AHAs) (34). Glycolic and lactic acids are the two AHAs that are most frequently used in moisturizers and cleanser products. At low to medium range of concentrations (2–10%) both of these fruit acids have profound inhibitory effects on corneocyte adhesion (35,36). This inhibitory effect promotes desquamation of the upper layers of stratum corneum, leading to gentle exfoliation which ultimately improves skin texture and roughness. Prescription products are available with higher concentrations of AHAs (>12%) for scaly skin. To treat severely photodamaged skin, higher AHA concentrations are generally employed to cause superficial necrosis, epidermolysis, and chemical peeling of the epidermis (37,38). In addition to its exfoliating effects, glycolic acid is used to provide synergy with other active ingredients in the products, for example, enhancing the wrinkle reduction activity of retinoids or skin depigmentation effects of hydroquinone-based products.

Salicylic acid, a beta-hydroxy acid, and other polyhydroxy acids are used in many cosmeceutical products to improve the appearance of acne. These acids concentrate in sebaceous glands, thereby explaining their beneficial effects on acne. They also lead to exfoliation of the stratum corneum, promoting a smoother skin. These acids also have an important utility in cosmeceuticals as these enhance the benefits of other active ingredients present in the formulation.

Wrinkle Reduction

In addition to changes in the skin texture, an important contributor to the look and feel of damaged skin is rhytides. Among cosmeceutical benefits, improvement of wrinkles is perhaps the most desired attribute for the consumer. However, the scientific definition of what constitutes a wrinkle is somewhat elusive; even histologically it is difficult to identify and quantify individual wrinkles. In general, the underlying damage to the dermal cytoskeleton involving collagen and elastin structural alterations seem to correlate with the surface appearance of fine lines and wrinkles of various depths.

Topical retinoids are the gold standard against which other products that claim treatment of photoaging and wrinkle reduction are compared. A claim to reduce or treat wrinkles falls under the drug claim according to the FDA regulations; on the other hand, reducing the appearance of wrinkles is considered a cosmetic or cosmeceutical claim. Topical retinoids, whether prescription or cosmeceutical, are built on the core structure of the naturally occurring retinol, vitamin A. Vitamin A is derived from the dietary component beta carotene following intracellular hydrolysis. The most commonly used retinoids in the cosmeceuticals marketplace for fine lines, wrinkles, and photodamaged skin include retinol and its esterified derivatives retinyl acetate, retinyl propionate, and retinyl palmitate. Compared with retinol, these ester derivatives are more stable to light and oxidation and have a better skin penetration profile. To achieve skin benefits, both retinol and its ester derivatives are thought to be metabolically converted to retinoic acid, the active metabolite (39).

The acid form of retinol, all-transretinoic acid (tretinoin) is the most active form and is classified as a drug by the FDA. The first topical application of tretinoin was in the treatment of acne as a prescription product Retin-A® (Ortho Dermatologics, Los Angeles, CA), and was later approved under the trade name RENOVA® (Ortho Dermatologics, Los Angeles, CA) for the treatment of photodamaged skin and wrinkles. The efficacy of topical tretinoin is well established for the treatment of rhytides and photodamaged skin (40–44). In addition to wrinkles, improvement in skin pigmentation, texture, and sallowness have been shown in several controlled clinical studies (45–49). Although tretinoin is the most studied (41,50) some studies indicate that isotretinoin (cis-retinoic acid) can also provide comparable benefits (51,52). Improvement in the appearance of fine lines and wrinkles in photodamaged skin has also been demonstrated by cosmeceutical formulations containing retinol (53,54), retinal/retinaldehyde (55,56), retinyl acetate, and retinyl palmitate (57). Small fine lines and wrinkles may also be due to or exacerbated by an excessive loss of water from the dermal layer. Therefore using hydrating formulations that have the ability to reduce transepidermal water loss can synergistically enhance the observed benefits of retinoids.

The biochemical mechanism of action and pharmacology of tretinoin is well studied, whereas for retinol and its esters their mechanism for skin repair is not as well established (53,58,59).

At the morphological level, topical retinoids stimulate proliferation and differentiation of keratinocytes, and increase production of glycosaminoglycans and collagen in the dermal layer. The net result at the macro level is epidermal and dermal thickening that smoothes out wrinkles (60–63). At the cellular level, retinoids are potent biochemical modulators capable of eliciting changes in the gene expression pattern by regulating the activity of transcription factors, as well as influencing epithelial cell proliferation and differentiation (64). The gene regulation by retinoids occurs via binding to heterodimer, nuclear receptor complexes from the retinoic acid receptor and the retinoid X receptor protein family. The activated receptor complex can then stimulate targeted gene expression by binding to the promoter region of select genes.

Recent studies have demonstrated other functions of retinoids, including direct anti-inflammatory effects and indirect antimicrobial effects in patients with acne. It is not known whether the anti-aging effect of topical retinoids is also through downregulation of inflammation found in skin; this remains an area of active investigation. Adapalene (Differin®, Galderma Laboratories, Fort Worth, TX) and tazarotene (Tazorac®, Allergan Inc, Irvine, CA), the two synthetic retinoids have been approved as prescription products for the topical treatment of acne. Of these, only tazarotene 0.1% cream has been approved for the treatment of photodamaged skin, fine lines, and wrinkles (65). In a vehicle-controlled study, tazarotene cream was shown to treat photodamaged skin and significantly improve mottled hyperpigmentation, fine lines and wrinkles, lentigines, pore size, and tactile roughness (66).

A significant side effect from topical retinoid use is a relatively high incidence of skin irritation, including erythema, scaling/peeling, and postinflammatory hyperpigmentation. These side effects, if they occur, generally subside following two to four weeks of continued use. Another problem commonly attributed to potent retinoids is photosensitivity. A progressive thinning of stratum corneum is probably a contributing factor to these dermal side effects.

REVERSING PIGMENTARY CHANGES AND IMPROVING SKIN TONE

Skin pigmentary disorders are an important and noticeable part of the aging process. Irregular hyperpigmentation may be discrete or diffuse, and clinically manifest as freckles, solar lentigines, melasma, dyschromia, or an ashy appearance of the skin. Unfortunately, these pigmentary changes are hallmarks of chronologically aged or photodamaged skin. Cosmeceutical and drug products in this category are aimed at skin lightening by reducing the appearance of hyperpigmented spots in order to achieve a more even skin tone.

Most of the depigmentation-active ingredients in marketed cosmeceuticals are natural derivatives that have activity against one or more of the skin melanogenesis processes, which are responsible for the formation and deposition of the melanin in human skin. Hydroquinone (1, 4-dihydroxybenzene), a phenolic compound, is a potent inhibitor of the rate-limiting enzyme tyrosinase, responsible for melanin formation. The molecule also causes inhibition of DNA and RNA synthesis and degradation of melanosomes and melanocytes. A 3–5% concentration is generally required to produce a significant level of depigmentation. In the United States, concentrations below 2% can be marketed as OTC items, whereas levels above 2% fall under the prescription category. Reported adverse effects include skin irritation and sensitization (67–69). Some of the dermal side effects can be reduced by adding topical corticosteroids (70) to the formulation. The combination products containing hydroquinone with a steroid, retinoid, and/or an alpha hydroxyl acid have been shown to provide an enhanced clinical efficacy while reducing the side effects (71–73). A triple combination first introduced by Kligman (74), containing hydroquinone, tretinoin, and dexamethasone (or another steroid) has been clinically proven to provide highly effective melasma treatment (71,72). A commercial product (Tri-Luma®, Galderma Laboratories, Fort Worth, TX) for treatment of moderate to severe melasma contains hydroquinone 4%, fluocinolone acetonide 0.01%, and tretinoin 0.05% in a cream base (72).

In addition to the prescription agent hydroquinone, there are several cosmeceuticals that contain natural derivatives with demonstrated mild to moderate skin-lightening effects. Azelaic acid, a naturally derived straight-chain dicarboxylic acid from the cultures of *Pityrosporum ovale* is a non–drug active ingredient that achieves its clinical effect by mechanism similar to hydroquinone, i.e., by inhibiting the enzyme tyrosinase. Even though it does not have the potency of hydroquinone, it seems to have sufficient efficacy for the treatment of hyperpigmented skin and melasma (75,76). Mild skin-lightening effects for melasma treatment have also been reported for the licorice extract that contains a flavonoid liquiritin (77). Kojic acid (5-hydroxymethyl-4H-pyrane-4-one), another naturally derived tyrosinase inhibitor, is widely used in skin-lightening cosmeceuticals and has been reported to have activity comparable to hydroquinone-based products (78).

NEWER ACTIVE INGREDIENTS FOR COSMECEUTICALS

Peptides

An emerging trend in cosmeceuticals is the inclusion of an active peptide to beneficially affect cellular functions. Several peptides have been designed to mimic the active amino acid sequence of type I collagen. The basic scientific rationale suggests that these molecules can induce a "wound healing response" which results in neocollagen synthesis. A number of small-molecular-weight peptides (typically 3–5 amino acids) have been demonstrated through in vitro fibroblast cultures to have biological responses that would be considered beneficial for skin health. One of the most widely used peptides in cosmeceuticals is a pentapeptide (Lys-Thr-Thr-Lys-Ser) linked to palmitic acid known as Pal-KTTKS (79,80). The peptide is designed to mimic the collagen type-1 fragment, and is thought to signal downregulation of collagenase, an enzyme responsible for collagen breakdown, and at the same time upregulate collagen synthesis. It is not clear how much of the topically applied peptide actually penetrates the skin and reaches the dermal layer where its biological function is expressed.

Another utility of peptides in cosmeceutical products is as a carrier molecule for copper and to facilitate copper uptake by cells. Copper is an essential cofactor for superoxide dismutase, an enzyme responsible for reducing the levels of free radicals in cells; copper is also a necessary cofactor for lysyl oxidase, a key enzyme in collagen and elastin formation. A tripeptide GHK–copper complex has been used in topical products to provide skin benefits.

Niacinamide

In addition to topical vitamins A, C, and E, niacinamide, a water-soluble member of the vitamin B complex, has more recently entered the cosmeceutical arena and provides skin benefits that have been shown to be similar to topical retinoids (39).Niacinamide is thought to work by restoring levels of NADH (Nicotinamide Adenine Dinucleotide hydride) and reduced NADPH (Nicotinamide Adenine Dinucleotide Phosphate) in keratinocytes and dermal fibroblasts in aged and photodamaged skin to levels seen in young skin. Topical preparations containing niacinamide can restore skin barrier function and reduce the appearance of wrinkles, blotchiness, and hyperpigmented spots in aging facial skin (81).

CONCLUSIONS

The field of cosmeceuticals is rapidly growing and constantly evolving. Although cosmeceuticals are not regulated as medications by the FDA and may not make marketing claims that are considered drug-like, they most certainly have a significant impact in helping patients achieve their ideals of beauty. Cosmeceuticals contain active ingredients that help to improve the appearance of wrinkles, provide an anti-aging effect by countering ROS and oxidative skin damage, enhance skin moisturization, and improve the appearance of skin tone and texture. It is therefore important for physicians to be aware of the utility of cosmeceuticals, incorporate them into their practice, discuss them with their patients, and make them an integral part of their patient's cosmetic regimen.

REFERENCES

1. Lavker RM, Zheng PS, Dong G. Morphology of aged skin. Dermatol Clin 1986; 4: 379–89.
2. Fenske NA, Lober CW. Structural and functional changes of normal aging skin. J Am Acad Dermatol 1986; 15: 571–85.
3. Kligman LH, Kligman AM. The nature of photoaging: its prevention and repair. Photodermatol 1986; 3: 215–27.
4. Kang S, Fisher GJ, Voorhees JJ. Photoaging: pathogenesis, prevention, and treatment. Clin Geriatr Med 2001; 17: 643–659.
5. Viña J, Borrás C, Miquel J. Theories of ageing. IUBMB Life 2007; 59: 249–54.
6. Wei YH, Lu CY, Wei CY, Ma YS, Lee HC. Oxidative stress in human aging and mitochondrial disease-consequences of defective mitochondrial respiration and impaired antioxidant enzyme system. Chin J Physiol 2001; 44: 1–11.
7. Oblong JE, Millikin C. Skin biology: understanding biological targets for improving appearance. In: Ahluwalia GS, ed. Cosmetic Applications of Laser and Light-Based Systems. New York: William Andrew, Inc., 2009: 37–48.
8. Alpermann H, Vogel HG. Effect of repeated ultraviolet irradiation on skin of hairless mice. Arch Dermatol Res 1978; 262: 15–25.
9. Bernstein EF, Chen YQ, Kopp JB, et al. Long-term sun exposure alters the collagen of the papillary dermis. Comparison of sun-protected and photoaged skin by northern analysis, immunohistochemical staining, and confocal laser scanning microscopy. J Am Acad Dermatol 1996; 34: 209–18.
10. Fisher GJ, Datta SC, Talwar HS, et al. Molecular basis of sun-induced premature skin ageing and retinoid antagonism. Nature 1996; 379: 335–9.
11. Harley CB, Vaziri H, Counter CM, Allsopp RC. et al. The telomere hypothesis of cellular aging. Exp Gerontol 1992; 27: 375–82.
12. Morley JE, Unterman TG. Hormonal fountains of youth. J Lab Clin Med 2000; 135: 364–6.
13. Yaar M, Gilcrest BA. Skin aging: possible mechanisms and consequent changes in structure and function. Clin Geriatr Med 2001; 17: 617–30.
14. Vessey DA. The cutaneous antioxidant system. In: Fuchs F, Packer L, eds. Oxidative stress in dermatology. New York: Marcel Dekker, 1993: 81–103.

15. Harman D. The free radical theory of aging. Antioxid Redox Signa 2003; 5: 557–61.

16. Baumann LS. A refresher on antioxidants. Skin Aller New 2004; 35: 31.

17. Bissett DL, Miyamoto K, Sun P. Topical niacinamide reduces yellowing, wrinkling, red blotchiness, and hyperpigmented spots in aging facial skin. Int J Cosmet Sci 2004; 26: 231–8.

18. Jacobson MK, Kim H, Kim M. Modulating NAD-dependent DNA repair and transcription regulated pathways of skin homeostasis: evaluation in human subjects 60th Annual Meeting of the American Academy of Dermatology, New Orleans, LA, Feb. 4–8, 2011.

19. Nachbar F, Korting HC. The role of vitamin E in normal and damaged skin. J Mol Med 1995; 73: 7–17.

20. Mayer P. The effects of vitamin E on the skin. Cosmet Toilet 1993; 108: 99–109.

21. Darr D, Combs S, Dunston S, et al. Topical vitamin C protects skin from ultraviolet radiation-induced damage. Br J Dermatol 1992; 127: 247–53.

22. Darr D, Dunston S, Faust H, et al. Effectiveness of antioxidants (vitamin C and E) with and without sunscreens as topical photoprotectants. Acta Derm Venerol (Stockh) 1996; 76: 264–8.

23. Dreher F, Denig N, Gabard B, et al. Effect of topical antioxidants on UV-induced erythema formation when administered after exposure. Dermatol 1998; 198: 52–5.

24. Dreher F, Gabard B, Schwindt DA, et al. Topical melatonin in combination with vitamins E and C protects skin from ultraviolet-induced erythema: A human study in vivo. Br J Dermatol 1998; 139: 332–9.

25. Eberlein-Konig B, Placzek M, Przybilla B. Protective effect against sunburn of combined systemic ascorbic acid (vitamin C) and d-alpha-tocopherol (vitamin E). J Am Acad Dermatol 1998; 38: 45–8.

26. Stoyanovsky DA, Osipov AN, Quinn PJ, Kagen VE. Ubiquinone dependent recycling of vitamin E radicals by superoxide. Arch Biochem Biophy 1995; 323: 343–51.

27. Bagchi D, Garg A, Krohn RL, et al. Oxygen free radical scavenging abilities of vitamins C and E, and a grape seed proanthocyanidin extract in vitro. Res Commun Mol Pathol Pharmacol 1997; 95: 179–89.

28. Katiyar SK, Ahmad N, Mukhtar H. Green tea and skin. Arch Dermatol 2000; 136: 989–94.

29. Baker CG. Moisturization: new methods to support time proven ingredients. Cosmet Toilet 1987; 102: 99–102.

30. Friberg SE, Ma Z. Stratum corneum lipids, petrolatum and white oils. Cosmet Toilet 1993; 107: 55–9.

31. De Groot AC, Weyland JW, Nater JP. Unwanted effects of cosmetics and drugs used in dermatology. Amsterdam: Elsevier, 1994: 498–500.

32. Spencer TS. Dry skin and skin moisturizers. Clin Dermatol 1988; 6: 24–8.

33. Neudecker BA, Maibach HI, Stern R. Hyaluronan: the natural skin moisturizer. In: Elsner P, Maibach HI, eds. Cosmeceuticals and Active Cosmetics. FL: Taylor and Francis Group, 2005: 373–406.

34. Uhoda E, Pierard-Franchimont C, Petit L, Pierard GE. Hydroxyacids. In: Elsner P, Maibach HI, eds. Cosmeceuticals and Active Cosmetics. FL: Taylor and Francis Group, 2005: 207–18.

35. Berardesca E, Maibach H. AHA mechanisms of action. Cosmet Toilet 1995; 110: 30–1.

36. Fartasch M, Teal J, Menon GK. Mode of action of glycolic acid on human stratum cornium: ultrastructural and functional evaluation of the epidermal barrier. Arch Dermatol Res 1997; 289: 404–9.

37. Murad H, Shamban AT, Premo PS. The use of glycolic acid as a peeling agent. Dermatol Clin 1995; 13: 285–307.

38. Rubin MG. Therapeutics: personal practice. The clinical use of alpha hydroxyl acids. Aust J Dermatol 1994; 35: 29–33.

39. Oblong JE. Wrinkles: Cosmetics, Drugs, and Energy-Based Systems. In: Ahluwalia GS, ed. Cosmetic Applications of Laser and Light-Based Systems. New York: William Andrew, Inc., 2009: 301–16.

40. Goldfarb MT, Ellis CN, Weiss JS, Voorhees JJ. Topical tretinoin therapy: its use in photoaged skin. J Am Acad Dermatol 1989; 21: 645–50.

41. Weiss JC, Ellis CN, Headington JT, et al. Topical tretinoin improves photoaged skin: a double-blind vehicle-controlled study. J Am Med Assoc 1988; 259: 527–32.

42. Davies PJA, Basilion JP, Haake AR. Intrinsic Biology of Retinoids in the Skin. In: Goldsmith LA, ed. Physiology, Biochemistry, and Molecular Biology of the Skin. New York: Oxford University Press, 1997: 1, 385–409.

43. Kligman AM, Grove GL, Hirose R, Leyden JJ. Topical tretinoin for photoaged skin. J Am Acad Dermatol 1986; 15: 836–59.

44. Griffiths CE, Finkel LJ, Tranfaglia MG, et al. An in vivo experimental model for effects of topical retinoic acid in human skin. Br J Dermatol 1993; 129: 389–94.

45. Samuel M, Brooke RC, Hollis S, Griffiths CE. Interventions for photodamaged skin. Cochrane Database Syst Rev 2005; 25: CD001782.

46. Gilchrest BA. A review of skin ageing and its medical therapy. Br J Dermatol 1996; 135: 867–75.

47. Olsen EA, Katz HI, Levine N, et al. Tretinoin emollient cream: a new therapy for photodamaged skin. J Am Acad Dermatol 1992; 26: 215–44.

48. Nyirady J, Bergfeld W, Ellis C, et al. Tretinoin cream 0.02% for the treatment of photodamaged facial skin: a review of two double blind clinical studies. Cutis 2001; 68: 135–42.

49. Kang S, Bergfield W, Gottlieb AB, et al. Long term efficacy and safety of tretinoin emollient cream 0.05% in the treatment of photodamaged facial skin: a two year randomized placebo controlled trial. Am J Clin Dermatol 2005; 6: 245–53.

50. Weinstein GD, Nigra TP, Pochi PE, et al. Topical tretinoin for treatment of photodamaged skin. Arch Dermatol 1991; 127: 659–65.

51. Cunningham WJ, Bryce GF, Armstrong RA, et al. Topical isotretinoin and photodamage. In: Saurat J-H, ed. Retinoids. 10 Years On. Basel: Karger, 1991: 182–90.

52. Sendagorta E, Lesiewicz J, Armstrong RB. Topical isotretinoin for photodamaged skin. J Am Acad Dermatol 1992; 27: S15–18.

53. Kang S, Duell EA, Fisher GJ, et al. Application of retinol to human skin in vivo induces epidermal hyperplasia and cellular retinoid binding proteins characteristic of retinoic acid but without measurable retinoic acid levels of irritation. J Invest Dermatol 1995; 105: 549–56.

54. Kafi R, Kwak HS, Schumacher WE, et al. Improvement of naturally aged skin with vitamin A (retinol). Arch Dermatol 2007; 143: 606–12.

55. Creidi P, Humbert P. Clinical use of topical retinaldehyde on photoaged skin. Dermatol 1999; 199S: 49–52.

56. Diridollou S, Vienne MP, Alibert M, et al. Efficacy of topical 0.05% retinaldehyde in skin aging by ultrasound and rheological techniques. Dermatol 1999; 199S: 37–41.

57. Oblong JE, Bissett DL. Retinoids (Chapter 6). In: Draelos Z, ed. Procedures in Cosmetic Dermatology Series: Cosmeceuticals. Elsevier Publishers, 2005: 37–44.

58. Duell EA, Derguini F, Kang S, et al. Extraction of human epidermis treated with retinol yields retro-retinoids in addition to free retinol and retinyl esters. J Invest Dermatol 1996; 107: 178–82.

59. Duell EA, Kang S, Voorhees JJ. Unoccluded retinol penetrates human skin in vivo more effectively than unoccluded retinyl palmitate or retinoic acid. J Invest Dermatol 1997; 109: 301–5.

60. Bhavan J. Short and long-term histologic effects of topical tretinoin on photodamaged skin. Int J Dermatol 1998; 37: 286–92.

61. Eichner R, Gendimenico GJ, Khan M, et al. Effects of long term retinoic acid treatment on epidermal differentiation in vivo: specific modifications in the program of terminal differentiation. Br J Dermatol 1996; 135: 687–95.

62. Fisher GJ, Esmann J, Griffiths EM, et al. Cellular, immunologic and biochemical characterization of topical retinoic acid-treated human skin. J Invest Dermatol 1991; 96: 699–707.

63. Griffiths EM, Russman AN, Majmudar G, et al. Restoration of collagen formation in photodamaged human skin by tretinoin. N Engl J Med 1993; 329: 530–5.

64. Varani J, Fisher GJ, Kang S, Voorhees JJ. Molecular mechanisms of intrinsic skin aging and retinoid-induced repair and reversal. J Invest Dermatol Symp Proc 1998; 3: 57–60.

65. Sefton J, Kligman AM, Kopper SC, et al. Photodamage pilot study: a double blind vehicle controlled study to assess the efficacy and safety of tazarotene 0.15 gel. J Am Acad Dermatol 2000; 43: 656–63.

66. Kang S, Leyden JJ, Lowe NJ, et al. Tazarotene cream for the treatment of facial photodamage: a multicenter, investigator masked, randomized, vehicle-controlled. Parallel comparison of 0.01%, 0.025%, 0.05% and 0.1% tazarotene cream with 0.05% tretinoin emollient cream applied once daily for 24 weeks. Arch Dermatol 2001; 137: 1597–604.

67. Grimes PE. Melasma: etiologic and therapeutic considerations. Arch Dermatol 1995; 131: 1453–7.

68. Fisher AA. Hydroquinone uses and abnormal reactions. Cutis 1983; 31: 240–50.

69. McEvoy GK. AHFS Drug Information. Bethesda, MD: American Society of Health System Pharmacist, 2001.

70. Engasser PG, Maibach HI. Cosmetic and dermatology: bleaching creams. J Am Acad Dermatol 1981; 5: 143–7.

71. Taylor SC, Torok H, Jones T, et al. Efficacy and safety of a new triple-combination agent for the treatment of facial melasma. Cutis 2003; 72: 67–72.

72. Torok HM, Jones T, Rich P, et al. Hydroquinone 4%, tretinoin 0.05%, fluocinolone acetonide 0.01%: a safe and efficacious 12-month treatment for melasma. Cutis 2005; 75: 57–62.

73. Penneys NS. Ochronosis-like pigmentation from hydroquinone bleaching creams. Arch Dermatol 1985; 121: 1239–49.

74. Kligman AM, Willis I. A new formula for depigmenting human skin. Arch Dermatol 1975; 111: 40–8.

75. Fitton A, Goa KL. Azelaic acid: a review of its pharmacological properties and therapeutic efficacy in acne and hyperpigmentary skin disorders. Drugs 1991; 41: 780–98.

76. Balina LM, Graupe K. The treatment of melasma: 20% azelaic acid versus 4% hydroquinone cream. Int J Dermatol 1991; 30: 893–5.

77. Amer M, Metwalli M. Topical liquiritin improves melasma. Int J Dermatol 2000; 39: 299–301.

78. Garcia A, Fulton JE. The combination of glycolic acid and hydroquinone or kojic acid for the treatment of melasma and related conditions. Dermatol Surg 1996; 22: 443–7.

79. Thornfeldt CR. Cosmeceuticals: separating fact from voodoo science. Skinmed 2005; 4: 214–20.

80. Lupo MP. Cosmeceutical peptides. Dermatol Surg 2005; 31(7 P 2): 832–6.

81. Matts PJ, Oblong JE, Bissett DL. A review of the range of effects of niacinamide in human skin Intl Fed Soc Cosmet Chem Mag. 2002; 5: 285–9.

Achieving healthy skin through a multimodality approach
Howard Murad

KEY POINTS

- The best methods to restore youthful-appearing skin implement a multimodality all-inclusive approach
- Best considered in a three-pillar approach: external care, internal care, and emotional care
- External care is a cornerstone of therapy that includes topical retinoids, aesthetic facials, topical antioxidants (particularly vitamin C), and topical peptides
- Internal care should include a properly balanced, nutritious diet, oral anti-inflammatories and antioxidants, as well as specific essential vitamins and nutrients
- Emotional care can be achieved through stress-reduction treatments, adequate sleep regimens, and relaxing physical activities
- By combining effective external, internal and emotional care, people can begin to achieve their look of healthy, youthful skin

---

The advancement in the digital revolution, rapid rate of communication, and high technology have produced a new level of collaboration across specialties. This collaboration has encouraged innovative thoughts in employing neutraceuticals, exercise, and therapies that address emotional composition to promote healthy skin through whole-body health. In other words, the merging of professions and research has offered cosmetic physicians a blended strategy to achieve healthy skin. This new way of thinking has brought about vast changes in traditional methods used in cosmetic medicine. Moreover, cosmetic investigators have continued their research below the dermis, contemplating all internal corporal aspects to unfold the precise mechanisms of inflammation, a wide range of diseases, hormonal imbalances, and their complex interactions with the epidermis. The simplest but most significant discovery from the research pursuits—and surely the greatest challenge to a healthy skin—is that all systems, organs, tissues, and emotions are indeed connected. In place of applying single therapies, implementing inclusive health protocols that address cellular health topically, internally and emotionally, has been found to produce ideal cosmetic results with the greatest longevity. As such, rather than being the exception, the multidisciplinary treatment has become the norm to achieve a healthy skin.

The philosophy behind an inclusive health approach represents the next logical step in the sequence of today's medical care. It includes all therapies and is based on a patient's specific needs. It offers an approach that is comprehensive with its goal being to stimulate the body to take care of itself. In essence, therapies work in tandem to create the most complete healthcare program for overall wellness and cosmetic concerns. By and large, skin care has become health care.

Generally, this approach can be accomplished using a three-pillar formula that addresses the mind, skin, and body through a systematic protocol, which includes programs that focus on external, internal, and emotional concerns. To summarize, it includes the following:

External care—to address the skin, the body's largest organ and the first line of defense. This includes topical treatments such as aesthetic facials, appropriate skin care regimens, and cosmetic medical services.

Internal care—to support all aspects of a healthy lifestyle. This includes nutrition, supplements, physical activity, and prescription medication.

Emotional care—to help patients achieve psychological and social balance. This includes the feel-good services that can be offered at spas, stress-reduction activities like exercise, and support groups to nurture the psyche.

EXTERNAL CARE

A thorough review of cosmeceuticals and their mechanism of action to prevent and/or reverse photoaging can be found in additional chapters in this section. One of the most important and widely used topical treatments for acne and anti-aging is topical retinoids, which are comedolytic and anti-inflammatory. Retinoids cause epidermal differentiation and normalize follicular hyperproliferation and hyperkeratinization. Retinoids work within the cells, unlike alpha hydroxyl acids (AHAs) which work in between the cells. In the right proportion, at the right time, retinoids can reduce inflammation and the overproduction of dead cells. Nevertheless, skin irritation with peeling and redness may be associated with their use, or rather misuse. It is fairly common for patients to overuse prescription retinoid products.

Nondrying cleansers and noncomedogenic moisturizers may help reduce this irritation. Alternate-day dosing may be considered if irritation persists. Topical retinoids thin the stratum corneum, and they have been associated with sun sensitivity, so patients must be instructed about sun protection. In addition, patients on retinoids need to take extra caution when waxing or undergoing similar services.

Aesthetic facial treatments have been found to be quite effective in addressing aging skin and reactive oxygen species (ROS) effects; thus they form an integral part of an inclusive protocol for healthy skin. The basic functions of facials performed by aestheticians are to repair, revitalize, and rehydrate skin. Aesthetic facials form the prelude to more invasive medical services and are beneficial in postoperative protocols.

Aesthetic facial treatments can be initiated and tailored based on information gathered at the patient consultation. The first step in facial treatment is to exfoliate dead skin cells and this can be done efficiently with a number of exfoliating products like alpha hydroxy acids (AHAs), which were truly the first cosmeceutical ingredients. AHAs initiate the repair process as they accelerate cell turnover and encourage healthy skin, unveiling an ever-greater improvement in skin texture, tone, and youthfulness with each treatment. AHAs also function well to prepare the skin to accept moisturizing ingredients and nutrients such as antioxidants, and they remain an essential part of professional and at-home skin care treatments.

Beyond exfoliation, facial treatments must infuse topical antioxidants to revitalize skin. An abundance of literature is available on topical antioxidants such as vitamins A, C, and E, which are documented to correct, protect, nourish, and condition newly exfoliated skin. Antioxidants, in general, have been found to stimulate collagen production, and, as such, they are key ingredients in anti-aging protocols.

It is important to note that of the topical antioxidants, one topical vitamin stands out—vitamin C. Vitamin C is a multitasker in the skin. In the epidermis, where there is five times more vitamin C than in the deeper skin layers, it performs several functions. It helps prevent water loss and therefore maintains the skin's barrier function. It is involved in collagen and elastin building. And it deactivates the unstable free radicals before they cause too much damage. There is also increasing evidence that vitamin C shields the skin from the sun's burning rays, especially when it is applied in high concentrations or combined with vitamin E, sunscreens, and skin soothers (Fig. 1.3.1). Because there is a limit to how much the body can absorb through food, researchers have discovered that topical application can increase the skin's vitamin C content more than 20 times. Stability issues have plagued vitamin C products; however, airtight packaging and anhydrous silicone-based formulations have been produced to protect the ingredient from oxidation and offer superior penetration.

Since the discovery of topical vitamin C, more powerful antioxidants have been discovered in goji berry fruit, pomegranate, and green tea. Studies continue to elucidate the ingredients' full potential both topically and internally.

Goji berry contains 500 times more vitamin C by weight than an orange. Goji berries contain more than 20 trace

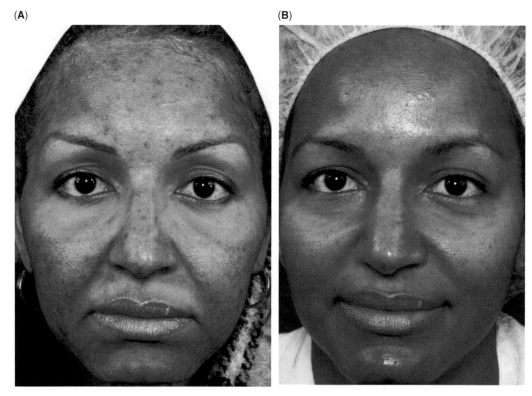

(A)   (B)

Figure 1.3.1 (**A**) Patient had trichloroacetic acid peel in another doctor's office and ended up with severe hyperpigmentation. We treated her for 2 months with in-office medical glycolic peels and vitamin C treatments, alternated weekly. Patient was put on a dietary supplement program with pomegranate extract, glucosamine, essential fatty acids, B vitamins, and antioxidants. Home use consisted of a daily application of a vitamin C treatment and sunscreen. (**B**) Appearance of the skin after 8 weeks.

minerals such as iron, copper, calcium, and zinc and they are rich in carotenoids. The berries upregulate cytokine expression (1).

Pomegranate contains ellagic acid, which is one of the most potent antioxidants as it effectively scavenges free radicals. It also stimulates an increase in the body's own built-in antioxidant, glutathione. Perhaps the most extraordinary benefit of this radically innovative ingredient is that it actually boosts the sun protection factor rating of topical sunscreens so that the same sun protection factor levels are maintained using less chemicals and more antioxidants. Research shows that ellagic acid found in pomegranate juice has powerful anti-aging properties and is currently being studied for its anti-cancer and healing benefits.

Green tea contains catechins, which are antioxidants that have been shown to reduce inflammation and inhibit cancer formations on skin. In laboratory studies, tea catechins were found to inhibit cancer growth by scavenging oxidants before cell injuries occur, reducing the incidence and size of chemically induced tumors and inhibiting the growth of tumor cells. In studies of liver, skin, and stomach cancer, chemically induced tumors were shown to decrease in size in mice that were fed green and black tea (2,3).

The final step in facial treatment is rehydration and this requires lipid replacement and skin barrier protection (Fig. 1.3.2). Many moisturizing products have been introduced to serve this function. Countless of them also incorporate sunscreen and antioxidants, which are critical in preventing new sun damage and free-radical damage to cellular membranes. For the most part, multifunctional products have become the standard, as have home care systems for daily care. Without daily home care, in between professional aesthetics services and more invasive medical treatments, results will be limited.

Peptides have also been another promising discovery for topical care. Peptides, which are long chains of amino acids, have been touted to reduce wrinkles and skin roughness among other things. Fundamentally, they help increase the communication between epidermal cells so the cells can do their jobs more efficiently. The benefits of new peptide technology offer alternative ways to stimulate cells to increase the rate of skin cell regeneration. In fact, work has been completed at the Scientific Center of State Research in St. Petersburg, Russia, to evaluate the immunostimulating properties of a newly discovered peptide called Nonapeptide-78. Nonapeptide-78 has been independently proven to encourage an immune response and stimulate growth factors. This isolated peptide, of algae origin, was demonstrated to effectively upregulate proliferative growth factors in healthy tissues and cell cultures. It demonstrated increases in keratinocytes as well, and it was shown to increase the expression of the genes of fibroblast, epidermal and endothelial growth factors.

There are a variety of peptides that produce different effects when applied topically. Peptide technology research for skin treatments is ongoing as interest continues to be extremely high. It is, therefore, part of an ever-expanding category of ingredients. Following are some of the peptides used in cosmetics and how they are believed to affect skin (4).

- Acetyl Hexapeptide-8 (Argireline®): Reduces the depth of expression wrinkles
- Hexapeptide-9 (Collaxyl®): Used for skin regeneration and anti-aging
- Decorinyl®: Improves skin suppleness and strength
- Dipeptide-2 and Palmitoyl Tetrapeptide-3 (Eyeliss™): Rejuvenates the eye area; paired with Regu®-Age for synergistic effects
- GHK-Cu (copper peptide or tripeptide-1): Skin healing; increases collagen production; hydrates skin
- Matrixyl-3000®: The next-generation Matrixyl; includes a combination of palmitoyl oligopeptide and palmitoyl tetrapeptide
- Dextran and Nonapeptide-1 (Melanostatine®-5): Inhibits the release of the alpha melanocyte stimulating hormone, therefore suppressing melanin production
- Hexapeptide-10 (Serilesine®): Improves cell adhesion to ensure proper skin nutrition and health; anti-aging effect
- Palmitoyl Oligopeptide (Dermaxyl®): Stimulates collagen; repairs skin
- Palmitoyl Oligopeptide and Palmitoyl Tetrapeptide-7 (Haloxyl™): Used to reduce dark under-eye circles
- Palmitoyl Pentapeptide-4 (Matrixyl®): Increases collagen production, plumps and thickens skin
- Palmitoyl Tripeptide (Biopeptide CL™): Thickens dermis; anti-wrinkle effect
- Palmitoyl Tetrapeptide-7 (Rigin™): Stops inflammation, smoothes, and regenerates skin; boosts collagen; mimics growth factors; reduces inflammation
- Palmitoyl Tripeptide-8 (Neutrazen™): Decreases inflammation in the skin
- Snap-8: Alters nerve signals to lessen muscle contractions
- Soy Peptides and Oxido Reductases (Regu®-Age): Rejuvenates the eye area
- Synthetic Tripeptide (Syn-Ake®): Reduces muscle contractions; called "synthetic snake venom"
- SYNiorage™: Improves the adhesion between epidermis and dermo-epidermal junction through collagen XVII; refines skin texture
- Palmitoyl Tripeptide-5 (Syn®-Coll): Promotes collagen; plumps skin
- Oligopeptides: Skin lightening peptides created to replace hydroquinone use

INTERNAL CARE

Perhaps the largest and most ever-expanding category of ingredients includes those used internally. After external care and in combination with daily home care, to promote healthy skin, an inclusive protocol must include a nutritional strategy. Topical skincare products will address approximately 20% of the epidermis. The remaining 80% requires an internal approach, feeding the skin the appropriate nutrients through foods and dietary supplements. In addition to increasing cellular water, adequately feeding the body nutrients will boost the body's immune system and its ability to fight invaders, and this can be useful to increase skin and body health in general.

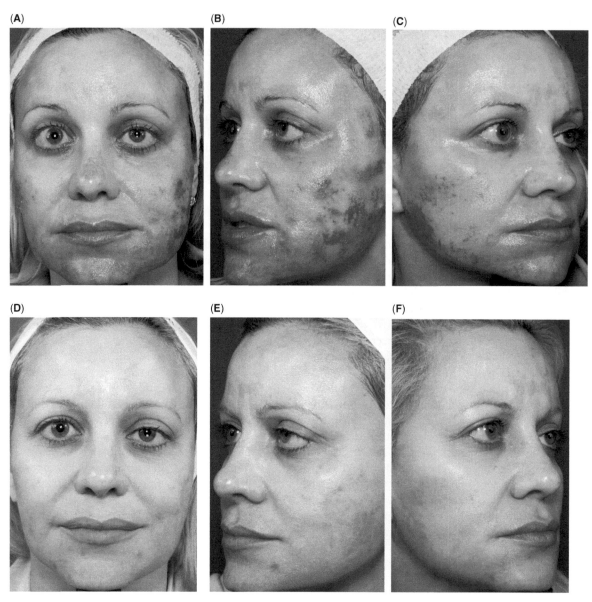

Figure 1.3.2 (**A, B, C**) Patient came to us with 2nd-degree burns from a laser treatment performed in another office. In-office vitamin C treatments and soothing, hydrating facials were performed with a plant-based lipid serum and hyaluronic acid serum and a final application of a skin soothing ointment. Patient was put on a dietary supplement program with pomegranate extract, glucosamine, essential fatty acids, B vitamins, key minerals, and antioxidants. Her home-use program consisted of a mild cleanser, lipid and hyaluronic acid serums, a vitamin C treatment and moisturizer, plus sunscreen. (**D, E, F**) Appearance of the skin after 6 months.

The benefits of oral neutraceutical supplementation have been studied. Specifically, a supplement containing antioxidants, glucosamine, essential amino acids, and minerals in reversing certain clinical features of cutaneous aging such as fine lines and wrinkles was shown to significantly reduce the number of wrinkles and fine lines by 34%, exclusive of epidermal hydration, in as little as six weeks. The oral supplement studied contained proline and glycine because they are normal components of collagen and elastic fibers; *N*-acetylglucosamine and glucosamine sulfate, which are modified sugars present in glycosaminoglycans; antioxidant vitamins C and E, in addition to selenium, copper, zinc, and manganese; and "naturally" available herbal products including quercetin, catechin-based preparations, and grape seed extract. Sixty-five subjects (12 controls) were involved in the study. Subjects were instructed, during a seven-day conditioning period before the study, to discontinue any moisturizing products, sunscreens, soaps, and makeup products and avoid excessive ultraviolet exposure. Subjects selected included Fitzpatrick skin types I–IV and had not used tretinoin, isotretinoin, or received facial peels, dermabrasion, or laser services within the last 12 months. Apart from the 34% reduction in skin wrinkling and fine lines, according to the data presented, supplementation did not provide any significant increase in epidermal hydration, which indicates that oral supplements do not obviate the need for topical skin treatment with moisturizers (5).

The inference is that a complete inclusive strategy that pairs topical therapies with oral supplements offers an optimal strategy to assist in repairing epidermal and dermal evidence of aging, while preserving and perhaps increasing skin hydration. Notwithstanding, daily intake of key foods will also offer additional benefits, supplementation is not a substitution for foods.

Nutrition scientists have recognized that Americans eat less than the ideal to maintain good health and that many overeat substances that can be harmful to every aspect of well being. In summary, Americans are overfed and undernourished and many suffer from obesity. As a direct result, the U.S. weight loss market was projected to grow from $58 billion to $69 billion by 2010 (6). While obesity is a problem, it is just one part of the issue. The major concerning factor is the suboptimal levels of nutrients including healthy fats, vitamins, and minerals. Nutrition can play three key roles in relation to degenerative disease: (*i*) poor nutrition accelerates their development; (*ii*) a healthful diet and optimal nutrition can help forestall, prevent, and even reverse them; and (*iii*) nutrition therapy can ease their impact if they do occur.

In general, patients should consume an anti-inflammatory, immune system–enhancing diet based on fruits and vegetables rather than starches. Refined grains and carbohydrates, high-calorie refined sugars, red meat, and other saturated fat meat products should be substituted with healthier alternatives. In addition, whole-fat dairy products and unhealthy fats and oils must be avoided.

Fruits and vegetables: We should eat more of these foods than any other: three or more servings a day of fruits and four or more servings of vegetables. One-half to one cup of chopped fruit or vegetables represents one serving. Fruits and vegetables are rich in the healing antioxidants the body needs. They also contain many of the trace minerals and B vitamins that the body uses to metabolize carbohydrates, fats, and protein, in addition to synthesizing DNA and new cells. Also, it is known that cruciferous vegetables contain some compounds that may have a cancer-inhibitory effect. Whenever possible, fruits and vegetables should be eaten raw.

Whole grains: The diet should contain four to eight servings of whole grains a day. One slice of whole-grain bread represents a serving. Whole grains contain the entire grain kernel—the bran, germ, and endosperm. Examples include whole-wheat flour, bulgur (cracked wheat), oatmeal, whole cornmeal, brown rice, and popcorn. Whole grains are sources of magnesium and selenium. Magnesium helps build bones and release energy from muscles. Selenium protects cells from oxidation and is also important for a healthy immune system.

Protein: The diet should consist of four to six servings of protein a day. About 3 ounces of fish or chicken represents one serving. Soy products should be substituted for dairy products. Beef and pork should be avoided because of their high levels of saturated fats. Complete foods including eggs, seeds, and beans, which are rich in embryonic material and lecithin, should be incorporated as well. Protein-rich foods—including omega-3-rich fish, white-meat chicken, eggs, soy foods, fat-free and low-fat dairy products, and beans—provide the essential amino acids needed to build collagen and elastin. Specifically, protein sources also provide sulfur amino acids. Early studies on sulfur in the diet have indicated that the element is detoxifying and anti-inflammatory. In addition, other studies have suggested that

sulfur compounds promote circulation, reduce pain, and enhance the immune system (7).

Fats: The diet should be limited to 3 to 4 servings of healthy fat a day. A teaspoon of oil represents one serving. "Healthy" fats are unsaturated, such as omega-3, -6, and -9 fatty acids, flaxseed oil, extra-virgin olive oil, canola oil, natural-style nut butters, and nuts. Hydrogenated oils or trans fats should be avoided. Essential fatty acids (EFAs) are found in cell membranes where they offer protection and prevent intracellular water from escaping, thus optimizing cellular functions. As such, in stratum corneum skin cells, EFAs play a role in maintaining the immune system. Omega-3 fatty acids contain alpha linoleic acid. It is recommended to take at least 2.2–4.4 g of alpha linoleic acid (omega-3 fatty acid) per day in a supplement form.

RECOMMENDED NUTRIENTS

Unhealthy skin cannot maintain the natural balance of bacteria and yeast normally found on skin, so it will become compromised. In patients with acne, cutaneous immunity is critical. Immune system–boosting foods can help increase the number of white cells in the immune system; these cells war against infection and disease. In addition, the nutrients contained can assist with neutralizing ROS. Some of the top nutrients to include in a diet that promotes healthy skin include:

Vitamin A: Vitamin A is an antioxidant that plays a large role in the repair of body tissues and is vital for good eyesight and healthy skin. Food sources for vitamin A include liver, sweet potatoes, carrots, goji berries, mangos, eggs, and milk. For vitamin A, the upper daily limit is 3000 mcg or 10,000 IU.

B Vitamins: There are eight B vitamins and these play a key role in metabolism—they help the body in releasing energy from protein, fat, and carbohydrates. B vitamins are also essential for a healthy nervous system. While most of these are consumed in foods, it is advisable to take a supplement with a B complex daily to ensure optimal metabolism.

- Vitamin B1 (thiamine): brewer's yeast, sunflower seeds, wheat germ, green peas, whole grains, and beans
- Vitamin B2 (riboflavin): low-fat and nonfat dairy products, dark green leafy vegetables, brewer's yeast, asparagus, broccoli, and whole grains
- Vitamin B3 (niacin): poultry, fish, mushrooms, nuts, brewer's yeast, green peas, whole grains, and beans
- Vitamin B5 (pantothenic acid): all plant and animal foods; especially salmon, chicken, avocado, mushrooms, sweet potatoes, low-fat and nonfat milk, eggs, soybeans, peanut butter, bananas, oranges, and whole grains
- Vitamin B6 (pyridoxine): watermelon, bananas, spinach, soybeans, brewer's yeast, fish, poultry, wheat germ, and whole grains
- Vitamin B7 (biotin): eggs, most vegetables, brewer's yeast, wheat germ, oatmeal, cereals, almonds, soybeans, bananas, grapefruit, and tomatoes

- Vitamin B9 (folate and folic acid): brewer's yeast, dark green leafy vegetables, asparagus, orange juice, beets, broccoli, and beans
- Vitamin B12 (cyanocobalamin): fish, poultry, low-fat and nonfat dairy products, fortified soy milk, eggs, and brewer's yeast

Vitamin C: Citrus fruits and goji berries are the best sources of vitamin C. Other sources include kiwi, mango, papaya, and black currents; however, virtually all fruits and vegetables contain this potent antioxidant. Vitamin C increases the production of infection-fighting white blood cells and increases the levels of interferon. For vitamin C, the upper daily limit is 2000 mg.

Vitamin D: While naturally present in very few foods, vitamin D can be found in the flesh of fish such as salmon, tuna, and mackerel and fish liver oils are among the best sources. Vitamin D is essential for promoting calcium absorption and plays a role in immune function and in reducing inflammation. Most people meet their vitamin D needs through exposure to sunlight. For vitamin D, the upper daily limit is 400 IU.

Vitamin E: Because vitamin E is a fat-soluble antioxidant, it can be stored in cell walls, ready to offer immediate protection from free radicals. Vitamin E helps the body use vitamin K. It is also important in the formation of red blood cells, which have been recently indicated to play a part in the body's immune response (8). Vitamin E stimulates the production of natural killer cells and enhances the production of B-cells. The ideal amount is 30–60 mg a day, which can be obtained from a diet rich in seeds, such as sunflower seeds and raw almonds.

Vitamin K: Vitamin K is known as the clotting vitamin, because without it blood cannot clot. Some studies indicate that it helps in maintaining strong bones in the elderly. Vitamin K is found in cabbage, cauliflower, spinach, and other green leafy vegetables, cereals, and soybeans. The bacteria that line the gastrointestinal tract are capable of making vitamin K. For vitamin K, the upper daily limit is 65 mcg for adult women and 80 mcg per day for adult men.

Alpha-linoleic acid: Alpha-linoleic acid (ALA) works together with antioxidants such as vitamins C and E. It is important for growth, helps prevent cell damage, and helps the body rid itself of harmful substances. The body needs ALA to produce energy. It plays a crucial role in the mitochondria. Its role in cellular health is very important to prevent the breakdown of cells leading to water loss. Although ALA is found in vegetables, beans, fruits, flaxseed oil, canola oil, wheat germ, brewer's yeast, walnut oil, and raw walnuts, obtaining ALA from supplements is the best way to get concentrated amounts of this antioxidant. ALA belongs to the omega-3 family of fatty acids.

Alpha lipoic acid: Healthy sources of alpha lipoic acid include spinach, broccoli, and brewer's yeast. Alpha lipoic acid is a powerful antioxidant that neutralizes free radicals and plays a crucial role in cellular functions. The body produces enough alpha lipoic acid to keep the cells going, but not enough for it to act as an antioxidant. The free-radical scavenger is said to prevent and treat age-related diseases like heart disease, diabetes, stroke, and Parkinson's and Alzheimer's

diseases. It boosts cellular energy, enhances immunity and muscle strength, and improves brain function. Alpha lipoic acid enhances the functions of other antioxidants such as vitamins C and E, as it improves cell growth and repair while it prevents cell damage. While there are no established recommended doses, for general support, a daily intake of 20–300 mg is recommended.

Carotenoids: Beta carotene increases the number of infection-fighting cells, natural killer cells, and helper T-cells. Beta carotene is the most familiar carotenoid, but it is only one member of a large family. Researchers believe that it is not just beta carotene that produces all these good effects, but all the carotenoids working together. For this reason, consuming carotenoids in the diet is ideal compared to taking supplements alone. The body converts beta carotene to vitamin A, which itself has anti-cancer properties and immune system–boosting functions. Foods rich in orange and yellow pigments such as apricots, carrots, papaya, cantaloupe, yams, and mangos contain high levels of carotenoids. Those taking a supplement form of vitamin A should avoid mega doses, which can be toxic. It is recommended that people start with 5000 IU per day.

Coenzyme Q10: Coenzyme Q10's benefits come from two major attributes. First, coenzyme Q10 is able to protect the mitochondria from free-radical damage. Second, it is necessary for the production of energy in all cells of the body. Even though coenzyme Q10 occurs in the cells of all plants and animals, dietary sources do not provide adequate levels of this nutrient; as a result, supplements are helpful.

Garlic: A member of the onion family, garlic is a powerful immune system booster that stimulates white blood cells and boosts natural killer cell activity. Garlic contains sulfur compounds such as allicin and sulfides; garlic is also an antioxidant that helps reduce free-radical buildups. Some cultures with a garlic-rich diet have a lower incidence of intestinal cancer. Garlic may be eaten raw or cooked, or taken in a supplement form at levels of 100 mg per day.

Glucosamine: Glucosamine is a prominent precursor in the biochemical synthesis of glycosylated proteins and lipids. Some research indicates that glycosylation may play a part in cell–cell adhesion (a mechanism used by immune system cells). Glucosamine is a precursor for glycosaminoglycans. It is recommended that 1200 mg of either glucosamine sulfate or glucosamine hydrochloride be taken every day.

Grape seed extract: This extract contains high levels of polyphenols and may help prevent and treat heart diseases such as high blood pressure and high cholesterol. It also contains EFAs and resveratrol. Resveratrol, an ingredient in red wine that has been linked to a lowered risk of heart disease, is a sirtuin stimulator. Sirtuins have been found to play a role in regulating aging. They are cellular enzymes that allow cells to survive damage and delay cell death. For this reason, many new anti-aging drugs that target sirtuins are being researched.

Lecithin: Lecithin is a vital component to any wellness and skin rejuvenation program. Main sources for lecithin include eggs and soy foods. Lecithin repairs tissues as it fills in and rebuilds cell walls. It is mainly comprised of phosphatidylcholine, which is a major component of cellular membranes. A lecithin supplement (2000–4000 mg) should be taken every day.

Mushrooms: Mushrooms have been an important food source and a potent medicinal ingredient for many cultures around the world. There are approximately 10,000 species of mushrooms, of which 200 species have been identified to have medicinal properties. Some of the most well known and researched include reishi, shiitake, and maitake, which have immunity-enhancing, infection-fighting properties. A diet that includes a variety of mushrooms is helpful for overall immunity.

Omega-3 fatty acids: These healthy, fatty acids help increase the activity of phagocytes. Omega-3 fatty acids are vital for preserving healthy cell membranes. Sources include cold water fish such as mackerel, tuna, or salmon. Healthful oils from avocados, olive oil, flaxseeds, and walnuts also provide omega-3 fatty acids.

Polyphenols: Many polyphenols are known to provide certain health benefits to the cardiovascular system and immune system. These chemicals help to downregulate the formation of free radicals. The strongest polyphenol is ellagic acid. The highest levels are found in raspberries, strawberries, and pomegranates. Other polyphenol food sources include nuts, whole-grain cereals, brightly colored fruits, vegetables, berries, soybeans, tea (especially green tea), red grapes, red wine, onions, and citrus fruits.

Quercetin: Quercetin is a bioflavonoid known for its antioxidant and anti-inflammatory benefits. It helps inhibit the manufacture and release of histamine and is often referred to as an anti-allergy nutrient. Eating a diet rich in apples, onions, red grapes, citrus fruits, cherries, raspberries, cranberries, and broccoli helps provide quercetin; alternatively, a dietary supplement of 1 g per day supports daily nutrition.

Selenium: This mineral helps increase natural killer cells. The best food sources are tuna, red snapper, whole grains, egg yolks, sunflower seeds, Brazil nuts, and brown rice. Selenium is also found in many vegetables; however, the amount varies depending on the amount of selenium in the soil. Selenium may also be taken in supplement form at 70 mcg per day.

Turmeric: Turmeric has antioxidant qualities and has been studied for use with liver functions, cholesterol, and in treating Alzheimer's disease. High in iron and manganese, it also contains vitamin B6. Curcumin, its primary component, has been shown to offer anti-inflammatory benefits.

Zinc: This valuable mineral helps increase the production of white blood cells to fight infection. Zinc may be obtained in lozenges, dietary supplements, and through food. The goal is to aim for 15–25 mg per day of zinc. Foods rich in zinc include beans, nuts, whole grains, oysters, beef, and dark meat turkey. Also, many whole-grain cereals are fortified with zinc.

EMOTIONAL CARE

Often, a patient's lifestyle is the single most important factor in determining his or her success rate with an inclusive program. Accordingly, stress is the largest factor that dominates poor lifestyle choices. In addition to affecting behavior, there are several ways in which stress affects hormone levels. Consequently, an inclusive strategy must incorporate stress reduction therapies.

Emotional distress adversely affects health. Digestive problems, constipation, diarrhea, high blood pressure, dizziness, tension headaches, chest pain, heart disease, panic attacks, and irregular periods might exist because of accumulated stress (9). Because all systems are connected, the epidermis suffers as well.

To ascertain a patient's stress level ask him or her this question: "What would you do tomorrow if you had no obligations?" Follow this up with another question: "Why can't you do or start that today?" The patient's answers will indicate his or her primary stressors. Clinically, we now categorize stress in three ways: acute stress, episodic acute stress, and chronic stress.

Acute stress: Acute stress is short-term and is the most common form of stress. This type of stress comes from things like taking a test or giving a speech. Once the test is over or speech is done, the stress goes away. It is the most treatable and manageable kind of stress.

Episodic acute stress: This type of stress happens to those who live in chaos. Those who experience this kind of stress seem to always be rushed, but ironically, they are habitually late.

Chronic stress: Chronic stress is debilitating. This is the stress that people feel when they cannot see a way out of a miserable situation, for example, an unhappy marriage, poverty or a horrible job.

While these three categories have been adequate for the last decades, so much has changed in the world, it has become necessary to add another subcategory, to describe the stress that is superimposed on all other stressors: cultural stress. This type of constant stress has much to do with who we are as a culture.

Cultural stress: Cultural stress is the result of human evolution. It includes everyday stressors that come from technology, commuting, over-scheduling, etc. From the advent of the digital revolution in the 1980s, to increased population and affluence, to the world-changing events on September 11, 2001, many of life's stressors have taken a more prominent and invasive position in our daily lives.

The hormones DHEA and cortisol have a direct link to stress levels and illustrate the clear relationship stress has with skin health. As an example, many physicians believe that every kind of stress negatively affects acne. Researchers at the Department of Dermatology, Stanford University School of Medicine conducted a study to illustrate this connection. Their objective was to clarify the possible relationship between stress and acne exacerbation by evaluating changes in acne severity during non-examination and examination times. Study volunteers consisted of 22 students (15 women and 7 men) with varying degrees of acne. Participants were evaluated by a dermatologist and had their acne rated for severity a month before a final examination and again right after they took the final examination. To further confirm the evaluation, a separate investigator verified the acne rating through photographs of each volunteer. The study conclusion confirmed that people with acne may experience even more breakouts during test time (10). Changes in acne severity correlate highly with increasing stress, suggesting that emotional stress from external sources does have an influence on acne.

A report in *Diabetes Research and Clinical Practice* discusses the results of a study that closely examined the benefits of yoga and meditation. The study showed that yoga and meditation, practiced for three months, reduced waist circumference, systolic blood pressure, fasting blood sugar, and triglyceride levels, and increased high-density lipoprotein (the good fats). In addition, at the end of the study period, feelings of anxiety, stress, and depression were significantly decreased, and optimism was significantly increased. The conclusion is that yoga not only helps in prevention of lifestyle diseases, but can also be a powerful adjunct therapy when diseases occur (11,12).

Another recent report revealed that tai chi, a type of mind–body practice that originated in China as a martial art, has exhibited positive health effects. According to research supported by the federally funded National Institute on Aging and National Center for Complementary and Alternative Medicine, tai chi may help older adults in avoiding contracting shingles as it increases immunity to the varicella-zoster virus and boosts the immune response to the varicella vaccine.

All things considered, touch therapies are exceptional at reducing stress levels. For skin care and spa professionals, their hands offer strong, healing medicine to the mind and body. Skin not only signals touch and temperature, it detects nuances in our environment and communicates them to the brain. Harvard University researchers have dubbed this connection the neuro-immuno-cutaneous-endocrine network or N.I.C.E. Loosely, everything that affects the skin, affects the body, and vice versa. The skin is connected to our brain, our nervous system, our hormones and our immune system.

In broader terms, it is a mind–skin link that reflects health as well as disease (13).

PATIENT MINDSET

Because everything is connected in the body, externally, internally, and emotionally, a patient seeking healthy skin must enter a new mindset. Skincare is health care and in order to achieve long-lasting goals, all aspects of health must be addressed. This revolutionary, all-embracing approach to health and anti-aging can only function if there is synergy between the team of medical, aesthetic, and lifestyle professionals as well as the patient. All parties must work side by side to address physical and emotional fitness and cosmetic treatments for skin health and rejuvenation.

In the medical office, to initiate an inclusive program, begin with a thorough analysis of the patient. Evaluate all aspects of his or her topical, internal and emotional concerns. Shortly after the first visit, consultation and evaluation, offer the patient a treatment roadmap that outlines the following:

External care—Provide a prescription for topical products and treatments and recommend a schedule of facial services, as well as any medical procedures that may ameliorate topical skin conditions.

Internal care—Provide a detailed dietary and nutritional menu listing the appropriate nutrients and quantities of foods necessary for the patient's body type, concerns and goals, in addition to a prescription for supplements and a recommendation for physical activity. Moreover, offer a discussion of any other prescription medication that may be necessary to correct internal issues such as hormonal imbalance or disease.

(A)   **(B)**

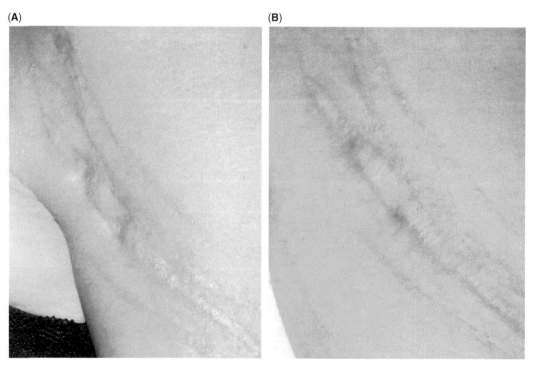

Figure 1.3.3 (**A**) Patient experienced a severe scar with hardened scar tissue on the left arm. In-office treatments consisted of weekly glycolic acid peels and vitamin C treatments. Patient was put on a dietary supplement program utilizing glucosamine, essential fatty acids, B vitamins, and antioxidants. Home use comprised of a daily soothing regimen to reduce redness, a cleanser with triclosan and licorice extract, followed by a treatment with azaleic acid, and a moisturizer with sunscreen. (**B**) Appearance of the skin after 5 weeks.

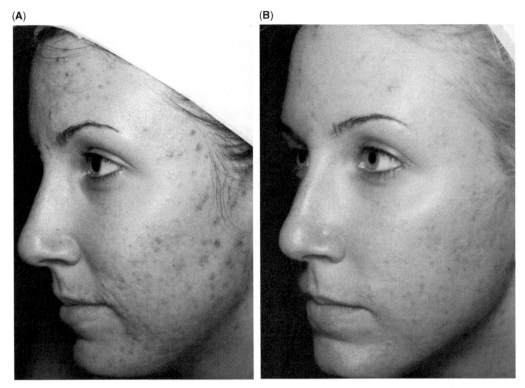

Figure 1.3.4 (**A**) Patient was experiencing inflamed papulopustular and pustular acne lesions. In-office medical facials consisted of 1 soothing facial, 6 glycolic peels, and 1 vitamin C facial. Patient was put on a dietary supplement program utilizing vitamin A, beta carotene, zinc, yellow dock, burdock root, curcumin, and various other antioxidants. Home use was comprised of a daily salicylic acid cleanser, a glycolic- and salicylic-based treatment, a soothing hydrating lotion, and an oilfree sunscreen. (**B**) Appearance of the skin after 8 weeks.

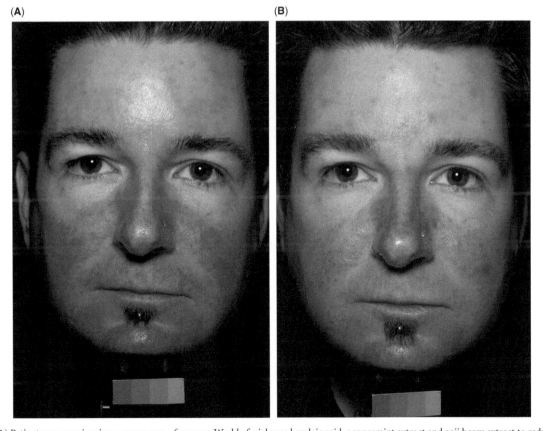

Figure 1.3.5 (**A**) Patient was experiencing a severe case of rosacea. Weekly facials used azaleic acid, peppermint extract and goji berry extract to reduce inflammation and redness. A soothing mask using seaweed, balm mint, and sodium PCA was applied. Patient was put on a dietary supplement program utilizing essential fatty acids, pomegranate extract, vitamin A, beta carotene, zinc, yellow dock, burdock root, curcumin, and various other antioxidants. Home use was comprised of a daily soothing regimen to reduce redness; a cleanser with triclosan and licorice extract followed by a treatment with azaleic acid and a moisturizer with sunscreen. (**B**) Appearance of the skin after 8 weeks.

Emotional care—Provide a service list of spa treatments for stress reduction such as massage and include a recommended frequency for treatments. Offer referrals to psychological counseling if necessary and/or social support groups that may be appropriate. Also, give the patient any literature that may be suitable for his or her specific conditions. Finally, recommend a physical activity schedule with exercise therapies like yoga, tai chi, walking, etc. that target stress-induced imbalances or behavior.

CONCLUSIONS

Following this protocol, much like Ponce De Leon, together, all parties will enter a new frontier—one that has brought us ever closer to the antidote for aging. Perhaps researchers will one day discover a way to defy cell mortality. In the meantime, our best solution is to soldier on and continue to present aging its toughest battle as new theories are explored. The best approach requires a knowledge and integration of external care, internal care, and emotional care to minimize and reverse skin damage and the aging process. This approach can help patients with extrinsically damaged skin (Fig. 1.3.3), those who are suffering from medical conditions such as acne and rosacea (Figs. 1.3.4, 1.3.5), or those who seek to rejuvenate and revitalize their skin. Drawing from what we already know and moving beyond the basic principles, we have been able to realize a new fountain of youth—one where aging and degenerative disease are not completely inevitable.

REFERENCES

1. Gan L, Zhang SH, Liu Q, Xu HB. A polysaccharide-protein complex from Lycium barbarum upregulates cytokine expression in human peripheral blood mononuclear cells. Eur J Pharm 2003; 471: 217–22.
2. Dufresne CJ, Farnworth ER. A review of latest research findings on the health promotion properties of tea. J Nutr Biochem 2001; 12: 404–21.
3. Hakim IA, Harris RB. Joint effects of citrus peel use and black tea intake on risk of squamous cell carcinoma of the skin. BMC Dermatol 2001; 1: 3.
4. Smith MS. Science in a Bottle. DAYSPA 2008; 3: 98–110.
5. Murad H, Tabibian M. The effect of an oral supplement containing glucosamine, aminoacids, mineral, and antioxidants on cutaneous aging. J Dermatol Treat 2001; 12: 47–51.
6. Marketdata Enterprises. "U.S. weight loss market to reach $58 billion in 2007." Press release: April 17, 2007. Marketdata Enterprises, Tampa, FL (Epub 18 June 2008).
7. Parcell S. Sulfur in Human Nutrition and Applications in Medicine. Altern Med Rev 2002; 7(1): 22–44.
8. "Red blood cells do more than just carry oxygen. New findings by NUS team show they aggressively attack bacteria too." The Straits Times, 1 September 2007. (Epub 24 May 2008).
9. Miller L, Smith A. The Stress Solution. New York: Pocket Books, 1993.
10. Chiu A, Chon SY, Kimball AB. The response of skin disease to stress: changes in the severity of acne vulgaris as affected by examination stress. Arch Dermatol 2003; 139: 897–900.
11. Khatri D, Mathur KC, Gahlot S, et al. Effects of yoga and meditation on clinical and biochemical parameters of metabolic syndrome. Diabetes Res Clin Pract 2007; 78: e9–10.
12. Hagins M, Moore W, Rundle A. Does practicing hatha yoga satisfy recommendations for intensity of physical activity which improves and maintains health and cardiovascular fitness? BMC Complementary Altern Med 2007; 7: 40.
13. O'sullivan RL, Lipper G, Lerner E. The Neuro-Immuno-Cutaneous-Endocrine Network: Relationship of Mind and Skin. Arch Dermatol 1998; 134: 1431–5.

2.1 Introduction to facial rejuvenation
Andrew L. DaLio

The desire to look more youthful is as old as civilization. The hieroglyphics of ancient Egypt depicted the painted faces of Pharaohs and commoners alike, and cosmetics have been a staple of every society ever since (1). The face is unique in that it is the very essence of one's identity. Unfortunately, the aging process on the face is as visible to others as it is to us every time we look in the mirror. When we begin to look too much like our grandparents and not enough like the youthful selves that we still feel ourselves to be, perhaps it is time to consider cosmetic procedures that can unwind a few years off the clock.

Most of us don't feel our age and even fewer of us wish to look it. Unfortunately, there is no cure for the aging process and no Fountain of Youth to restore youth. Modern science has brought us Botox, dermal fillers, lasers, and surgeries all in an attempt to slow down time's razor edge. By utilizing these technologies either alone or in combination, it is absolutely possible to slow down the aging process, soften its effects, and hold on to our youthful good looks for as long as possible.

REFERENCE

1. Oumeish OY. The cultural and philosophical concepts of cosmetics in beauty and art through the medical history of mankind. Clin Dermatol 2001; 194: 375–86.

2.2   The aging process on the face
Andrew L. DaLio

KEY POINTS

- The aging process follows a relatively predictable pattern on most patients
- The first signs of aging develop in the late 30s, with dynamic rhytides and the nasolabial folds beginning to develop
- As the aging process continues, the malar fat pad atrophies. This loss of central facial volume results in deeper nasolabial folds and the development of jowls
- Eventually, patients develop platysmal neck bands, dermatochalasis of the upper and lower eyelids, and brow ptosis

Certainly age takes its toll on every part of the human body, but the face is perhaps unique in that it is the one part of our body that is always visible to others—it is the very visage of our identity—and it is where the effects of our aging are as visible to others as they are when we look in the mirror. When those effects become too pronounced, patients turn to their physicians to help soften the aging process.

The first visible signs of aging begin to reveal themselves sometime between the late 30s and mid-40s. The nasolabial folds, the lines that run from the sides of the nose to the corners of the mouth and separate the cheek from the upper lip, begin to deepen during this time period. The cheeks slowly begin to sag in a process called jowling, as we lose volume from the malar cheek fat pads. Lateral orbital commissure lines—crow's feet—begin to form around the outside corners of the eyes. Dynamic rhytides, or wrinkles, begin to appear in the forehead and glabellar region of the face. These early changes represent some of the first signs of aging and are a common cosmetic reason for patients to present for rejuvenation.

The aging process continues through the 50s. The nasolabial folds deepen and become more distinct; the jowling of the cheeks also becomes more pronounced. The dynamic rhytides, previously present only upon contraction of muscles, begin to become apparent at rest as static lines. Platysmal bands of contracted muscle and excessive skin begin to form around the neck. Finally, marionette lines, creases of skin perpendicular to the corners of the mouth, begin to appear.

In the 60s and 70s, the face loses significantly more of the underlying fat that gives it its shape and volume. This loss of volume helps to drive the aging process. The midface ultimately begins to sag. The malar fat pad, which in youth gives the cheeks their definition, descends. This loss of the malar fat pad adds sharp prominence to the nasolabial folds and allows the cheeks to fall over the jaw line forming distinct jowls. The platysmal bands around the neck become more prominent and the redundancy of sagging skin erases the cervicomental angle (the line that distinguishes the neck from the lower portion of the jaw). Surface rhytides—wrinkles and worry lines—become more apparent and appear "etched" into the skin.

Unfortunately, from there it gets only worse. Facial aging can result in brow ptosis: a sagging, uneven brow line. Dermatochalasis of the upper and lower eyelid develops, resulting in a redundancy of skin, fat, and muscle that causes the eyelid to sag and can impair vision. Many patients ultimately develop lower eyelid bags. Finally, around our mouth, the upper lip will atrophy, and wrinkles around the corner of the mouth known as perioral rhytides will form.

The common sequela for facial aging includes the following:
- Forehead and glabellar rhytides and brow ptosis
- Upper and lower eyelid dermatochalasis and rhytides
- Volume loss and infraorbital hollowing
- Mid-face laxity and ptosis with an accentuation of the nasolabial fold
- Lateral commissure rhytides and marionette lines
- Jowling
- Submental skin redundancy, platysmal bands, and obscuration of the cervicomental angle

The skin also undergoes predictable changes as it ages:
- Solar lentigines and hyperpigmentation of the skin develop
- Elastosis of the skin occurs
- Flattening of the epidermal–dermal junction
- Decreased levels of skin collagen
- Decreased levels of hyaluronic acid

As long as humans have been aging, they have been attempting to cheat the clock. Cosmetics and makeup have been around since the time of ancient Egypt. Fortunately, today, patients have more options at their disposal than ever before to attempt to slow the aging process. Skin creams, chemical peels, and lasers can diminish the visible signs of sun damage and aging. Botulinum toxin can be used to reduce the appearance of dynamic wrinkles. Injectable soft tissue fillers can be used to restore some of the face's lost volume, giving it a more youthful contour. And when noninvasive methods have failed to achieve the desired results, patients can undergo a facelift or brow lift for a long-term lifting procedure.

Each one of the procedures we discuss in this section targets a specific aspect of the aging process. Unfortunately, there is no single "magic bullet" which reverses all of these signs of aging. Instead, cosmetic physicians need to incorporate each of these modalities to help patients achieve their ideal youthful, beautiful appearance. Throughout this section, we will focus on this multimodality approach to rejuvenation.

2.3 Laser rejuvenation
H. Ray Jalian and Andrew Nelson

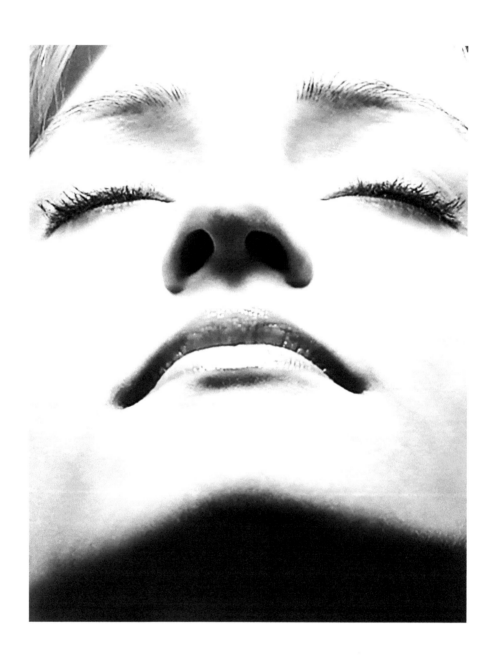

> **KEY POINTS**
>
> - Several different laser technologies are available and effective in rejuvenating the skin. The ideal laser depends on the patient and their treatment goal
> - Pulsed dye lasers (PDLs) and intense pulsed light are effective in treating facial erythema and telangiectasias, as these devices target hemoglobin and blood vessels
> - Dyschromia and pigmented conditions, such as lentigines, can be effectively treated with high-energy, short pulse duration Q-switched lasers. The exact Q-switched device depends on the color of the pigment being targeted, as well as its location within the epidermis or dermis
> - Noninvasive devices have been reported to improve skin wrinkling and induce mild skin tightening. Devices such as PDL, 1320-nm neodymium:yttrium-aluminum-garnet and 1450-nm diode laser, radiofrequency (RF) devices, and combination devices incorporating laser and RF, have all been reported to be effective
> - Fractional devices represent the newest technologies for skin rejuvenation. These devices treat only a portion of the skin surface to result in clinical efficacy with the least downtime and lower risks of side effects. Ablative and nonablative fractional devices exist for the treatment of facial rejuvenation, texture, rhytides, dyspigmentation, and scar treatment
> - The best cosmetic outcomes typically occur following the use of multiple laser technologies, particularly if the patient has extensive extrinsic and intrinsic aging processes. Furthermore, adjuvant botulinum toxin and fillers may further enhance the efficacy of these treatments

As we age, our skin is subjected to numerous intrinsic and extrinsic causes of damage. Ultimately, these insults lead to rhytides, dyschromia, telangiectasias, erythema, and poor skin texture and elasticity. While none of us want to look our age, there remains no perfect treatment to reverse the signs of aging.

In truth, the best treatment option for these changes is preventing them from developing in the first place. All patients should be counseled on the use of broad spectrum sunscreens, including a physical blocking agent such as titanium dioxide or zinc oxide. Furthermore, cosmetic physicians should emphasize the utility of long-term topical retinoid use, as these compounds have been shown to improve wrinkles, facial texture, and photoaging (1). Finally, patients should consider the use of topical antioxidants and other neutraceuticals to slow down the aging process (2), as discussed in chapter 1.2. These interventions are the first step in helping patients to slow down and reverse facial aging. Unfortunately, for many patients, these simple topical remedies are not effective enough to help them achieve their ideal of beauty; patients often then turn to their physicians or aestheticians to improve photodamage, facial rhytides, dyspigmentation, and skin texture.

Traditional treatments for photoaged skin work by ablating the epidermis and inducing dermal tissue damage. Such treatment modalities include ablative lasers, chemical peels, and dermabrasion. These therapies result in the improvement of clinical manifestations of photoaged skin. Many of these treatments produce dermal collagen remodeling in response to the dermal tissue injury, and this remodeling may well explain the noticeable reduction in facial rhytides and elasticity (3,4). However, these traditional modalities also lead to ablation of the epidermis and thus require one to three weeks or more of healing, the so-called "downtime." In addition, these procedures can result in complications such as persistent erythema, hyperpigmentation, hypopigmentation, scarring, and infection (5).

In the last several years, patients have increasingly sought efficacious treatments with minimal downtime and lower risk for post-procedure complications; as a result, nonablative laser resurfacing modalities have largely replaced ablative treatments. The goal of nonablative laser rejuvenation is to reverse or minimize as many of the signs of aging as possible. Fundamentally, this requires multiple therapeutic modalities, as each treatment targets different clinical imperfections (6). These laser therapies have emerged as a promising alternative for facial rejuvenation, and are at present one of the most commonly performed cosmetic procedures in the United States.

THE MECHANISMS OF LASERS

Lasers (light amplified stimulated emission of radiation) have several important characteristics that are utilized in rejuvenation. First, lasers emit monochromatic light, or light with a single wavelength. Second, laser light is directional implying that is a tight, strong, concentrated beam. Third, it is coherent, meaning that it is organized into uniform emitted wave fronts. Finally, it is of high intensity (7). Lasers are classified according to the wavelength of the photons they emit, which is in turn determined by the medium of the laser. Aesthetic physicians use lasers with different wavelengths for different purposes; ranging from visible light [pulsed dye laser (PDL), 585–595 nm], to infrared portions of the electromagnetic spectrum (750–10,600 nm).

The field of lasers was revolutionized with the concept of selective photothermolysis (8). In essence, the theory states that in order to target a specific structure, proceduralists must select the proper laser and treatment parameters. In general, there are three main parameters when utilizing a laser to influence its clinical outcome: (*i*) wavelength, which is fixed and determined by the medium of the laser; (*ii*) fluence, which represents the quantity of energy produced by the laser; and (*iii*) pulse duration, which represents the amount of time the tissue is exposed to the laser energy.

In the skin, there are three main chromophores (targets): melanin (pigment), hemoglobin, and water (9). These different chromophores absorb light at different wavelengths (Fig. 2.3.1). Depending on which chromophore the cosmetic surgeon is attempting to target, a laser that produces energy at the corresponding wavelength of the chromophore is selected. Once the proper laser is determined, the proceduralist then must select an ideal fluence and pulse duration.

As the chromophore absorbs energy, heat is produced, which is responsible for the clinical outcome. A sufficiently high fluence is necessary to generate heat for the clinical effect (10); however, utilizing too high of a fluence can result in thermal injury such as scarring (11). There exists, therefore, a treatment window where a sufficient fluence results in an ideal clinical outcome, without the risk of significant adverse effects.

Finally, proceduralists must select the proper pulse duration to achieve a desired clinical outcome without side effects.

As tissue targets are heated, the heat will diffuse into surrounding tissues. In general, proceduralists wish to heat the targeted tissue faster than the rate at which this energy diffuses into surrounding, unintended targets in order to result in selective, localized treatment. The thermal relaxation time is defined as the time necessary for the heated, targeted tissue to lose half of its heat to the surrounding tissues (12). This thermal relaxation time is a function of the size and shape of the chromophore. Larger chromophores, including hair follicles, have longer thermal relaxation times compared to smaller chromophores, such as tattoo and pigment particles. The ideal pulse duration for a laser is slightly shorter than, or equal to, the thermal relaxation time of the target.

Selective photothermolysis states that by selecting a laser with a wavelength preferentially absorbed by the chromophore, sufficient energy fluence, and appropriate pulse duration, it is possible to selectively target and heat tissue while sparing the surrounding areas. This concept guides most clinical decision making in laser rejuvenation. Rather than listing each laser individually, throughout the remainder of this chapter, we will group the lasers by which chromophore they target and their clinical effects.

TELANGIECTASIA AND ERYTHEMA

As the skin ages, people develop dilated and twisted blood vessels, clinically apparent as telangiectasias and diffuse background erythema. Facial erythema and dilated vessels are one of the most common cosmetic complaints of patients.

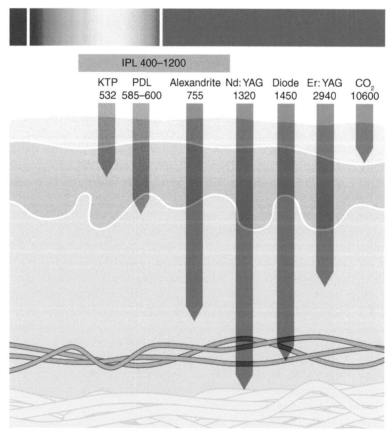

Figure 2.3.1 Absorption spectra for the three main chromophores in the skin (wavelengths are represented in nanometers).   *Abbreviations*: KTP, potassium-titanyl-phosphate; IPL, intense pulsed light; PDL, pulsed dye laser.

In order to treat these vessels, it is necessary to target the oxyhemoglobin inside the vessels. The hemoglobin is heated with the energy from the laser; this heat then diffuses from the hemoglobin to the blood vessel walls. As the vessel walls are heated, they constrict, resulting in an improvement in the clinical appearance of erythema and telangiectasias. If the vessels are heated rapidly and with sufficient energy, purpura (bruising) can develop. Many patients prefer to be treated with lower, subpurpuric energies in order to avoid any temporary bruising; however, purpuric energy levels may be necessary to result in clinical improvement in certain situations.

Various laser and light sources are available to effectively target oxyhemoglobin as a chromophore. The two most commonly utilized treatments are the pulsed dye laser (PDL) and intense pulsed light (IPL). Both modalities provide substantial improvement in both discrete telangiectatic vessels and diffuse erythema.

Pulsed Dye Light

PDL with wavelengths between 585 and 595 nm is the most frequently used device for treating ectatic blood vessels. This laser was first used to treat vascular defects such as port-wine stains, hemangiomas, and facial telangiectasias (13); it remains the gold-standard treatment for these conditions. Today, the PDL's usefulness has expanded beyond just the treatment of congenital vascular malformations, as it is now used for a wide range of dermatologic conditions. The most common cosmetic uses of the PDL include the treatment of individual telangiectatic vessels, diffuse facial erythema, and photorejuvenation (Fig. 2.3.2).

The PDL effectively targets oxyhemoglobin within blood vessels. As the oxyhemoglobin absorbs energy, heat is generated which ultimately results in the clinical improvement. After treatment with the PDL, individual blood vessels have been demonstrated to contain agglutinated erythrocytes, fibrin, and thrombi. Four weeks after this treatment, the damaged blood vessels have been shown to be replaced by normal appearing vessels (14).

Historically, PDL devices employed ultra-short pulse durations, ranging from 0.45 msec to 1.5 msec. These short pulse durations are shorter than the thermal relaxation time of most facial vessels, and result in the clinical appearance of purpura after treatment (15). While this purpura outbreak is not permanent, it can require up to two weeks to fully resolve. Purpura can be difficult for patients to conceal, and as a result, may not be suitable for all patients. More recently, longer pulsed PDL devices have been developed, with pulse durations ranging from 0.45 msec to 40 msec. As the pulse duration is lengthened, the vessels are heated slowly and more uniformly, decreasing the likelihood of purpura. Longer pulse durations with lower energy fluences, commonly referred to as nonpurpuric settings, have been shown to be similarly effective in the treatment of erythema and telangiectasia (16). In general, pulse durations longer than 6 msec are nonpurpuric, while pulse durations shorter than 3 msec result in purpura. As the energy fluence is increased, the risk of purpura increases. When treating diffuse background erythema, in our experience, we find that nonpurpuric settings are typically as effective as purpuric settings; however, patients should be counseled that multiple treatments will probably be necessary. Individual dilated telangiectatic vessels, on the other hand, may respond better to purpuric doses; nonpurpuric settings can be effective if multiple treatments are performed approximately every four to six weeks. Manufacturers of PDLs produce tables of recommended treatment parameters for their specific device. The exact energy fluence and pulse duration will depend on the clinical indication, and the experience of the proceduralist.

Side effects of PDL vary and depend on the location, energy, skin type, and pulse duration. Notably, transient erythema and edema are commonly observed side effects. At higher fluences and shorter pulse widths, purpura is an expected complication.

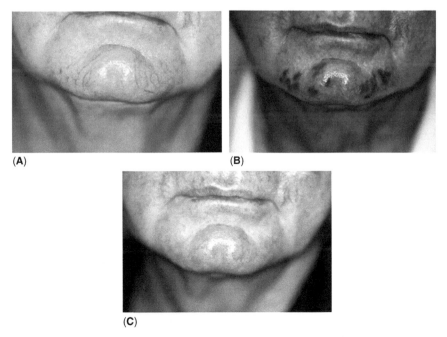

(A)   (B)

(C)

Figure 2.3.2 Clinical improvement in the appearance of the telangiectasia on the chin treated with 595-nm pulsed dye laser (**A**) prior to treatment (**B**) immediately postoperative at standard purpuric settings, and (**C**) 1 month after treatment.   *Source*: Photos courtesy of Gary Lask, MD.

(A)   **(B)**

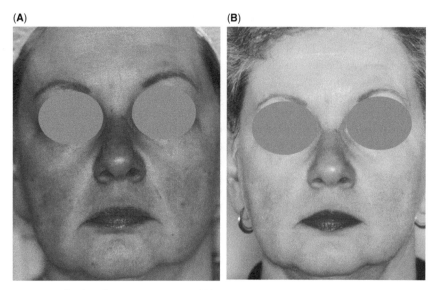

Figure 2.3.3 Clinical improvement in facial erythema, pigmentation, and skin texture (**A**) before and (**B**) after treatment with intense pulsed light.   *Source*: Photos courtesy of Gary Lask, MD.

Crusting, blistering, and pigment alterations have also been observed, as well as rare incidence of scarring (17).

Intense Pulsed Light

IPL is another commonly used technology for the treatment of facial erythema and telangiectasias. IPL is actually a non-laser light source, emitting a continuous spectrum of wavelengths from 500 to 1200 nm. Although it emits multiple wavelengths of light, it is not a true laser. IPL wavelengths can be limited by using a variety of filters. These filters block out all the wavelengths of light below the filter. For instance, if a 560-nm filter is used, all wavelengths below 560 nm are blocked while all the wavelengths from 560 to 1200 nm are allowed to pass. Depending on which filter is used, it is possible to target hemoglobin, melanin, and water, or a combination of the three chromophores.

Due to its wide spectrum of light produced, IPL is not as specific or targeted as PDL lasers. However, as the wavelength spectrum encompasses the peak absorption of hemoglobin, IPL can be used to improve facial erythema, flushing, and telangiectasias (Fig. 2.3.3) (18,19). IPL devices have the advantage of a large treatment size (~8 × 35 mm), which is useful when treating diffuse facial erythema or poikiloderma on the neck and upper chest. Additionally, as IPL produces a spectrum of light, it can also be used to target multiple chromophores at once. This is particularly useful when treating patients with both lentigines and telangiectasias, or for the management of poikiloderma.

Initial IPL treatment consists of four to five monthly treatment sessions, with maintenance treatments performed every six months. In general, IPL is very well tolerated; however, extra care must be taken with sensitive and sun-damaged skin such as the neck and chest. As with all laser and light sources, caution must be taken to use the right setting to avoid the risks of hyper and hypopigmentation of the skin, erythema, and crusting. Judicious sun protection must be emphasized to patients, both before and after treatment, as this can reduce the risk of complications.

DYSCHROMIA AND SKIN TEXTURE

In addition to vascular changes, uneven distribution of pigment and rough texture characterize photoaged skin. On a histologic level, the dyschromia is due to irregular distribution of epidermal melanin. Thus, when attempting to improve dyschromia, physicians target the epidermal melanin. The absorption spectrum for melanin extends broadly (Fig. 2.3.1). Unfortunately, it can be difficult to target the abnormal epidermal melanin causing dyschromia, while avoiding damage to the surrounding normal skin and melanin. Thus, physicians should be cautious when treating these lesions; we encourage the use of test spots (i.e., treating a small area of noncosmetically sensitive skin) in order to evaluate for any potential adverse events prior to performing full face or extensive treatments. Despite the potential challenges of treating dyschromia, several lasers are available which, when utilized properly, can result in significant improvement.

Q-Switched Lasers

One of the most commonly used technologies to target pigment particles, including melanin, is Q-switched lasers (Fig. 2.3.4). These lasers deliver high-intensity energy in extremely short pulse durations; the short pulse durations allow the laser to selectively target small molecules, such as individual melanocytes or tattoo particles (20). The absorption of this high-intensity energy leads to dispersion and destruction of the pigment particle. Clinically, this manifests as an immediate whitening of the pigment particle, which then slowly returns to its previous color over the next minutes or hours (21). The destroyed and dispersed pigment is then absorbed and eliminated by phagocytes in the skin, gradually reducing the color and intensity of the pigment over the next several weeks. For heavily pigmented areas, such as tattoos, multiple treatments are likely necessary every six to eight weeks.

Multiple Q-switched devices are available. These devices typically employ one of four common wavelengths: the frequency doubled neodymium: yttrium-aluminum-garnet

(A)   **(B)**

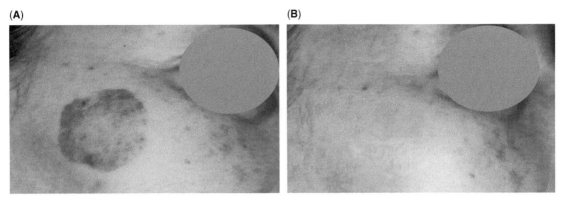

Figure 2.3.4 Clinical resolution of a lentigo on the cheek of a woman (**A**) before and (**B**) after treatment with a Q-switched Nd:YAG Laser.   *Source*: Photos courtesy of Gary Lask, MD.

(Nd:YAG) (532 nm), ruby (694 nm), alexandrite (755 nm), and Nd:YAG (1064 nm). Again, based on selective photothermolysis, the appropriate laser wavelength is selected. The frequency-doubled Nd:YAG, due to its relatively shorter wavelength, does not penetrate as deeply into the skin; it is therefore useful when treating epidermal and superficial pigments such as lentigines and freckling. On the other hand, longer wavelengths such as the Nd:YAG (1064 nm) penetrate much deeper into the dermis, and are useful for deeper pigments such as tattoos and dermal melanocytosis. Furthermore, the ideal laser to be utilized depends on the color of the pigment being targeted. Blue or black colors tend to be effectively treated with any of the above wavelengths. Red and yellow colors, on the other hand, tend to respond best to the frequency-doubled Nd:YAG (532 nm) wavelength; green colors can be effectively treated with either the ruby (694 nm) or alexandrite (755 nm) wavelengths (22). Finally, the proceduralist must consider the skin type of the patient being treated. Patients with darker skin types, and therefore greater concentrations of epidermal melanin, should be treated with longer wavelengths to decrease the likelihood of adverse events. The Nd:YAG (1064 nm) is considered the safest of these Q-switched devices in darker skin types (Fitzpatrick IV–VI).

Once the device to be utilized is determined, the proceduralist must then decide on the energy fluence. The energy fluence necessary depends on the skin type of the patient, as well as the color and density of the pigment particle. The denser the pigment is, the lower the fluence that will be required. Utilizing too high of a fluence will result in excess heat production and will increase the risk of adverse events including pigmentary alterations and scarring. The pulse durations of Q-switched lasers are fixed and do not need to be determined by the proceduralist.

Many physicians advocate for the use of a test-spot laser treatment prior to a full treatment. The test spot should be performed on a noncritical, less visible lesion or portion of the tattoo or pigmented lesion; the patient should then return to have the area examined in two to four weeks. If the patient has developed any signs of hypopigmentation or scarring, the patient either should be tested again at significantly lower energy fluences or should not be treated at all. While the test spot can help the proceduralist to determine whether a full treatment will be efficacious, the greatest utility is in reducing

the risk of adverse effects. This practice will greatly reduce the risk and incidence of potentially serious adverse effects from Q-switched laser treatments.

Intense Pulsed Light

As discussed previously, IPL is actually a light source which emits multiple different wavelengths of light. This can be extremely useful in the treatment of dyschromia, as IPL can simultaneously target both melanin and hemoglobin. IPL can therefore potentially improve both dyspigmentation and erythema with a single treatment modality. Additionally, since large spot sizes are available, IPL treatments can target a greater surface area with each pulse than laser treatments; this is particularly useful for treating off-face areas such as chest, hands, and extremities.

In clinical trials, IPL has demonstrated significant improvement in dyspigmentation and telangiectasia. Histologically, decreased melanin is observed at the dermal-epidermal junction following IPL treatments. IPL can also result in targeting the underlying dermal collagen by stimulating collagen synthesis and forming more compact collagen fibers in the papillary dermis. In clinical trials, IPL improves the appearance of skin texture and rhytides. Numerous other studies have quantified the efficacy of IPL in specific aspects of photoaging, including facial erythema, flushing, dyspigmentation, and fine wrinkles (9,19,23). Patient satisfaction with this device is high, presumably because of the rapid improvements notable in the color hues of photoaged skin, minimal downtime, and few adverse effects.

Typically, either the 515-nm or 550-nm cutoff filters are utilized for the IPL machine when treating patient's dyschromia. However, if a patient with darker skin tone is to be treated (skin type IV or greater), longer pulse durations with a 550-nm or 570-nm cutoff filter should be utilized to reduce the risk of damage to the patient's normal melanin, which can result in hyper or hypopigmenation (24). IPL treatments for dyschromia are typically a series of 4 to 6 treatments performed approximately once every four to six weeks. The exact energy and pulse duration settings will vary depending on the specific IPL device and manufacturer; typically, manufacturers provide a listing of suggested treatment parameters for their specific device.

Addition of Topical Aminolevulinic Acid

Application of photosensitizing agents, such as aminolevulinic acid (ALA), prior to PDL treatment has shown enhanced efficacy in the treatment of photoaging (25–27), presumably by preferentially targeting photodamaged cells. The observed clinical improvement is predominantly attributed to textural improvement and the removal of actinic keratosis, lentigines, and fine rhytides. ALA in conjunction with PDL has also been shown to increase collagen I and III production, increase epidermal proliferation, and enhance dermal remodeling at the molecular level (28).

Photodynamic therapy, combining ALA with IPL treatments has also been demonstrated to be more efficacious than IPL alone. A randomized, blinded, split-face clinical study of 20 patients comparing ALA followed by IPL to IPL treatment alone demonstrated that after two monthly treatments, there was greater improvement in erythema, dyspigmentation, and fine rhytides on the side receiving ALA plus IPL (29). In this study, both treatments were equally well tolerated. However, it is important to exercise caution when using a combination of ALA and IPL, as clinical responses vary and there is a risk of side effects. There have been reports of significant crusting with IPL treatments after one- to two-hour incubation with ALA (30); caution should therefore be exercised in treating photoaging with these combination regimens. In general, it is recommended to begin with low fluences designed for photorejuvenation when combining these technologies with ALA.

RHYTIDES

Over the last decade, many new noninvasive technologies have been developed to improve the appearance of rhytides. The traditional facelift remains the gold standard for wrinkle reduction, but many patients prefer to avoid a surgical procedure and its downtime to achieve these goals. As a result, a rapid development of noninvasive devices designed to tighten skin, promote new collagen formation, and improve the appearance of rhytides has occurred.

Pulsed Dye Lasers

Early research demonstrated histologic collagen remodeling in hypertrophic scars and striae distensae following PDL treatments. An early, preliminary study demonstrated significant improvement in the clinical appearance of periorbital and perioral rhytides following a single pass PDL (585 nm), at nonpurpuric fluence, and 0.45-msec pulse duration. Nine of the 10 patients with mild wrinkling reported a 50% improvement, and 40% of patients with moderate to severe wrinkling were noted to have clinical improvement. Histologic evidence of increased elastin and collagen staining, cellularity, and mucin deposition in the papillary dermis was also demonstrated (31). Despite the initial encouraging results, subsequent studies have failed to demonstrate significant clinical improvements. The PDL, utilizing nonpurpuric fluences and a 0.5-msec pulse duration, was reported to be ineffective in improving periorbital rhytides (32). A double blind study using PDL technology demonstrated only 18% improvement in photoaging (33), with the observed improvement mainly attributed to the targeting of telangiectasia (34).

Although biochemical and histologic evidences demonstrate quantifiable alterations in procollagen I, procollagen III, and TNF-a (35), following PDL treatments, these changes have not been shown to reliably correlate with clinical improvements. While there remain conflicting reports of the utility of PDL for the improvement of rhytides, the device has nonetheless gained U.S. Food and Drug Administration (FDA) approval for the treatment of photodamage.

Infrared Lasers

Infrared lasers, operating with wavelengths from 700 nm to 2000 nm target the water within tissues. When used in conjunction with epidermal cooling devices, selected infrared lasers can function as nonablative modalities for photorejuvenation. These devices have been reported to result in mild to moderate improvement in rhytide appearance. This modest efficacy of these devices may be related to the fact that they only induce dermal changes, and therefore having little effect on patient's epidermal photodamage (e.g., dyspigmentation, erythema). These devices are therefore best suited for patients with predominantly dermal photoaging and with relatively little epidermal photodamage. Of the available infrared lasers, the most commonly used for the treatment of photoaging include the 1320-nm long-pulse neodymium:yttrium-aluminum garnet (Nd:YAG) laser and the 1450-nm diode laser. Other devices are available with similar wavelengths and similar mechanisms of action.

Nd:YAG Laser (1320 nm)

The archetype of the nonablative infrared laser is the Nd:YAG, with a 1320-nm wavelength, 200-μsec pulse duration, and 10-mm treatment spot size. This device was designed for the purpose of treating acne and acne scarring, improving rhytides, and improving overall skin texture. The Nd:YAG uses a cryogen cooling system so that while thermal damage occurs within the dermis, there is minimal resulting epidermal damage. It is thought that the Nd:YAG targets water within the dermis, thereby generating heat and damage in the dermis. This damage ultimately will result in collagen remodeling, as well as neocollagenesis, to improve the appearance of rhytides.

This mechanism of action has been supported by histologic studies. Neocollagenesis has been demonstrated histologically on biopsy specimens six months post treatment (36). More recently, studies have shown that one hour after resurfacing with the Nd:YAG laser, skin displays epidermal spongiosis as well as basal cell edema (37). Three days following treatment microthrombi, sclerosis of blood vessels, and dermal neutrophilic infiltrates appear (38). These findings have led researchers to postulate that the immediate epidermal edema may lead to the recruitment of cytokines and other inflammatory mediators necessary to induce neocollagenesis.

Numerous clinical studies have been conducted evaluating the efficacy of the long pulsed Nd:YAG laser in the treatment of facial rhytides. One study using fluences from 28 to 38 J/cm^2 demonstrated mild to moderate reproducible improvement in facial rhytides in 10 of 10 patients, as assessed by the patient. However, of these 10 patients, only six of them were felt by the investigator to show definitive improvement (39). Another study with similar parameters demonstrated mild but statistically significant improvement after three biweekly treatments of mild, moderate, and severe rhytides. At 24 weeks post treatment, an appreciable clinical improvement was sustained in those patients with severe rhytides (40). In addition, one small case series demonstrated the efficacy of the 1320-nm Nd:YAG in reducing photoaging on the hands of patients (41). It should be noted that most studies have shown mild to moderate improvement using Nd:YAG laser and that multiple treatments are needed for optimal clinical improvement of photoaged skin.

Advantages of the Nd:YAG include minimal patient discomfort, relatively short downtime, and the ability to be safely used on all skin types. In general, the higher the fluence used, the greater the degree of improvement. Expectedly, higher fluence is more uncomfortable for patients and probably increases the risk of adverse effects such as thermal burns. Other adverse effects including transient hyperpigmentation and pinpoint pitted scarring have been reported with higher fluences (42). Finally, it is important to set reasonable patient expectations with this device. Most likely the patient will experience mild to moderate improvement in the appearance of the rhytides, albeit after a series of treatments; it is important to set this level of expectation prior to initiating treatment.

Diode Laser (1450 nm)

The 1450-nm diode laser has a similar mechanism of action to 1320-nm Nd:YAG laser. Light is absorbed in the dermis by the chromophore water; this energy is converted to heat, with the thermal effect being responsible for the clinical improvement. A cryogen spray cooling system in either a 4- or 6-mm spot is incorporated into the device to protect the epidermis from thermal damage. This effectively isolates the thermal heating to the dermis in an effort to prevent adverse effects.

The 1450-nm diode laser has demonstrated mild to moderate efficacy in the treatment of rhytides, similar to that of the 1320-nm Nd:YAG. The first study to demonstrate the efficacy of this treatment evaluated split-face treatments of periorbital and perioral rhytides in comparison to cryogen cooling alone (43). Mild to moderate clinical improvement was noted in 12 of the 16 study participants; histological specimens demonstrated neocollagenesis with diminution of sebaceous glands. A subsequent study demonstrated 35% percent improvement in rhytides in a split-face single blinded trial of nine patients (44).

Radiofrequency Tightening

Monopolar radiofrequency (RF) devices use volumetric heating to achieve a clinically evident "tightening effect." The flow of electrical current within an electric field generates heat due to the electrical resistance of the dermal and subcutaneous tissue; this ultimately results in controlled volumetric heating of the dermis. Simultaneously, epidermal cooling devices are utilized to prevent heating and damage of the epidermal tissue. The isolated deep dermal tissue heating results in collagen damage and subsequent new collagen formation. Both immediate and sustained long-term effects have been observed with RF treatment. Immediate results are attributed to a shortening of collagen bundles, while the long-term effects are thought to be secondary to the induced inflammatory cascade, an increase in type I collagen gene expression and neocollagenesis.

RF has shown clinical efficacy in the treatment of periorbital rhytides, upper and lower face laxity. In one blinded, prospective study, 83% of patients treated in the lateral canthal and forehead areas demonstrated clinical improvement in periorbital rhytides six months after a single pass treatment with energies ranging from 52 to 220 J. The investigators also reported a modest increase in eyebrow lift following treatments. A similar split-face treatment study reported a mild eyebrow elevation, superior palpebral crease elevation, and lateral eyebrow elevation following RF treatments (45). Similarly, skin tightening has been reported following RF treatment to the cheeks and neck (46).

In clinical practice, some proceduralists and patients have found the results to be less convincing than in these initial studies. A study used patient self-assessment to determine the efficacy of RF treatments; of the 16 patients treated, 10 found the results unsatisfactory while five were satisfied. While RF tightening can be a great treatment option for patients, proceduralists should bear in mind that the results may be modest. Patients should view these treatments as an option for minimally invasive tightening, but should also bear in mind that the results will likely not be as significant as a traditional facelift.

Adverse effects of RF are generally limited. Most patients will experience transient erythema and edema following the treatment. There have also been reports of transient tenderness along the jawline, as well as temporary anesthesia of the earlobe. Previously higher energy treatment protocols resulted in the observation of indurated subcutaneous nodules along the jawline and localized fat atrophy (47). The use of multiple pass lower-fluence treatment protocols have been associated with a marked reduction in these observed adverse effects, a more favorable clinical outcome, and greater patient satisfaction.

Combination Devices

Recent advances in rejuvenation include the introduction of combination of nonablative lasers and monopolar RF, referred to as electro-optical synergy. The use of two forms of energy allows for lower energy fluences from the laser device, which is then supplemented by RF energy. The laser optical energy initially heats the target, thus lowering its resistance and attracting RF energy to further heat the selective target. This synergism theoretically allows for treatments with greater clinical efficacy while reducing the likelihood of adverse events.

Limited studies have been conducted to determine the efficacy of these combination devices, comprised of RF coupled with infrared lasers (900- to 915-nm diode) or IPL (500–1200 nm). The conclusions of these studies demonstrate that the devices appear safe and effective for the treatment of mild to moderate facial rhytides and skin laxity. One study demonstrated improvement in wrinkle reduction, erythema, telangiectasia, and hyperpigmentation. Another study demonstrated a greater than 50% improvement in the subjective appearance of wrinkles on the face and neck in the majority of study participants (48). In addition, skin laxity was also shown to improve following combined RF and diode laser treatments (49). Adverse effects in these limited studies included mild to moderate pain, transient post-treatment erythema, and edema. A small minority of patients experienced vesiculation and superficial blistering which resolved within a week without any sequelae. No pigmentary alterations or scarring have been reported to date.

While the premise of a combined device utilizing reduced energies of both optical and thermal energy logically will result in less adverse side effects, the proposed synergistic action of these devices have not been conclusively proven. To date, no head to head comparisons of these combination laser/RF or IPL/RF devices to either optical or RF alone have been performed.

SKIN RESURFACING AND FRACTIONAL TECHNOLOGIES

Traditionally, skin resurfacing was performed by utilizing fully ablative laser technologies, predominantly with either a CO_2 (10,600 nm) or an Er:YAG (2940 nm) device. The target chromophore for these devices is water, specifically epidermal and superficial dermal water. As these lasers do not penetrate deeply into the dermis, their primary effects are due to removal (ablation) of the epidermis. While these devices can obviously result in significant clinical improvements due to this tissue ablation, they also have resultant limitations. These devices require significant downtime, as patients require nearly two weeks to heal and re-epithelialize the treated area. During this time, the barrier function of the epidermis is inhibited; potentially serious bacterial and viral infections can develop. Patients should be treated with prophylactic antibiotic and antiviral agents. Even once the area re-epithelializes, persistent erythema may result, lasting several months. In the long term, while the devices can result in significant improvement in facial rejuvenation, persistent hypopigmentation and scarring can develop. In short, these devices can be extremely useful in the treatment of patients with significant rhytides and discoloration. In fact, they remain the gold standard for improvement in these areas. However, given the downtime and healing associated with the treatment, many proceduralists and patients elect to pursue more minimally invasive technologies. Fractionated technologies represent an attempt to balance the benefits of ablative resurfacing with the reduced downtime of nonablative techniques.

Fractional Photothermolysis

Fractional photothermolysis is a relatively novel concept, in which only a microscopic portion of the skin is treated for rejuvenation, while the surrounding skin is left undamaged to stimulate faster healing and recovery (50). Columns of energy, known as microthermal zones (MTZs) treat both the epidermis, as well as the underlying dermis, creating targeted areas of thermal damage. The MTZs are surrounded by areas of spared, intact epidermis and dermis which facilitates rapid repair and healing. As a result, higher energy fluences may be delivered to targeted tissue depths, resulting in greater clinical efficacy. Furthermore, by only treating a portion of the skin's surface, the risk of adverse effects would also be greatly reduced.

In general, there are two main treatment parameters when utilizing fractional devices. The first is the treatment density. A higher treatment density implies closer grouping of the MTZs, and therefore a greater percentage of the skin surface being treated with the device. The second parameter is the energy fluence. This parameter dictates the depth to which the MTZ penetrates. The higher-energy fluence implies greater penetration into the tissue. The exact treatment parameters depend on the specific device being utilized; suggested treatment paradigms and parameters are typically suggested by the manufacturer of the device.

Nonablative Fractional Devices

The original nonablative fractional device was a 1550-nm erbium doped laser. Since the development of this initial device, several nonablative or minimally ablative fractional devices have been developed using different laser wavelengths, including 1440 nm, 1540 nm, and 1550 nm. These devices have been reported to be efficacious in the treatment of many conditions, including facial tone and texture, rhytides, photodamage, dyspigmentation, melasma, lentigines, acne, striae, and scarring (Figs. 2.3.5 and 2.3.6) (51). In addition to these facial treatments, nonablative fractional technologies also have been used to rejuvenate non-facial sites including neck, chest, and hands.

Histologic studies have demonstrated the ability of these devices to induce localized microscopic columns of both epidermal and dermal damage, which correlate with the MTZs. Epidermal damage is usually limited to the lower half of epidermal keratinocytes. Twenty-four hours post treatment there is a migration of cells from the periphery of the columns into the treatment areas (52). Over the next three to seven days, there is transepidermal extrusion of thermally damaged debris comprised of damaged epidermal and dermal cells along with melanin and elastin. Immunohistochemical analysis during this period demonstrates neocollagenesis, manifested by the expression of collagen III, proliferating cell nuclear antigen, and alpha smooth muscle actin (53). Additionally, one day after fractional photothermolysis, heat shock protein 70 can be detected, suggesting the induction of a wound healing response (53). These histologic changes likely account for the clinical effects of nonablative fractional photothermolysis, as well as the time necessary for the full clinical effect and neocollagenesis to develop.

Patients should be counseled that the full effect of these treatments may not be seen for one to two months after the treatment, once collagen remodeling and neocollagenesis have occurred. Furthermore, the ideal clinical effects are typically only achieved after a series of four to six treatments, conducted approximately every six weeks. It is important to emphasize the clinical time frame in order for the patients to make an informed decision regarding their treatment. Once the decision to proceed with a nonablative fractional device is made, the choice of laser parameters varies depending on the intended clinical target. For lentigines, dyschromia, or melasma, lower fluences with a higher-density setting have been shown to be effective when using the 1550-nm fractional system. For deeper rhytides and scarring, higher-energy fluences are necessary. These higher-energy fluences can increase the risk of adverse effects as a result of bulk heating. This risk can be reduced by decreasing the density setting. Lower treatment density can be compensated for by performing more treatment passes (54); however, proceduralists should allow sufficient time between passes when treating smaller surface areas to avoid the effects of bulk heating.

In general, adverse side effects following nonablative fractional rejuvenation are mild and transient. Topical anesthesia

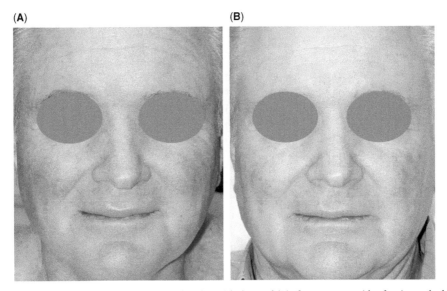

Figure 2.3.5 Clinical improvement erythema, pigmentation, and fine rhytides (**A**) before and (**B**) after treatment with a fractionated erbium:glass 1550-nm device. *Source*: Photos courtesy of Gary Lask, MD.

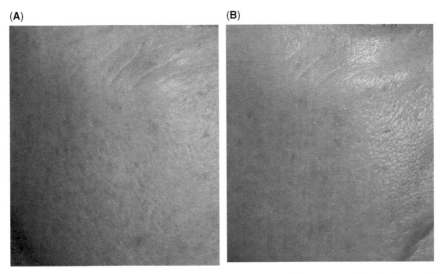

Figure 2.3.6 Clinical improvement erythema, pigmentation, and fine rhytides (**A**) before and (**B**) after treatment with a fractionated erbium:glass 1550-nm device. *Source:* Photos courtesy of Gary Lask, MD.

is suggested in order to make the procedure more comfortable. Additionally, the use of a cooling device is suggested to reduce the likelihood of bulk heating, increase patient comfort, and increase efficacy of the treatment. Despite the overall safety of these devices, patients may experience a constellation of mild side effects following treatment. In one study, all patients reported erythema and 82% reported facial edema (55). In addition, patients should be counseled regarding other potential complications including postoperative discomfort, transient bronzing, flaking, pruritus, and xerosis. Blistering and crusting can rarely occur and acneiform eruption has been seen when high energy was used, particularly around the perioral skin (56). As with any laser, post-inflammatory hyperpigmentation can occur, particularly with darker skin types. When treating darker skin patients, the authors recommend utilizing lower energy fluences and decreasing the number of treatment passes to avoid bulk heating of the epidermis. Serious side effects are uncommon when appropriate treatment parameters are used. Hypertrophic scarring following

nonablative fractional rejuvenation has also been reported, particularly in small treatment areas where bulk heating can occur, possibly due to higher-energy fluences and multiple treatment passes.

Ablative Fractional Technologies

While nonablative fractional rejuvenation is effective in improving multiple skin conditions, in general the results are not as remarkable as traditional ablative technologies. However, the decreased downtime associated with these nonablative fractional technologies make them desirable to patients. Recently, fractional technology has been applied to traditional ablative lasers (CO_2 and erbium). These ablative fractional laser devices offer clinically notable improvement in photodamage, acne scarring, facial rhytides, and skin tightening after a single treatment, with less downtime compared with traditional fully ablative technologies (Figs. 2.3.7, 2.3.8, 2.3.9) (57).

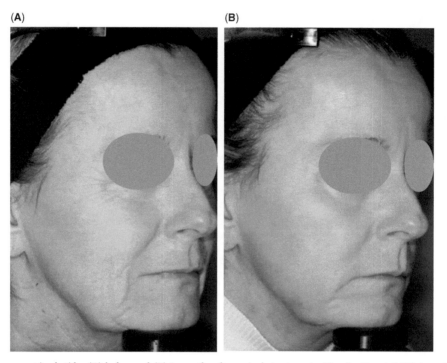

Figure 2.3.7 Clinical improvement in rhytides (**A**) before and (**B**) 3 months after a single treatment with a fractionated CO_2 laser. Note the improvement in periorbital rhytides and tightening of the jawline.   *Source*: Photos courtesy of Chris Zachary, MD.

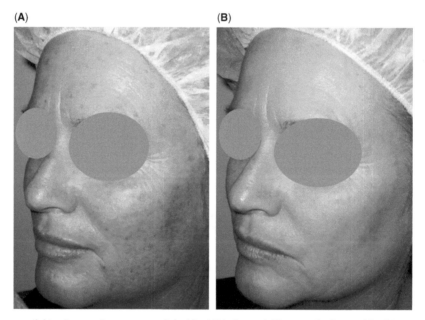

Figure 2.3.8 Clinical improvement of skin pigmentation, texture, and rhytides (**A**) before and (**B**) 1 month after combined intense pulsed light and erbium:YAG laser.   *Source*: Photos courtesy of Gary Lask, MD.

Studies have demonstrated a greater than 75% percent improvement in the treatment of wrinkles, epidermal pigmentation, or solar elastosis following a single ablative fractional treatment. Due to the fact that these fractional technologies only treat a portion of the skin surface, the results may not equal that of conventional ablative technology. However, the post-treatment recovery time is diminished, and the risk of hypopigmentation or permanent scarring appears to be reduced. Ablative fractional photothermolysis may also provide more significant efficacy in the improvement of facial rhytides and photodamage than nonablative fractional lasers. Ablative fractional resurfacing has also proven effective in the treatment

of acne scarring, demonstrating at least 25–50% improvement in texture, atrophy, and scar depth in patients (58). As of yet, there have been no significant clinical trials comparing traditional ablative lasers with fractional ablative lasers.

Fractional ablative technologies are well tolerated by patients when performed properly. Topical anesthesia is necessary, and nerve blocks of facial nerves may be of benefit. Patients may also be more comfortable with the administration of an oral anxiolytic, if the proceduralist desires. Following the treatment, meticulous topical care of the treated area is necessary, as the barrier function of the epidermis is impaired due to tissue ablation. Patients need to apply topical moisturizer or

(A) (B)

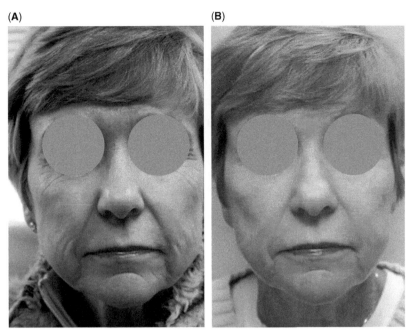

Figure 2.3.9 Clinical improvement of rhytides (**A**) before and (**B**) after two treatments with a fractionated erbium:YAG device.　*Source*: Photos courtesy of Michael Gold, MD.

other occlusive type products in order to promote wound healing and prevent formation of crusting during the healing process. Although the healing process is faster with fractional ablative technologies, patients will likely need to continue this topical care for one to two weeks following treatment until the skin has completely re-epithelialized. Prior to beginning this treatment, it is important that patients understand that while there is significantly faster healing than traditional ablative lasers, it still requires downtime.

Theoretically, the risk of side effects should be decreased with fractional ablative technologies compared with traditional ablative lasers. Immediately following the treatment, the skin is erythematous, and there may be focal areas of pinpoint bleeding. The patient's skin then flakes and sloughs for the next several days. Once the skin has re-epithelialized, which typically takes approximately one week, the treated area may remain erythematous for the next several weeks. Finally, there remains a risk of long-term hypopigmentation and scarring, although this appears to be less likely than with traditional ablative lasers.

CONCLUSIONS

Recent advances in laser and light therapy have enabled aesthetic physicians to both selectively target specific molecular chromophores, as well as offer global improvements in the appearance of a photodamaged skin. However, the clinician must remain cognizant of several important aspects when performing photorejuvenation using these treatment modalities. First, it is the clinician's obligation to address prevention of further photodamage and to provide information on topical regimens aimed at improving the skin's appearance. Second, the clinician must decide which treatment modality will be most effective for achieving the patient's desired goals. Third, it is imperative to realize and to convey to patients that one type of laser cannot fix all; rather, a combination of different modalities may be optimal in many clinical situations.

Fourth, the judicious use of dermal fillers, botulinum toxin, and other rejuvenation techniques should be utilized concomitantly to offer a global improvement in aspects of both intrinsic and extrinsic aging of the skin.

REFERENCES

1. Samuel M, Brooke RC, Hollis S, Griffiths CEM. Interventions for photo-damaged skin. Cochrane Database Syst Rev 2005; 25: CD001782.
2. Bruce S. Cosmeceuticals for the attenuation of extrinsic and intrinsic dermal aging. J Drugs Dermatol 2008; 7 (2 suppl): s17–22.
3. Kirsch K, Zelickson B, Zachary C, Tope W. Ultrastructure of collagen thermally denatured by microsecond domain pulsed carbon dioxide laser. Arch Dermatol 1998; 134: 1255–9.
4. Kirsch K, Zelickson B, Zachary C, Tope W. Ultrastructure of collagen thermally denatured by microsecond domain pulsed carbon dioxide laser. Arch Dermatol 1998; 134: 1255–9.
5. Alster TS, Lupton JR. Treatment of complications of laser skin resurfacing. Arch Facial Plast Surg 2000; 2: 279–84.
6. Tierney EP, Hanke CW. Recent advances in combination treatments for photoaging: review of the literature. Dermatol Surg 2010; 36: 829–40.
7. Carroll L, Humphreys TR. LASER-tissue interactions. Clin Dermatol 2006; 24: 2–7.
8. Anderson RR, Parrish JA. Selective photothermolysis: precise microsurgery by selective absorption of pulsed radiation. Science 1983; 220: 524–7.
9. Hirsch RJ, Wall TL, Avram MM, Anderson RR. Principles of laser-skin interactions. In: Bolognia JL, Jorizzo JL, Rapini RP, eds. Dermatology. New York (NY): Mosby Elsevier, 2008: 2089–97.
10. Polla BS, Anderson RR. Thermal injury by laser pulse: protection by heat shock despite failure to induce heat shock response. Lasers Surg Med 1987; 7: 398–404.
11. Hirsch RJ, Wall TL, Avram MM, Anderson RR. Principles of laser-skin interactions. In: Bolognia JL, Jorizzo JL, Rapini RP, eds. Dermatology. New York (NY): Mosby Elsevier, 2008: 2089–97.
12. Hruza GJ, Geronemus RG, Dover JS, et al. Lasers in dermatology. Arch Dermatol 1993; 129: 1026–33.
13. Glassberg E, Lask GP, Tan EM, et al. The flashlamp-pumped 577-nm pulsed tunable dye laser: clinical efficacy and in vitro studies. J Dermatol Surg Oncol 1988; 14: 1200–8.
14. Tan OT, Carney M, Margolis R, et al. Histologic responses of port-wine stains treated by argon, carbon dioxide, and tunable dye lasers. Arch Dermatol 1986; 122: 1016–22.

15. Garden JM, Tan OT, Kershcmann R, et al. Effect of dye laser pulse duration on selective cutaneous vascular injury. J Invest Dermatol 1986; 87: 653–7.

16. Bernstein EF, Kligman A. Rosacea treatment using the new-generation, high-energy, 595 nm, long pulse-duration pulsed-dye laser. Lasers Surg Med 2008; 40: 233–9.

17. Gaston DA, Clark DP. Facial hypertrophic scarring from pulsed dye laser. Dermatol Surg 1998; 24: 523–5.

18. Angermeier MC. Treatment of facial vascular lesions with intense pulsed light. J Cutan Laser Ther 1999; 1: 95–100.

19. Brazil J, Owens P. Long-term clinical results of IPL photorejuvenation. J Cosmet Laser Ther 2003; 5: 168–74.

20. Polla LL, Margolis RJ, Dover JS, et al. Melanosomes are a primary target of Q-switched ruby laser irradiation in guinea pig skin. J Invest Dermatol 1987; 89: 281–6.

21. Dover JS, Margolis RJ, Polla LL. Pigmented guina pig skin irradiated with Q-switched ruby lasers. Arch Dermatol 1989; 25: 43–9.

22. Alexiades-Armenakas MR, Dover JS, Arndt KA. Laser therapy. In: Bolognia JL, Jorizzo JL, Rapini RP, eds. Dermatology. New York (NY): Mosby Elsevier, 2008: 2099–120.

23. Trelles MA, Allones I, Velez M. Non-ablative facial skin photorejuvenation with an intense pulsed light system and adjunctive epidermal care. Lasers Med Sci 2003; 18: 104–11.

24. Negishi K, Tezuka Y, Kushikata N, Wakamatsu S. Photorejuvenation for Asian skin by intense pulsed light. Dermatol Surg 2001; 27: 627–31; discussion 632.

25. Alexiades-Armenakas MR, Geronemus RG. Laser-mediated photodynamic therapy of actinic keratoses. Arch Dermatol 2003; 139: 1313–20.

26. Alexiades-Armenakas MR, Geronemus RG. Laser-mediated photodynamic therapy of actinic cheilitis. J Drugs Dermatol 2004; 3: 548–51.

27. Alexiades-Armenakas M. Aminolevulinic acid photodynamic therapy for actinic keratoses/actinic cheilitis/acne: vascular lasers. Dermatol Clin 2007; 25: 25–33.

28. Orringer JS, Hammerberg C, Hamilton T, et al. Molecular effects of photodynamic therapy for photoaging. Arch Dermatol 2008; 144: 1296–302.

29. Dover JS, Bhatia AC, Stewart B, Arndt KA. Topical 5-aminolevulinic acid combined with intense pulsed light in the treatment of photoaging. Arch Dermatol 2005; 141: 1247–52.

30. Hall JA, Keller PJ, Keller GS. Dose response of combination photorejuvenation using intense pulsed light-activated photodynamic therapy and radiofrequency energy. Arch Facial Plast Surg 2004; 6: 374–8.

31. Zelickson BD, Kilmer SL, Bernstein E, et al. Pulsed dye laser therapy for sun damaged skin. Lasers Surg Med 1999; 25: 229–36.

32. Reynolds N, Thomas K, Baker L, Adams C, Kenealy J. Pulsed dye laser and non-ablative wrinkle reduction. Lasers Surg Med 2004; 34: 109–13.

33. Rostan E, Bowes LE, Iyer S, Fitzpatrick RE. A double-blind, side-by-side comparison study of low fluence long pulse dye laser to coolant treatment for wrinkling of the cheeks. J Cosmet Laser Ther 2001; 3: 129–36.

34. Goldberg D, Tan M, Dale Sarradet M, Gordon M. Nonablative dermal remodeling with a 585-nm, 350-microsec, flashlamp pulsed dye laser: clinical and ultrastructural analysis. Dermatol Surg. 2003; 29: 161–3.

35. Orringer JS, Voorhees JJ, Hamilton T, et al. Dermal matrix remodeling after nonablative laser therapy. J Am Acad Dermatol 2005; 53: 775–82.

36. Goldberg DJ. Non-ablative subsurface remodeling: clinical and histologic evaluation of a 1320-nm Nd:YAG laser. J Cutan Laser Ther 1999; 1: 153–7.

37. Fatemi A, Weiss MA, Weiss RA. Short-term histologic effects of nonablative resurfacing: results with a dynamically cooled millisecond-domain 1320 nm Nd:YAG laser. Dermatol Surg 2002; 28: 172–6.

38. Fatemi A, Weiss MA, Weiss RA. Short-term histologic effects of nonablative resurfacing: results with a dynamically cooled millisecond-domain 1320 nm Nd:YAG laser. Dermatol Surg 2002; 28: 172–6.

39. Goldberg DJ. Full-face nonablative dermal remodeling with a 1320 nm Nd:YAG laser. Dermatol Surg 2000; 26: 915–18.

40. Kelly KM, Nelson JS, Lask GP, Geronemus RG, Bernstein LJ. Cryogen spray cooling in combination with nonablative laser treatment of facial rhytides. Arch Dermatol 1999; 135: 691–4.

41. Sadick N, Schecter AK. Utilization of the 1320-nm Nd:YAG laser for the reduction of photoaging of the hands. Dermatol Surg 2004; 30: 1140–4.

42. Kelly KM, Nelson JS, Lask GP, Geronemus RG, Bernstein LJ. Cryogen spray cooling in combination with nonablative laser treatment of facial rhytides. Arch Dermatol 1999; 135: 691–4.

43. Hardaway CA, Ross EV, Paithankar DY. Non-ablative cutaneous remodeling with a 1.45 micron mid-infrared diode laser: phase II, J. Cosmet. Laser Ther. 2002; 4: 9–14.

44. Paithankar DY, Clifford JM, Saleh BA, et al. Subsurface skin renewal by treatment with a 1450-nm laser in combination with dynamic cooling. J Biomed Opt 2003; 8: 545–51.

45. Nahm WK, Su TT, Rotunda AM, Moy RL. Objective changes in brow position, superior palpebral crease, peak angle of the eyebrow, and jowl surface area after volumetric radiofrequency treatments to half of the face. Dermatol Surg 2004; 30: 922–8; discussion 928.

46. Alster TS, Tanzi E. Improvement of neck and cheek laxity with a nonablative radiofrequency device: a lifting experience. Dermatol Surg 2004; 30: 503–7; discussion 507.

47. Weiss RA, Weiss MA, Munavalli G, Beasley KL. Monopolar radiofrequency facial tightening: a retrospective analysis of efficacy and safety in over 600 treatments. J Drugs Dermatol 2006; 5: 707–12.

48. Sadick NS, Alexiades-Armenakas M, Bitter P Jr, Hruza G, Mulholland RS. Enhanced full-face skin rejuvenation using synchronous intense pulsed optical and conducted bipolar radiofrequency energy (ELOS): introducing selective radiophotothermolysis. J Drugs Dermatol 2005; 4: 181–6.

49. Doshi SN, Alster TS. Combination radiofrequency and diode laser for treatment of facial rhytides and skin laxity. J Cosmet Laser Ther 2005; 7: 11–15.

50. Manstein D, Herron GS, Sink RK, et al. Fractional photothermolysis: a new concept for cutaneous remodeling using microscopic patterns of thermal injury. Lasers Surg Med 2004; 34: 426–38.

51. Sherling M, Friedman PM, Adrian R, et al. Consensus recommendations on the use of an erbium-doped 1,550-nm fractionated laser and its applications in dermatologic laser surgery. Dermatol Surg 2010; 36: 461–9.

52. Hantash BM, Bedi VP, Sudireddy V, et al. Laser-induced transepidermal elimination of dermal content by fractional photothermolysis. J Biomed Opt 2006; 11: 041115.

53. Laubach HJ, Tannous Z, Anderson RR, Manstein D. Skin responses to fractional photothermolysis. Lasers Surg Med 2006; 38: 142–9.

54. Manstein D, Zurakowski D, Thongsima S, Laubach H, Chan HH. The effects of multiple passes on the epidermal thermal damage pattern in nonablative fractional resurfacing. Lasers Surg Med 2009; 41: 149–53.

55. Fisher GH, Geronemus RG. Short-term side effects of fractional photothermolysis. Dermatol Surg 2005; 31: 1245–9; discussion 1249.

56. Graber EM, Tanzi EL, Alster TA. Side effects and complications of fractional laser photothermolysis: experience with 961 treatments. Dermatol Surg 2008; 34: 301–7.

57. Hunzeker CM, Weiss ET, Geronemus RG. Fractionated CO2 laser resurfacing: our experience with more than 2000 treatments. Aesthet Surg J 2009; 29: 317–22.

58. Chapas AM, Brightman L, Sukal S, et al. Successful treatment of acneiform scarring with CO2 ablative fractional resurfacing. Lasers Surg Med 2008; 40: 381–6.

Eyes, lashes, and brows! Approaches to periorbital rejuvenation
Joseph F. Greco, Anastasia Soare, Frederick Beddingfield, and Jenny Kim

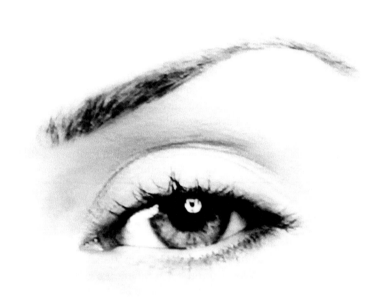

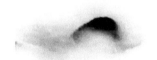

KEY POINTS

- The periocular area is one of the most significant aspects of our appearance. It is also unfortunately, one of the areas with the most significant ultraviolet exposure and volume loss, contributing to the aging process
- Multiple treatment options exist for rejuvenating the periorbital region
- Botulinum toxin can be utilized to improve dynamic and static lines in the periocular area by treating muscles, including procerus, corrugators, depressor supercilii, orbicularis oculi, frontalis, and nasalis
- Loss of volume also contributes to the aged appearance of the face. There are three main periorbital hollows, the "orbital rim hollow," "zygomatic hollow," and "septal confluence hollow" which create the tear trough. Soft tissue fillers should be placed deeply into the submuscular or epiperiosteal layers to result in the best outcomes for filling these hollows
- Topical bimatoprost can be applied to the upper eyelid margin to lengthen, thicken, and darken eyelashes resulting in a rejuvenated appearance
- Multiple lasers can be utilized to rejuvenate the periorbital skin, including nonablative lasers such as pulsed dye laser and infrared lasers. Ablative technologies, such as CO_2 and Erbium:YAG, can also be used to effectively resurface periorbital skin
- The best outcomes are achieved with combination treatments, including botulinum toxin, soft tissue fillers, and laser resurfacing, as the effects appear to be synergistic.

Eyes! lashes! and brows! … three distinguished components of the periorbital complex that bestow elements of physical beauty which is capable of captivating the attention of others. The eyes, metaphorically described as "the window to our soul" offer visual clues into our emotional well being. It should follow then, that periorbital aging may dramatically alter not only physical attributes, but also the perceptions into one's emotional state or past life experience.

PERIORBITAL AGING

Periorbital aging results from the interplay of many factors over time. Causative factors include the chronic effects of ultraviolet (UV) radiation, the gravitational descent of soft tissue, chronic contraction of underlying musculature, and localized loss of soft tissue and osseous volume. Chronic sundamage leads to regional nonspecific surface textural irregularities, dryness, brown dyschromia, vascular ectasia, and loss of collagen and elastic tissue. The chronic movement of periorbital muscles, in combination with sun damage, creates static and dynamic lines of the glabellar complex, nasal root, lateral orbit, and eyelid skin. Laxity of supporting ligaments lessens the body's ability to counter the gravitational pull, resulting in a descent of the periorbital soft tissue creating wrinkles, hollowed appearances, and redundant skin. Descent of the globe itself displaces infraorbital fat pads anteriorly forming fatty bags that suggest a tired appearance. Localized loss of soft tissue volume along the orbital rims reveals the underlying contours of deeper structures. The combination of gravitational descent and volume loss accentuate the angles of underlying structures and alter the refractive index of light. This creates a shadowing effect that enhances the perception of depth and color contrast as we age.

The above etiologies and a host of cutaneous manifestations are often the first unwanted signs of aging. These signs may be perceptually misattributed to fatigue, sadness, stress, and emotional hardship as well. Consequently periorbital rejuvenation has become a focal point of cosmetic procedures. The past decade has witnessed an unabated surge in minimally invasive cosmetic procedures as patients seek no downtime procedures to reverse the aging process; however, the requisite for maximum improvement has hardly changed. This poses a challenge to achieve results with minimally invasive procedures near or equal to those obtained after more invasive surgical measures.

The combination of two or more minimally invasive procedures can be a safe and reliable means to target the multiple manifestations of periorbital aging. With this approach, the physician can optimize the treatment design by choosing therapies with mechanisms of action that target different etiologies of periorbital aging. The synergistic approach of combination therapy seems logical to target the various effects that genetics and photoaging play on the periorbital skin. The chapter focuses on currently available minimally invasive procedures that have been demonstrated alone, or in combination, to successfully improve aspects of periorbital aging. A detailed and comprehensive discussion on the eyebrows, including the use of botulinum toxin in this area is included. Topical chemotherapeutics and various over-the-counter preparations are an essential component of periorbital rejuvenation; however, this matter will be covered in detail in other chapters.

PERIORBITAL ANATOMY

Our approach to periorbital rejuvenation begins with an understanding of the relevant structural anatomy. The foundation of this region is the bony orbit, a recessed socket housing and protecting the eyes. The frontal, maxillary, and zygomatic bones all equally share in the formation of the palpable margins of the orbital rim. Immediately superior to each supraorbital rim lays a bony crest known as the superciliary arch. The arches converge medially onto a rounded eminence of the frontal bone known as the glabella. Immediately inferior to the glabella lay the nasal bones.

The periorbital muscles of facial expression overlie the bony orbit and include the frontalis, orbicularis oculi, corrugators, depressor supercilii, procerus, and nasalis muscles. The frontalis is the lone brow elevator while the remaining muscles, minus the nasalis, serve to depress the brow.

The superficial muscular aponeurotic system is a fibrofascial network that envelops the muscles of facial expression and connects to the skin via a network of fibrous strands. Together the musculofascial and fibrocutaneous connections of the superficial muscular aponeurotic system unite to synchronize facial expressions in this region.

The skin overlying the muscle and bone of the periorbital region has variability in thickness, density of adnexal structures, and volume of subcutaneous and dermal tissue. Periorbital aging results from alterations in the inherent characteristics of the epidermis and dermis, in addition to the actions of underlying musculature, loss of bone, and redistribution of fat.

PERIORBITAL AGING OF THE SKIN

Periorbital aging results from the interaction between intrinsic and extrinsic factors over time. Intrinsic or innate factors are under genetic and hormonal influence. Manifestations are best seen in those areas protected from the sun. The skin typically appears smooth, fair, and evenly pigmented in these areas. Fine lines may develop from focal volume loss. Extrinsic aging on the other hand, occurs predominantly from UV light; however, smoking, diet, temperature extremes, pollution, illness, and disease also play a role. Most often, extrinsic factors are superimposed on the intrinsic factors thereby accelerating the cutaneous aging process. This is certainly the case with respect to the periorbital region which has ample exposure to sunlight.

The effects of UV light on the skin are numerous and additive. Nucleic acids and epidermal and dermal proteins serve as tissue chromophores absorbing damaging photons of light. Dimer formation and a clonal expansion of mutated cells may proliferate and form actinic keratoses and skin cancer. Free-radical formation, primarily from UVA light and cigarette smoking, adds to the insult creating elastosis of the upper dermis. A decrease in dermal glycosaminoglycans reduces the skin's water carrying capacity. UV light upregulates the matrix metalloproteinases collagenase, gelatinase, and stromolysin-1, which lead to degeneration of collagen, elastic fibers, and connective tissue matrix. In sum, the cumulative effects from UV light manifest cutaneously as brown dyschromia, vascular proliferation, ectasia, dryness, textural roughness, sagging skin, wrinkles, folds, and creases.

Among the first manifestations of periorbital aging are the rhytides of the glabellar and lateral periorbital region. At first, fine dynamic lines appear secondary to the chronic movement of the underlying orbicularis oculi, corrugators, depressor supercilii, procerus, and nasalis muscles. Characteristic rhytides are the vertical and horizontal glabellar frown lines, inferomedially oriented diagonal "bunny lines" overlying the nasal

bone, lateral periorbital radiating "crow's feet" line, and horizontal lower eyelid lines. At times a smaller crescent or comma shaped crease may appear just superolateral to the brow arch. With time the lines become static, pronounced, and may progress to deeper creases and folds. Subsequent collagen and elastic tissue degradation decreases the resiliency of the skin and leads to sagging and redundant tissue, notably over the upper and lower eyelids.

Fat redistribution and subcutaneous volume loss manifest as a hollowed appearance of the periorbital complex, which contributes to the aging process. The tear trough deformity is an anatomical designation given to the sunken basin over the medial infraorbital bony margin formed from volume loss in this region. Subsequent changes in the refractive index of light create shadows due to the accentuated contour irregularities from bony prominences with rounded or sharper angles. At times this is misattributed to an increase in pigmentation rather than volume loss.

TECHNIQUES FOR PERIORBITAL REJUVENATION

Improving Dynamic Rhytides with Periorbital Botulinum Toxin

Dynamic and static lines of the periorbital region result from the combined effects of photodamage and the chronic contraction of underlying musculature. Periorbital rhytides are often the initial presenting sign of aging around the eyes and may take the form of vertical or horizontal glabellar lines, laterally radiating periorbital crow's feet, horizontal lower eyelid lines, and inferomedially radiating nasal bunny lines. Botulinum neurotoxin type-A has been proven to consistently and safely reduce or eliminate periorbital rhytides with high levels of patient satisfaction. It is no surprise then that botulinum toxin injections remain at the top of the list of most performed cosmetic treatments in the nation.

Botulinum neurotoxins are synthesized as single-chain polypeptides that undergo enzymatic cleavage to yield a 150-kD di-chain toxin composed of a 100-kD heavy chain and a 50-kD light chain linked by disulfide bonds. The heavy chain functions as the binding and translocation region of the toxin while the light chain functions as its catalytic domain. Once the botulinum toxin is introduced into the body, the presynaptic motor nerve terminal hosts a series of events that lead to weakening or paralysis of target muscles. Through a multistep process of attachment, internalization, and blockade, botulinum toxins derail the normal sequence of events leading to muscle contraction. A key step in this process is the enzymatic cleavage of a specific protein of the SNARE (Soluble NSF Attachment Protein Receptor) complex preventing aggregation, docking, and fusion of the acetylcholine-containing vesicles. Subsequent acetylcholine release is blocked and muscular contraction is prevented.

Botox® (Allergan, Irvine, California, U.S.A.) is presently the prototypical and most widely used botulinum toxin for the treatment of periorbital rhytides. This is in part due to its high effectiveness, consistent results, minimal side effects, and relative ease of use for both patients and physicians. The glabellar muscular complex consists of the procerus, corrugators, and depressor supercilii and to a lesser degree, medial orbicularis oculi and inferomedial frontalis fibers. Starting dosages according to the Consensus guidelines on the use of botulinum toxin type-A published in 2004 for the glabellar complex and vertical frown lines are 20–30 units in women and 30–40 units in men distributed over five to seven injection sites. Care must be taken to avoid accidental drooping of the eyebrow from placement too close to the brow's superior margin or injecting the frontalis muscle with too high of a dose as the frontalis is the major brow elevator.

Laterally based crow's feet lines result from the chronic movement of the sphincteric orbicularis oculi muscle. Consensus guidelines recommend starting doses of 8–16 units in women or 12–16 units in men over two to five injection sites. Injections should be placed 1–1.5 cm lateral to the orbital rim in this region to avoid affecting the function of the lower eyelid musculature. Drooping of the lateral lower eyelid and accentuation of pre-existing fat herniations of the lower lid are potential complications if injections are placed too medial. Orbicularis fibers lie superficially and insert onto the thin skin of the lateral periorbital region. With the needle directed away from the eye, a superficial intradermal or subdermal placement creating a bleb is desired for a maximum botulinum toxin effect. Superficial placement under adequate lighting is also desirable to avoid the rich plexus of blood vessels around the eyes. Because the orbicularis muscle is a lateral brow depressor, treatment may result in lateral brow elevation. Horizontal lower eyelid lines form from contraction of the orbicularis muscle as well. Concomitant treatment of the lateral crow's feet and lower eyelid may have a synergistic effect. Two to 4 units placed 2–3 mm below the inferior eyelid margin along the mid-pupillary line targets these lines and may serve to open the eyes and create a more cheerful expression. Care should be taken not to inject too inferiorly as this may affect zygomaticus and result in the drooping of the lower lip on that side.

Bunny lines are diagonally oriented wrinkles running inferomedially over the bony nasal bridge resulting from the contraction of the underlying nasalis muscle and procerus muscles. They can be accentuated with the scrunching of the nose as if one is experiencing an offending odor. The administration of 1–2.5 units superficially on each side of the bony nasal bridge is typically enough to reduce or eliminate these lines.

The short-term efficacy of botulinum toxin when administered immediately prior to nonablative laser procedures was assessed in a group of 19 patients. Patients received bilateral nonablative facial resurfacing with a pulsed dye laser (PDL), intense pulsed light (IPL) device, or radiofrequency (RF) device within 10 minutes of administering botulinum neurotoxin type-A to one side of the periorbital and/or glabellar area. No loss of efficacy of the botulinum neurotoxin was noted at follow-up 2–3 weeks post treatment. Although the long-term efficacy was not directly studied, 18 of the 19 patients reported maintaining their results for more than three months.

Restoring Lost Periorbital Volume with Filler Products

As mentioned previously, soft tissue volume loss creates hollowed zones notable over the inferior periorbital region. Goldberg has nicely delineated a triad of such zones, the three periorbital hollows. They are the orbital rim hollow, the zygomatic hollow, and the septal confluence hollow. Of note, the medial portion of the orbital rim hollow is also known as the "tear trough" depression or nasojugal fold. The tear trough is bounded superiorly by the infraorbital fat protuberance and inferiorly by the suborbicularis fat, malar fat pad, and skin of the upper cheek.

Proper injection technique involves multiple, thread-like layers of the filler agent placed in a submuscular plane. As the skin overlying the periorbital hollows is relatively thin and transparent, too superficial of an injection may result in a blue-grayish appearance of hyaluronic acid fillers due to the Tyndall effect. Overcorrection and an uneven deposition are discouraged, as lumping of the filler agent will produce easily visible contour irregularities. Bruising and swelling are common and sometimes unavoidable. Care must be taken to avoid superfluous injections through the highly vascular orbicularis muscle. While feathering or fanning injections, the needle should be retracted and redirected in the submuscular plane rather than driving it repeatedly through and through the muscle. The application of ice packs before and after injections may minimize the occurrence of bleeding. In a retrospective case review by Goldberg using hyaluronic acid gel to fill the periorbital hollows, 89% of patients seen on follow-up exam were satisfied with the cosmetic improvement of the treatment areas. The most common side effects noted were bruising, color change, fluid accumulation, lumps, and contour irregularities.

In addition to restoring volume to the periorbital hollows, collagen or hyaluronic acid preparations may be injected to improve rhytides of the glabellar complex and crow's feet, and to create a subtle lift of the superolateral brow margin. In this setting, dermal or subcutaneous placement is desired and overcorrection is acceptable.

The lifetime of a volumizing agent is influenced by the activity of underlying musculature. High muscular activity, as seen over the periorbital and perioral areas is associated with a shorter lifetime of the filler agent. As such, pretreatment with botulinum toxins acts to reduce the underlying muscular activity and subsequently prolong the duration of effect of the fillers. A prospective, randomized parallel group study of 38 adult women evaluated the effectiveness of botulinum toxin plus non–animal sourced hyaluronic acid (Restylane®, Medicis Aesthetics, Scottsdale, Arizona, U.S.A.) compared with Restylane alone in the treatment of severe glabellar rhytides. The combination treatment demonstrated a better response at rest and on maximum frown when compared with botulinum toxin alone. The duration of effect for the combination was longer as well. Risks of injecting volumizing agents into the glabellar region include vascular occlusion and tissue necrosis from a direct introduction of the material into the vessel or from a tamponade of the vasculature from excessive product. One case of retinal artery occlusion leading to blindness has been reported as well using bovine collagen. Care must be taken while injecting the drug into the proper plane, and small-volume injections are encouraged to decrease the risk of these adverse events. Volumizing agents for crow's feet are generally reserved for those lines or hollows that remain after botulinum toxin has taken maximum effect. Primarily this involves the lower periorbital region where use of botulinum toxin injection runs the risk of paralyzing the mouth elevators.

Reshaping the Eyebrows

The remarkable impact that eyebrows have on overall facial appearance is undeniable. Though the eyes are called "the window to the soul," it is the eyebrows that are responsible for revealing inner emotions through the slightest changes in their shape and position. Hollywood teaches us all to take note of eyebrow position at a young age, creating its villains with sharply peaked brows that markedly slant toward the medial epicanthus; while in contrast, its young female heroines are often portrayed with over-elevated brows to create an appearance of innocence and awe. While these striking looks may be ideal for movie characters, cosmetic practitioners understandably strive for different objectives when initiating eyebrow recontouring consultations.

The definition of what constitutes "ideal" eyebrow shape has evolved over the ages and even today, numerous methodologies may be found for constructing "the perfect brow." Attempts to validate specific aesthetic rating scales have also occurred, though contrasting conclusions have been drawn and no one system has emerged superior. However, there is a consensus that the ideal brow for any given patient will vary based upon his/her bone structure, desired aesthetic effects, and unique features. The goal in eyebrow shaping is to create a look that will complement individual attributes and this will likely translate into a slightly different shape for each patient. What follows is one method, accepted widely throughout the cosmetic world, for first approaching brows.

The Ideal Eyebrows

The Golden Ratio, denoted by the Greek letter φ (phi), is a mathematical constant used by artists and architects throughout time because of the inherently pleasing aesthetic effects it confers. The Golden Ratio of measurements is achieved when the ratio between the sum of two distances and the larger of the two distances is the same as the ratio between the larger and the smaller distances. The Golden Ratio is found in the proportions of the human body as well. For instance, the ratio between one's height and the distance from navel to head approximates The Golden Ratio. In many people, The Golden Ratio may also be found when examining distances between facial features—the ratio between the distance from the top of the head to the chin and the width of the head = φ; the ratio between the length of the lips and the width of the nose = φ; the ratio of the distance between the outer eyes and the length of the lips = φ.

This ratio may be applied to brow shaping to create a harmonious, natural look. Initially, three precise points on a patient's face should be identified: (*i*) The Inner End Point (which lies on an imaginary line running vertically through the middle of the nostril), (*ii*) The High Point (which is the highest point on the eyebrow arch, and lies relatively closer to the temple), and (*iii*) The Outer End Point (which lies on an imaginary line running through the edge of the corresponding nostril through the outer edge of the eye). The High Point should then be placed on the eyebrow arch at the exact point where it will form a Golden Ratio with the two end points—on a "Golden Ratio" face this High Point is to be found on an imaginary line connecting the tip of the nose to the center of the iris.

Next, the type of eyebrow arch must be noted. Eyebrow stencils are available for different arch types (Petite Arch, Slim High Arch, Medium Arch, High Arch, or Full Arch) and grooming differs depending on the classification. For instance, in patients with high arches, care must be taken not to overpluck for fear of creating a sharp curve that appears severe. Hair should not be removed from the middle of the arch as this will establish added space between the eyelid and brow producing a hollow-eyed look. In those with low brow arches the key in shaping is to use restraint. There is a false assumption that the appearance of a higher arch may be created by increased plucking, while instead, this strategy can add an unappealing fullness to the face. In men, brows are naturally in a lower position with noticeably less arch than in women. This contributes to a masculine countenance and care should be taken to create a neatly groomed appearance without manipulating the fundamental character of the brows.

Other factors to be considered are brow color and brow width. Although the use of dyes to darken eyebrows has become commonplace, the goal of coloring should be to complement skin tone, not to match hair color. As a general rule, eyebrows should be tinted only one to two shades lighter or darker. This may be accomplished with the use of semipermanent eyebrow tints or temporary eyebrow pencils.

Probably the most widespread mistake in regards to eyebrow grooming is to create brows that are too thin. Overplucking throughout time can lead to permanent hair loss creating the all too common, yet unattractive, visage of older women with penciled-in brows. Skinny brows can also create the undesirable appearance of a heavier face. A helpful strategy to avoid this pitfall is to remember to concentrate on the face as a whole, remembering that the eyebrow is not an isolated unit. Overattention to each individual hair in the brow, rather than the brow as a whole, will not produce the desired effects.

Techniques for Shaping the Eyebrows

Cosmetologists, dermatologists, plastic surgeons, and patients themselves may all play a role in the eyebrow-contouring process. The available methods for manipulation are numerous and include waxing, tweezing, threading, trimming, tattooing, laser hair removal, hair transplant, Botox injections, and surgical brow lifts. For the average young women, a regimen involving visits to a cosmetologist for periodic grooming every three weeks, with supplementary home tweezing and smoothing, should be sufficient. As patients age and their brows begin to sag, cosmetologists may refer them to a plastic surgeon or dermatologist for a more significant alteration.

Although large alterations in brow position have traditionally been performed with blepharoplasty, recent advances in the use of botulinum toxin have decreased the need for many invasive procedures. Brow position is governed by a combination of the elevating frontalis muscle and the depressing procerus, corrugator, depressor supercilii, and lateral orbicularis oculi muscles. Each brow depressor has slightly different effects; for instance, the procerus is an inferomedial depressor that when activated, causes horizontal rhytides over the nasal bridge; the corrugator and depressor supercilii (positioned deep to the corrugator) also depress inferomedially but cause vertical glabellar rhytides, and the lateral orbicularis oculi, amongst other things, is responsible for periocular rhytides. Injections may be utilized to treat acquired or innate brow asymmetries and other imperfections, and may be beneficial as an adjunct to surgical procedures.

Brow position may be manipulated by selectively injecting specific muscles with varying doses of botulinum toxin. For instance, brow ptosis is increasingly common with progressing age. By weakening muscular brow depressors with botulinum toxin injections, the effects of the frontalis muscle are left unopposed and the brows elevate, achieving a more youthful appearance. In addition, when botulinum toxin is used to treat horizontal forehead furrows, resultant brow ptosis may be pre-empted by concurrently injecting brow depressors. Specific asymmetries may also be targeted; for example, lateral eyebrow ptosis may be improved by injecting the orbital component of the orbicularis while medial ptosis will be better treated with injections to the glabellar region. In brows that have been iatrogenically elevated to unappealing heights, injections into the frontalis muscle can be beneficial. In this instance, care should be taken not to inject below the lowest forehead rhytide as this may cause overdepression.

New innovations in eyebrow shaping have recently been explored for patients with more severe, acquired, or genetic brow abnormalities. Although overplucking is self-induced and the most common cause of eyebrow loss, other insults such as burns, surgical excisions, and trauma may have the same effect. Traditionally, reduced or missing eyebrow hair has been treated with surgical flaps and grafts taken from hair-bearing areas. Although these techniques are successful in the placement of hair, the resultant brows often have a brush-looking appearance and the hairs are not oriented in the same direction as a natural brow. Recently published studies have reported immense success in re-creating natural-appearing brows in burn victims with a dense packing of one to two hair grafting techniques. This method, though tedious, can be completed in one office visit and also offers a reasonable option for eyebrow reconstruction in those with hair loss from overplucking.

All the above points should be combined to create a unique eyebrow shape that complements a given patient's natural features and produces the desired aesthetic effect (Figs. 2.4.1 and 2.4.2). Although styles may evolve, and what society considers visually appealing may change, the clinician may be confident that the above general principles will always remain relevant.

Enhancing and Thickening the Eyelashes

Historically, eyelashes may have had a functional role related to the protection and lubrication of the eye. However, eyelashes also have a significant cosmetic and psychological impact; long and thick eyelashes are considered to be a sign of beauty. There are various techniques to enhance the appearance of eyelashes, such as the use of artificial eyelashes, mascara, and eyeliner which have been in practice for many years. More recently, an interesting side effect was noted in clinical studies regarding the use of prostaglandin and prostamide analogs for the reduction of intraocular pressure in glaucoma; patients were growing longer, thicker, and darker eyelashes as a side effect of the treatment. In large randomized clinical trials studying the effect of bimatoprost on intraocular pressure, about 42.6–53.6% of

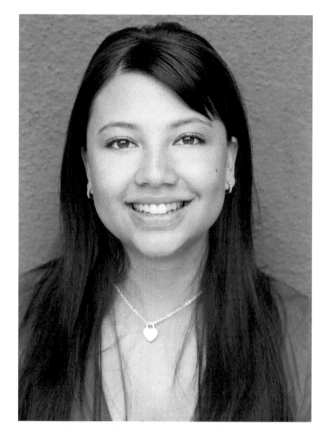

Figure 2.4.1 Patient prior to eyebrow shaping.

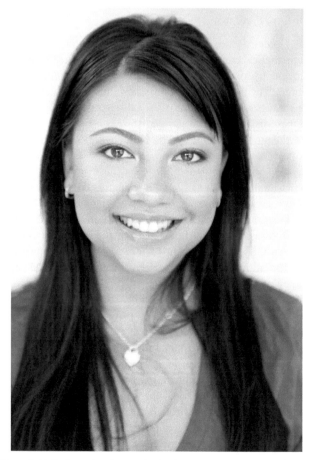

Figure 2.4.2 Patient after her eyebrow shaping treatment. Note that the eyebrow has only slightly been thinned. Also note the characteristics of this ideal brow, namely the inner end point, the outer end point, and a gentle arch at the high point.

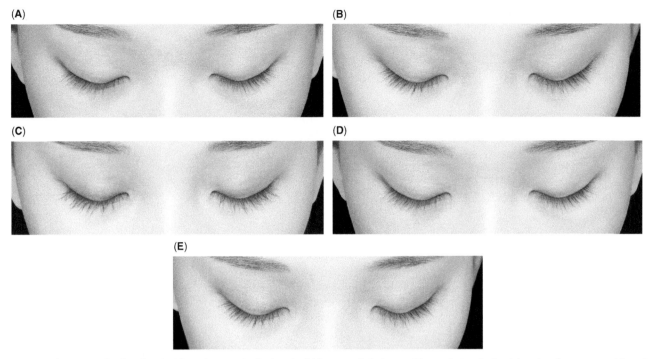

Figure 2.4.3 The patient developed a significant increase in the length, thickness, and darkness of her eyelashes during 16 weeks of treatment with topical bimatoprost (Latisse). (**A**) baseline, (**B**) 4 weeks into treatment, (**C**) 8 weeks into treatment, (**D**) 12 weeks into treatment, and (**E**) 16 weeks into treatment.

patients reported an increased eyelash growth. While initially this was reported as an adverse effect of the medication, the cosmetic utility of this effect was soon recognized.

Bimatoprost, a synthetic prostamide $F_{2\alpha}$ analog (Latisse®, Allergan, Irvine, California, U.S.A.) is now FDA approved for the treatment and enhancement of eyelashes, which increases the growth of the patient's lashes. Bimatoprost is applied once daily to the upper eyelid margin at the base of the eyelashes using the included single-use, sterile applicators. In a large, phase 3 trial of 278 patients, after 16 weeks of treatment, patients utilizing bimatoprost had, on an average, a mean increase of 1.39 mm of eyelash length (a 24% increase) compared with a mean increase of 0.11 mm (a 2% increase) for the placebo group. Additionally, a 106% improvement in the thickness of the eyelashes was observed following 16 weeks of bimatoprost treatment, compared to 12% increase in the placebo group. Finally, patients treated with bimatoprost were noted to have an 18% increase in eyelash darkness, compared to a 3% increase in the placebo group. All these results were statistically significant. A final measure, a Global Eyelash Assessment, was developed for the study. A significantly greater number of patients treated with bimatoprost demonstrated improvements in eyelash prominence compared with placebo (Fig. 2.4.3A–E, Fig. 2.4.4A–E). The exact mechanism of action of bimatoprost in increasing eyelash growth has not been definitively established; however, in mouse models, following two weeks of topical bimatoprost application, a greater number of eyelash follicles were noted to be in the anagen (growth) phase and that the duration of the anagen phase was prolonged which likely contributed to the increased length of the eyelashes. Furthermore, the dermal papilla and hair bulb diameters were increased in the early anagen phase, which may be associated with the increased thickness of the eyelashes. Finally, increased melano-

genesis was noted in the animal studies, with an increase in the number of melanin granules, which likely causes the eyelash darkening noted with bimatoprost therapy.

In the clinical trials, bimatoprost has been safe and well tolerated. Conjunctival hyperemia has been a reported adverse effect of the treatment, with an incidence of 3.6%. Intraocular pressure is reduced as a result of using bimatoprost, but this decrease is thought not to be of any clinical significance. Importantly, iris pigmentation has been reported as a side effect of bimatoprost eyedrops, with an incidence of 1.5%; however, no cases of iris pigmentation have been reported when applying the bimatoprost to the eyelid margin.

Bimatoprost is a safe, effective and well-tolerated treatment option to help lengthen, thicken, and darken eyelashes. These changes can help our patients to draw attention to their eyes, creating a beautiful, rejuvenated look (Fig. 2.4.5A–E, Fig. 2.4.6A–E). It is therefore a valuable, new option to help rejuvenate the periorbital area of patients.

RESURFACING THE SKIN TO IMPROVE TEXTURE AND DYSCHROMIA

Nonablative Laser Resurfacing Techniques

Pulsed Dye Laser (585 nm, 595 nm)

The 585-nm and 595-nm pulsed dye lasers (PDLs) have demonstrated variable success with nonablative periorbital rejuvenation in a number of studies. The mechanism of action is unknown; however, it has been proposed to be through a wound healing and wound remodeling response to microvasculature absorption of laser light. Histologically, studies have shown variable increases in expression of type I collagen mRNA, type III procollagen, chondroitin sulfate, fibroblasts, and thickened superficial

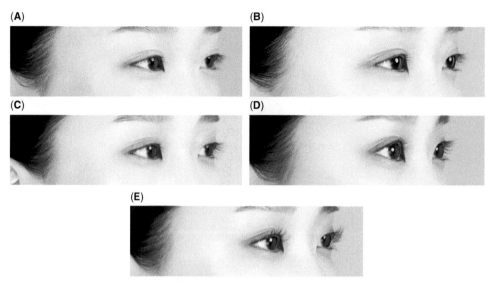

Figure 2.4.4 This is the same patient as in Figure 2.4.3, showing the dramatic improvement in eyelash length, thickness, and darkness associated with topical bimatoprost usage, from an angled profile view. (**A**) baseline, (**B**) 4 weeks into treatment, (**C**) 8 weeks into treatment, (**D**) 12 weeks into treatment, and (**E**) 16 weeks into treatment.

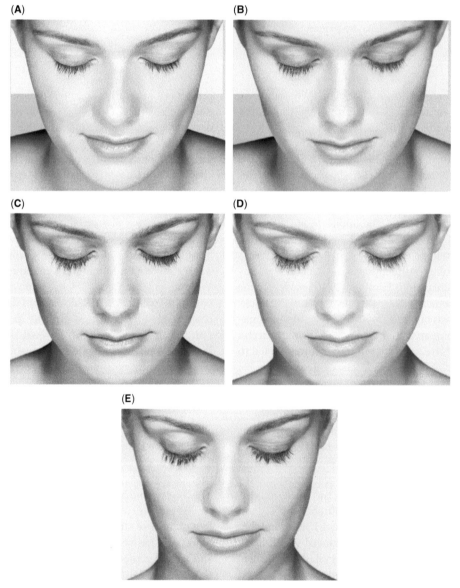

Figure 2.4.5 This patient developed noticeably longer, thicker, and darker lashes, which help to rejuvenate her entire face, with application of topical bimatoprost. (**A**) baseline, (**B**) 4 weeks into treatment, (**C**) 8 weeks into treatment, (**D**) 12 weeks into treatment, and (**E**) 16 weeks into treatment.

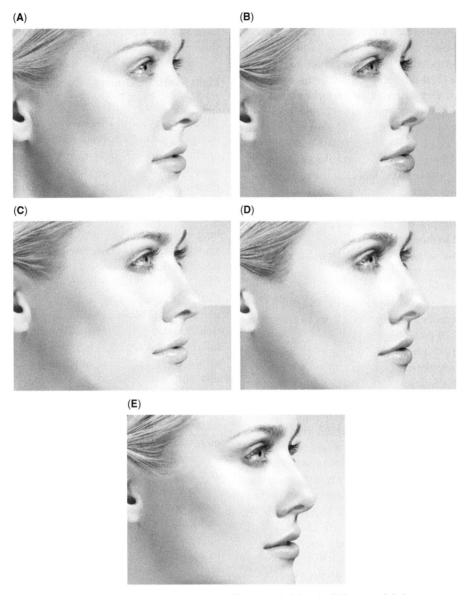

Figure 2.4.6 This is the same patient as in Figure 2.4.5, showing the dramatic effect on eyelash length, thickness, and darkness associated with the application of topical bimatoprost, shown from an angled profile view. (**A**) baseline, (**B**) 4 weeks into treatment, (**C**) 8 weeks into treatment, (**D**) 12 weeks into treatment, and (**E**) 16 weeks into treatment.

collagen layers after one or multiple treatments with the 585-nm or 595-nm PDLs. Clinical improvement with the above response is, however, variable. In a study using the 585-nm PDL to treat periorbital and perioral areas of 20 patients with mild to severe rhytides, 13 of the patients noted observable improvement. Hsu et al, conducted a split face comparison of 58 patients receiving one or two unilateral periorbital treatments with the 585-nm PDL, and patients demonstrated a mild, but statistically significant improvement in surface roughness over the treated sides. Increases in collagen, chondroitin sulfate, and grenz-zone thickness were observed in the treated sides as well. A further study documented detectible improvements in periorbital rhytides on photographic assessment in slightly over 50% of patients at 6 and 9 months post treatment with a 585-nm PDL. While other studies have failed to show any statistically significant improvement in periorbital treatment, nonablative rejuvenation with the 585-nm or 595-nm PDL is possible. Although results may be more subtle and variable, they can be achieved in a relatively safe manner with minimal side effects.

Infrared Lasers

The infrared laser devices used for periorbital rejuvenation include the Q-switched 1064-nm Nd:YAG, 1320-nm Nd-YAG, 1450-nm diode, and 1540-nm erbium (Er)-doped glass. The idea behind infrared lasers is to deliver controlled dermal heating in order to initiate neocollagenesis through an inflammatory and wound-healing response. The epidermis is to be protected and spared from the high temperatures and thus the clinical benefit periorbitally will focus on potential wrinkle reduction. Epidermal protection is generally achieved through cryogen spray or direct contact cooling.

The Q-switched 1064-nm Nd:YAG mid infrared laser has demonstrated effectiveness in improving periorbital rhytides. In a split-face study of 11 patients comparing treatment of one periorbital area with the 1064-nm Nd:YAG laser with the treatment of the contralateral periorbital area using 10,600-nm CO_2 laser, improvement in periorbital rhytides was seen in 9 of 11 patients with the 1064-nm Nd:YAG and in 11 of 11 patients with the CO_2 laser. Healing times with the Nd:YAG were shorter than the CO_2-treated side. Interestingly, three patients treated with the 1064-nm Nd:YAG had results identical to their respective CO_2-treated side. A multicenter trial of 35 patients evaluated the 1320-nm Nd:YAG laser in three sequential treatments at two-week intervals for periorbital rhytides. A statistically significant improvement in rhytides was seen in the mild, moderate, and severe groups at 12 weeks and in the severe rhytide group at 24 weeks after the last treatment. In separate studies, Goldberg showed clinical improvement in facial rhytides and a histological evidence of new collagen formation six months after treatment with the 1320-nm Nd:YAG laser (four treatments over 16 weeks) for full-face rejuvenation. Overall, clinical improvement with the infrared Nd:YAG lasers has shown mild to moderate improvement in periorbital rhytides with tolerable side effects which included transient erythema and hyperpigmentation, petechiae, pinpoint bleeding, and pinpoint scarring.

The 1450-nm diode laser is another infrared device designed to achieve dermal remodeling through subsurface heating. A split-face study of 20 patients with class I and II rhytides evaluated the 1450-nm diode laser plus cryogen spray cooling to cryogen spray cooling alone over a total of two to four treatments. A 6-month evaluation revealed clinical improvement in 13 of 20 patients on the treatment side compared with none on the control. Another study by Tanzi and colleagues treated 25 patients with mild to moderate periorbital and perioral rhytides with four successive treatments using a 1450-nm diode laser. Photographic assessment revealed mild to moderate improvement in rhytides in all 25 patients and new collagen formation was histologically seen at 6 months after the last treatment. Patient satisfaction was similar. Kopera and colleagues reported treatment of 9 patients with class I and II periorbital rhytides using a 1450-nm diode laser for three treatments at three-week intervals. While all patients reported mild to moderate improvements, pre- and post-treatment photographic evaluation by 23 of 25 independent dermatologist evaluators found no such improvement.

Nonablative periorbital rejuvenation with the 1540-nm Er:glass laser has been evaluated in a study of 60 patients receiving four treatments over six-week intervals. In addition to subjective improvements noted by all patients, objective measures like ultrasound imaging demonstrated a 17% increase in dermal thickness and a histological analysis revealed an increase in new collagen formation.

Nonablative Radiofrequency (RF) Rejuvenation

Nonablative RF rejuvenation devices have been developed with the goal of tissue tightening. The RF systems utilize high-frequency electrical energy to create collagen remodeling through heating of the dermis and superficial subcutaneous fat. In a study by Abraham and colleagues of 35 healthy adults with facial photodamage undergoing a monopolar RF treatment, increase in vertical brow height as well as improvement in skin laxity, wrinkles, clarity, and pore size were measured. A statistically significant increase in a mean vertical brow height of 1.6–2.4 mm was observed 12 weeks after treatment. Improvements in brow height were also observed in a study by Nahm and coworkers in 10 patients treated with RF to the left side of the face. Elevation in mid papillary and lateral canthal brow position was seen three months post treatment over the treatment side, as assessed through digital photography measurements.

Light Source Treatments

Intense pulsed light (IPL; 550–1200-nm) and broad band light (BBL; 400–1400-nm) technology use an incoherent, continuous, polychromatic band of wavelengths to target various signs of photoaging during a single-treatment session. Melanin and oxyhemoglobin are targeted as the primary tissue chromophores. As a result, both pigmented and vascular lesions may be treated simultaneously while nonspecific bulk heating of the dermis stimulates collagen remodeling. In a study by Goldberg evaluating histological changes after four treatment sessions with an IPL source, new papillary dermal collagen was noted on tissue biopsy six months after the final treatment. Clinically, this correlates with a concomitant reduction of erythema, telangiectasia, and melanin containing pigmented lesions as well as the potential for mild to modest softening of fine rhytides. Cutoff filters are used to define and limit the lower end of the wavelength spectrum depending on the clinical lesions to be treated. In treating photoaging with dyschromia and telangiectasias, a 515-nm filter is used to permit increased absorption of lower wavelengths by pigmented lesions. Alternatively, a 590-nm filter may be chosen to protect melanin-containing lesions and allow a more selective treatment of erythema and telangiectasia. The ability to use higher wavelength cutoff filters permits safer treatments in pigmented skin. Negishi and colleagues evaluated clinical and histological improvements in Asian skin after a series of five IPL treatments spaced three weeks apart. Improvements in skin texture, pigmentation, telangiectasia reduction, and overall global improvement were noted one month after the final treatment. In addition, there was histological evidence of an increase in type I and type III collagen in the dermis. The advantage of the IPL and BBL devices over the above-mentioned nonablative, infrared dermal remodeling systems is their ability to provide a more global improvement in photodamage.

We have found that the sequential combination treatment of a broadband light source followed by a superficial Er:YAG microlaser peel safely and effectively reduces multiple aspects of photodamage in a single or relatively few treatment sessions. The broadband light targets the nonspecific brown dyschromia and redness, while the Er:YAG microlaser peel reduces textural irregularities, as well as fine to moderate lines of the periorbital complex (Figs. 2.4.7, 2.4.8, 2.4.9, 2.4.10).

Ablative Resurfacing (CO_2 and Er:YAG Lasers)

Ablative laser resurfacing remains a highly effective method of periorbital rejuvenation through tissue vaporization, most commonly using the 10,600-nm CO_2 and 2940-nm Er:YAG lasers. The CO_2 and Er:YAG ablative lasers target intracellular water as the tissue chromophore. Vaporization of tissue occurs after laser light absorption elevates tissue temperatures above 100°C.

CO_2 Laser

The CO_2 laser emits a monochromatic wavelength of light at 10,600 nm producing a primary zone of tissue vaporization as

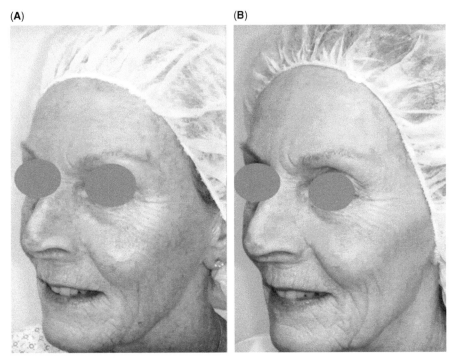

Figure 2.4.7 Patient before (**A**) and 1 week after (**B**) a combination treatment of broad band light source with an Er:YAG microlaser peel. Note the significant improvement in erythema, dyspigmentation, and lentigines.

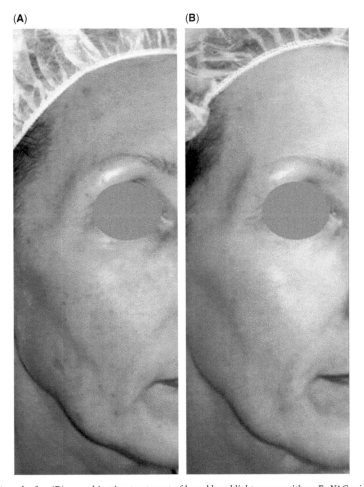

Figure 2.4.8 Patient before (**A**) and 1 week after (**B**) a combination treatment of broad band light source with an Er:YAG microlaser peel. Note the improvement in dyspigmentation and lentigines.

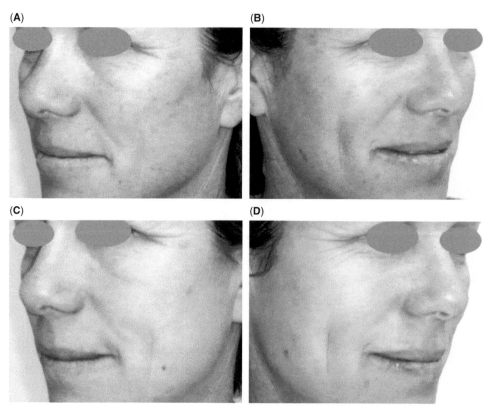

Figure 2.4.9 Patient before (**A & B**) and 1 week after (**C & D**) a combination treatment of broad band light source with an Er:YAG microlaser peel. Note the improvement in erythema, telangiectasias, dyspigmentation, and lentigines. There also appears to be mild skin tightening and reduction in the appearance of rhytides.

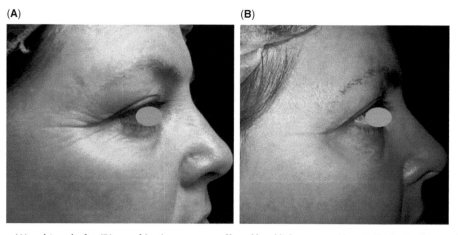

Figure 2.4.10 Patient before (**A**) and 1 week after (**B**) a combination treatment of broad band light source with an Er:YAG microlaser peel. Note the improvement in periocular rhytides and mild skin tightening following the treatment.

well as a peripheral zone of thermal diffusion. Within the secondary zone of thermal injury there is evidence of immediate collagen contraction, thermal coagulation, and associated dermal inflammatory wound-healing response. The zone of thermal diffusion increases with subsequent overlapping passes. The per-pass depth of ablation ranges from 20 to 60 μm with the secondary thermal diffusion reaching depths of 100–200 μm. As the periorbital skin is relatively thin compared with that of the remainder of the face, a single pass with the CO_2 laser may completely ablate the epidermis and have collateral thermal effects reaching the reticular dermis. Should multiple passes be used, the necrotic debris or char created from the initial ablation should be removed manually with wet gauze; otherwise, it

would limit the penetration of laser light. Advantages of the CO_2 laser include the ability to simultaneously ablate tissue while stimulating short- and long-term collagen contraction as well as thermal coagulation.

The clinical effectiveness of CO_2 laser resurfacing in the periorbital area is well known. Multiple studies demonstrate significant improvements in photodamage, periorbital rhytides, dermatochalasis, and folds after one or more passes. A study by Alster and Bellew of 67 patients with mild to severe dermatochalasis and periorbital rhytides showed a significant improvement after periocular ablative CO_2 resurfacing with minimal side effects limited to erythema and transient hyperpigmentation. A comparative split-face study evaluating two separate pulsed CO_2 lasers in the treatment of periorbital rhytides among 10 patients revealed mean improvements of 63% and 82% in periorbital rhytides between the systems. A retrospective review of 47 patients by Waldorf and colleagues revealed good to excellent cosmetic results in periorbital and glabellar rhytides as determined by photographic evaluation and/or chart review. Side effects with CO_2 ablation include temporary or persistent erythema, hyper and hypopigmentation, milia formation, irritant dermatitis, infection, scarring, and ectropion.

Er:YAG Laser

The Er:YAG laser emits a monochromatic wavelength of light at 2,940 nm which precisely approximates water's peak absorption at 3,000 nm. This effectively results in a highly precise tissue ablation with a more efficient absorption of laser energy than seen with the CO_2 laser. Ablation is achieved with short pulse durations with an approximate depth of ablation of 3–4 µm of tissue for every J/cm². The highly precise and immediate absorption of light, combined with short pulse durations, significantly reduces the secondary zone of thermal diffusion to approximately 20– 50 µm. The per pass ablation depth will be shorter than with CO_2 and consequently more passes will be required to achieve equivalent depths. However, as the proteinaceous debris is minimal, it is not necessary to remove this debris between sequential passes.

The advantage of the Er:YAG laser is in its highly precise ablation characteristics with minimal collateral damage. Superficial peels may be performed with heating limited to the epidermis and upper papillary dermis. However, this high precision with the short-pulsed Er:YAG laser is a disadvantage when dermal effects are desired. The absence of a larger secondary zone of thermal diffusion as seen with the CO_2 lasers limits the ability to stimulate a marked dermal wound healing response for neocollagenesis or to provide adequate hemostasis during deeper ablation. As a result, dual pulsed erbium lasers were developed. These incorporate a long pulse duration to permit a larger zone of thermal diffusion in conjunction with the short pulse ablative beam to maintain the precise ablation. The dual pulsed Er:YAG lasers now have the combined advantage of precise ablation and dermal heating to stimulate a wound healing response, collagen contraction, and thermal coagulation.

Improvement in mild, moderate, and deep periorbital rhytides has been demonstrated with the Er:YAG 2,940-nm laser. A study by Teikemeier of 20 patients undergoing Er:YAG facial resurfacing showed an improvement in superficial periorbital rhytides in all 20 patients two months after treatment. Perez and colleagues demonstrated varying degrees of improvement in superficial to medium-depth periorbital rhytides after a single to multiple passes with the Er:YAG laser with fluences of 4–5 J/cm². Their study also illustrated histologically that 3–4 passes with the erbium laser were needed for ablation of the epidermis at the noted fluences. In an evaluation of class III rhytides, Goldberg demonstrated the effectiveness of the Er:YAG laser after a series of three treatments. Twenty patients were each treated with 4 passes of an Er:YAG laser at a fluence of 5 J/cm² on three separate sessions spaced at three-month intervals. Mild to excellent improvement in deep rhytides was achieved six months after the final laser treatment.

The overall clinical benefits between erbium resurfacing and CO_2 resurfacing have been demonstrated to be similar with an overall improvement in wrinkle reduction being somewhat better with CO_2 resurfacing. Due to the different absorption characteristics, multiple passes with the erbium laser are required to provide near-equivalent results. The side effect profile with both the CO_2 and Er:YAG lasers are similar but more favorable with the Er:YAG laser at equivalent ablation depths due to the smaller zone of thermal diffusion. With deeper ablation, the risks of complications rise. Potential side effects include persistent erythema, hyper and hypopigmentation, acneiform eruptions, eczematous dermatitis, infection, and scarring. The postoperative healing times and side effect profile between the Er:YAG and CO_2 laser have been directly studied. Tanzi and Alster performed a retrospective chart review and photographic assessment of 100 patients undergoing either single-pass CO_2 resurfacing or multiple-pass long pulsed Er:YAG resurfacing. The rate of re-epithelialization, duration of erythema, and presence of complications were similar between the two groups with the erbium-treated group having slightly more favorable results.

The combined use of the CO_2 laser and short-pulsed Er:YAG laser has been reported by some authors. The thought is that the initial ablation is achieved with the CO_2 laser taking advantage of a greater depth of ablation on first pass and a larger zone of thermal diffusion within which hemostasis, collagen contraction, and remodeling may take place. A subsequent pass with the short pulse Er:YAG laser is performed to remove the superficial portion of thermally denatured tissue to hasten the postoperative healing time. Similar results may be achieved, however, using the dual pulsed Er:YAG systems which utilize both a short ablative pulse width as well as a longer coagulative pulse simultaneously.

The use of botulinum toxin as an adjunctive treatment prior to erbium and CO_2 resurfacing of the periorbital area has been shown to have a greater improvement in rhytides and other aspects of photodamage when compared with resurfacing alone. In a split-face, randomized, placebo controlled study of 33 patients, Yamauchi and colleagues concluded that the adjunctive use of botulinum toxin to the crow's feet area two to six weeks prior to erbium laser resurfacing provided more significant reduction in rhytides at rest and at maximum contraction when compared with the control side receiving saline injections prior to erbium resurfacing. Other signs of photodamage such as textural irregularities and pigmentation were more significantly improved on the botulinum toxin pretreated side as well. The adjunctive use of botulinum toxin one to three months after periorbital CO_2 resurfacing was demonstrated by West and Alster to prolong the effects on movement associated rhytides of the forehead, crow's feet, and glabella. It is postulated that the reduction of underlying muscular activity creates a static environment that provides a more favorable wound-healing environment for re-epithelialization, collagen remodeling, and even wound closure. In this respect botulinum toxin therapy in both pretreatment as well as maintenance therapy after cutaneous resurfacing may prolong the effects of rhytidosis.

Fractional Resurfacing: Ablative and Nonablative Technologies

Fractional resurfacing is a novel laser technology that delivers variable depth microscopic columns of thermally coagulated or

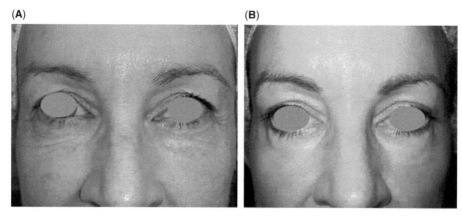

Figure 2.4.11 Patient before (**A**) and 1 month after (**B**) a combination treatment of broad band light source, with an Er:YAG microlaser peel, and a fractional ablative treatment with an Er:YAG 2940-nm device. This patient was also treated with adjuvant botulinum toxin (Botox). Note the improvement in the appearance of the patient's dyspigmentation and lentigines. The patient also achieved significant tightening of the lower eyelid skin, as well as substantial improvement in the "crow's feet" rhytides.

ablated tissue designed to volumetrically remove sun-damaged tissue. The microscopic columns are separated by large areas of healthy, viable tissue that serve as a biological reservoir to rapidly heal the zones of coagulation or ablation. In this manner, the skin is rejuvenated a fraction at a time which dramatically reduces the side effect profile. Deep tissue ablation or coagulation can be achieved safely as the intervening areas of untreated tissue provide healthy fibroblasts to initiate a wound remodeling response. Fractional resurfacing of the lateral periorbital area has been studied in a group of 30 subjects receiving four treatments over a two- to three-week period with a nonablative fractional resurfacing prototype device. Mild to moderate improvement in wrinkles and skin texture was demonstrated after one and three months after the last treatment. An 18% improvement in the wrinkle score was noted three months after the last treatment. Enhanced rete ridge patterning and increased mucin deposition in the upper dermis were noted on histology at three months. Improvement in periocular rhytides was also demonstrated in a study of 16 patients receiving one to three treatments with a combination fractional laser device.

Fractional resurfacing is commonly performed over a series of three to five treatments spaced one to four weeks apart for the nonablative devices. Clinical improvement in rhytides is mild to modest and certainly is less efficacious when compared with the results from fully ablative CO_2 and Er:YAG devices. Improvements in skin texture and dyschromia are more reliable (Fig. 2.4.11). However, the relatively short downtime and fewer side effects make this an attractive alternative to ablative resurfacing even though improvements are less dramatic. The creation of ablative fractional resurfacing devices using CO_2 or Er:YAG lasers may provide more significant clinical improvements. Several studies are in progress evaluating such benefits.

CONCLUSIONS: PUTTING IT ALL TOGETHER

Currently, our approach to global periorbital rejuvenation is through the combination of topical, injectable, laser and light source treatments spread over multiple visits to achieve a gradual and additive improvement. Recently, we treated a small series of patients with the above modalities over three distinct sessions. The first session involved the sequential treatment with a full face broadband light source followed immediately by an Er:YAG microlaser peel with emphasis on the periorbital area. On selected patients, a periorbital ablative fractional resurfacing procedure was also performed immediately after the microlaser peel. The target of this session was brown dyschromia, redness, static lines, and redundant skin. The second session was performed one week later and targeted dynamic periorbital rhytides with botulinum toxin injections. The final treatment session, performed three to six weeks after the initial session focused on volume replacement and static rhytides with collagen and hyaluronic acid dermal fillers.

We found the multi-session combination therapy with multiple minimally invasive procedures demonstrated a significant improvement in Fitzpatrick type I–III periorbital photoaged skin (Figs. 2.4.12,2.4.13,2.4.14). Their distinct mechanisms of action are additive and target various pathologies of chronic sun damage from the epidermal surface to the reticular dermis, in safe, reproducible, and relatively quick and comfortable procedures. Clinically we found this combination treatment to significantly improve dyschromia, skin texture, erythema, fine and moderate rhytides, volume loss, and redundant skin after the three distinct treatment sessions. Side effects and downtime were minimal and included erythema, edema, and peeling. Although our cases suggest that significant clinical improvement can safely be achieved with minimal downtime through the combination of various minimally invasive procedures, larger well-controlled studies are required to determine the true efficacy of these combination approaches for periorbital rejuvenation.

As the effects of botulinum toxin injections on periorbital rhytides are well known, we chose to evaluate the effectiveness of the combination BBL/MLP with or without ablative fractional resurfacing without any prior treatment. For this reason we performed the laser and light therapy first. However, as mentioned previously in the chapter, an adjunctive use of botulinum toxin one to two weeks prior to laser resurfacing may prolong the effects due to the creation of a more favorable, static wound-remodeling environment. In the same way,

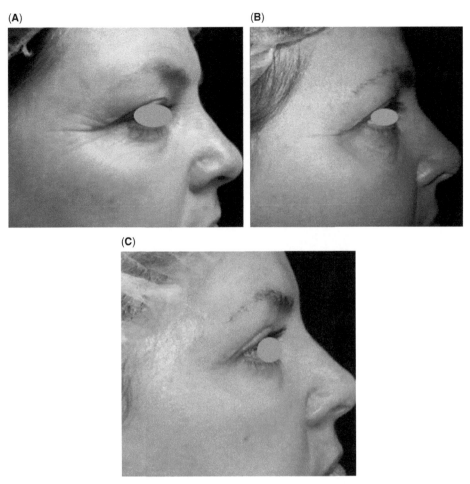

(A)

(B)

(C)

Figure 2.4.12 This is the same patient as in Figure 2.4.10, [baseline photo shown in **A**, results 1 month after combination treatment with broadband light source, Er:YAG microlaser peel and fractional ablative treatment shown in **B**] who has now undergone additional treatment with Botox to the periorbital "crow's feet" and collagen treatment to the tear trough area (**C**). Note the improvement in the appearance of her periocular rhytides and softening of the eye hollow appearance with the refilling of the tear troughs.

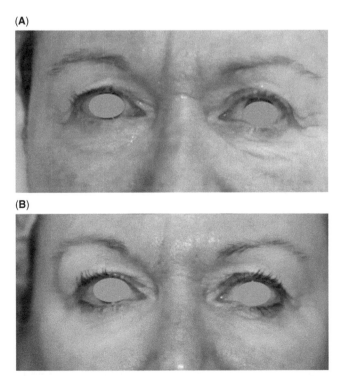

(A)

(B)

Figure 2.4.13 Patient before (**A**) and after (**B**) combination treatment with a broad band light source, Er:YAG microlaser peel, and fractional ablative treatment with an Er:YAG 2940-nm device. The patient was also treated with adjuvant Botox to the periorbital "crow's feet" and collagen treatment to the tear trough area. Note the improvement in the appearance of the dyspigmentation and lentigines, as well as tightening of the lower eyelid skin, improvement in periocular "crow's feet" rhytides, and refilling of the tear trough hollows.

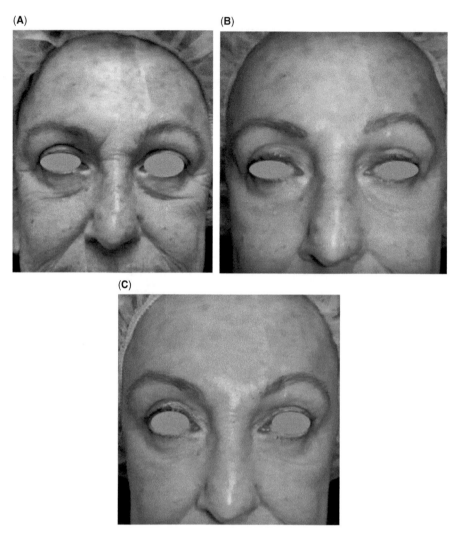

Figure 2.4.14 Patient before (**A**) and after (**B**) combination treatment with a broad band light source, Er:YAG microlaser peel, and fractional ablative treatment with an Er:YAG 2940-nm device. The patient was also treated with adjuvant Botox to the periorbital "crow's feet" and collagen treatment to the tear trough area (**C**).

pretreatment with botulinum toxin around areas of high muscular activity will prolong the lifetime of dermal fillers. With this in mind, it seems prudent to pretreat patients with botulinum toxin during the initial visit, then perform laser, light source, and dermal fillers on subsequent visits to prolong the clinical results. Spacing the treatments over three visits permits a gradual rejuvenation process with minimal downtime. This is desired when patients prefer more a subtle, steady clinical improvement rather than immediate and obvious and dramatic changes seen with invasive cosmetic and surgical procedures.

BIBLIOGRAPHY

Abraham MT, Chiang SK, Keller GS, et al. Clinical evaluation of non-ablative radiofrequency facial rejuvenation. J Cosmet Laser Ther 2004; 6: 136–44.

Alexiades-Armenakas MR, Dover JS, Arndt KA. The spectrum of laser skin resurfacing: nonablative, fractional, and ablative laser resurfacing. J Am Acad Dermatol 2008; 58: 719–37; quiz 738–40.

Alster TS, Bellew SG. Improvement of dermatochalasis and periorbital rhytides with a high-energy pulsed CO$_2$ laser: a retrospective study. Dermatol Surg 2004; 30: 483–7.

Balikian RV, Zimbler MS. Primary and adjunctive uses of botulinum toxin type A in the periorbital region. Otolaryngol Clin North Am 2007; 40: 291–303.

Bosniak S. Combination therapies: a nonsurgical approach to oculofacial rejuvenation. Ophthalmol Clin North Am 2005; 18: 215–25.

Bosniak S, Cantisano-Zilkha M, Purewal BK, Zdinak LA. Combination therapies in oculofacial rejuvenation. Orbit 2006; 25: 319–26.

Carruthers A, Carruthers J, Hardas B, et al. A validated brow positioning grading scale. Dermatol Surg 2008; 34(Suppl 2): S150–4.

Carruthers J, Fagien S, Matarasso SL, Botox Consensus Group. Consensus recommendations on the use of botulinum toxin type a in facial aesthetics. Plast Reconstr Surg 2004; 114(6 Suppl): 1S–22S.

Cohen JL. Enhancing the growth of natural eyelashes: the mechanism of bimatoprost-induced eyelash growth. Dermatol Surg 2010; 36: 1361–71.

Fagien S. Botulinum toxin type A for facial aesthetic enhancement: role in facial shaping. Plast Reconstr Surg 2003; 112(5 Suppl): 6S–18S.

Finn JC, Cox S. Fillers in the periorbital complex. Facial Plast Surg Clin North Am 2007; 15: 123–32.

Freund RM, Nolan WB 3rd. Correlation between brow lift outcomes and aesthetic ideals for eyebrow height and shape in females. Plast Reconstr Surg 1996; 97: 1343–8.

Glavas IP, Purewal BK. Noninvasive techniques in periorbital rejuvenation. Facial Plast Surg 2007; 23: 162–7.

Goldberg DJ. Non-ablative subsurface remodeling: clinical and histologic evaluation of a 1320-nm Nd:YAG laser. J Cutan Laser Ther 1999; 1: 153–7.

Goldberg DJ. New collagen formation after dermal remodeling with an intense pulsed light source. J Cutan Laser Ther 2000; 2: 59–61.

Goldberg DJ, Cutler KB. The use of the erbium:YAG laser for the treatment of class III rhytids. Dermatol Surg 1999; 25: 713–5.

Goldberg RA. The three periorbital hollows: a paradigm for periorbital rejuvenation. Plast Reconstr Surg 2005; 116: 1796–804.

Goldberg RA, Fiaschetti D. Filling the periorbital hollows with hyaluronic acid gel: initial experience with 244 injections. Ophthal Plast Reconstr Surg 2006; 22: 335–41.

Griffiths CE. The clinical identification and quantification of photodamage. Br J Dermatol 1992; 127(Suppl 41): 37–42.

Gunter JP, Antrobus SD. Aesthetic analysis of the eyebrows. Plast Reconstr Surg 1997; 99: 1808–16.

Ha RY, Nojima K, Adams WP Jr, Brown SA. Analysis of facial skin thickness: defining the relative thickness index. Plast Reconstr Surg 2005; 115: 1769–73.

Hantash BM, Gladstone HB. A pilot study on the effect of epinephrine on botulinum toxin treatment for periorbital rhytides. Dermatol Surg 2007; 33: 461–8.

Higginbotham EJ, Schuman JS, Goldberg I, et al. for the Bimatoprost Study Groups 1, 2. One-year, randomized study comparing bimatoprost and timolol in glaucoma and ocular hypertension. Arch Ophthalmol 2002; 120: 1286–93.

Hsu TS, Zelickson B, Dover JS, et al. Multicenter study of the safety and efficacy of a 585 nm pulsed-dye laser for the nonablative treatment of facial rhytides. Dermatol Surg 2005; 31: 1–9.

Jones D. Enhanced eyelashes: prescription and over-the-counter options. Aesthetic Plast Surg 2011; 35: 116–21.

Kopera D, Smolle J, Kaddu S, et al. Nonablative laser treatment of wrinkles: meeting the objective? Assessment by 25 dermatologists. Br J Dermatol 2004; 150: 936–9.

Manaloto RM, Alster TS. Periorbital rejuvenation: a review of dermatologic treatments. Dermatol Surg 1999; 25: 1–9.

Nahm WK, Su TT, Rotunda AM, et al. Objective changes in brow position, superior palpebral crease, peak angle of the eyebrow, and jowl surface area after volumetric radiofrequency treatments to half of the face. Dermatol Surg 2004; 30: 922–8.

Negishi K, Wakamatsu S, Kushikata N, et al. Full-face photorejuvenation of photodamaged skin by intense pulsed light with integrated contact cooling: initial experiences in Asian patients. Lasers Surg Med 2002; 30: 298–305.

Perez MI, Bank DE, Silvers D. Skin resurfacing of the face with the Erbium:YAG laser. Dermatol Surg 1998; 24: 653–8.

Semchyshyn NL, Kilmer SL. Does laser inactivate botulinum toxin? Dermatol Surg 2005; 31: 399–404.

Shook BA, Hruza GJ. Periorbital ablative and nonablative resurfacing. Facial Plast Surg Clin North Am 2005; 13: 571–82.

Tanzi EL, Williams CM, Alster TS. Treatment of facial rhytides with a nonablative 1,450-nm diode laser: a controlled clinical and histologic study. Dermatol Surg 2003; 29: 124–8.

Teikemeier G, Goldberg DJ. Skin resurfacing with the erbium:YAG laser. Dermatol Surg 1997; 23: 685–7.

Trautinger F. Mechanisms of photodamage of the skin and its functional consequences for skin ageing. Clin Exp Dermatol 2001; 26: 573–7.

Waldorf HA, Kauvar AN, Geronemus RG. Skin resurfacing of fine to deep rhytides using a char-free carbon dioxide laser in 47 patients. Dermatol Surg 1995; 21: 940–6.

Wang J, Fan J. Cicatricial eyebrow reconstruction with a dense-packing one- to two-hair grafting technique. Plast Reconstr Surg 2004; 114: 1420–6.

Weiss RA, Harrington AC, Pfau RC, Weiss MA, Marwaha S. Periorbital skin resurfacing using high energy erbium:YAG laser: results in 50 patients. Lasers Surg Med 1999; 24: 81–6.

West TB, Alster TS. Effect of botulinum toxin type A on movement-associated rhytides following CO_2 laser resurfacing. Dermatol Surg 1999; 25: 259–61.

Woodward JA, Haggerty CJ, Stinnett SS, Williams ZY. Bimatoprost 0.03% gel for cosmetic eyelash growth and enhancement. J Cosmet Dermatol 2010; 9: 96–102.

Yamauchi PS, Lask G, Lowe NJ. Botulinum toxin type A gives adjunctive benefit to periorbital laser resurfacing. J Cosmet Laser Ther 2004; 6: 145–8.

Zimbler MS, Holds JB, Kokoska MS, et al. Effect of botulinum toxin pretreatment on laser resurfacing results: a prospective, randomized, blinded trial. Arch Facial Plast Surg 2001; 3: 165–9.

2.5 Midface rejuvenation: Fillers for augmentation of the cheeks and nasolabial folds

Derek Jones and James C. Collyer

> **KEY POINTS**
>
> - Loss of volume in the midface and cheeks contributes to the appearance of nasolabial folds, and is a significant component of the aging process
> - It is important to have strong knowledge of the anatomic structures of the face to re-create the lost volume
> - Aesthetic physicians should be familiar with the vascular networks on the face, as injection into a blood vessel or injecting too much filler product in a high-risk area can result in skin necrosis
> - Multiple injectable dermal fillers are available to correct this loss of volume through soft tissue augmentation
> - Fillers can be of two types: temporary and permanent. Temporary fillers include hylauronic acid, calcium hydroxylapatite, poly-L-lactic acid, and porcine collagen. Permanent fillers include liquid injectable silicone and polymethylmethacrylate
> - Depending on the specific filler product utilized, the ideal depth and location at which to place the filler will vary. Additionally, there are multiple specific injection techniques which can be employed when perfoming soft tissue augmentation with fillers
> - This chapter reviews the most common filler products, their proper injection techniques, and associated potential side effects

The popularity of injectable dermal fillers for facial rejuvenation and soft tissue augmentation has exploded over the past two decades. Historically, the use of fillers for soft tissue augmentation began over ten decades ago with autologous fat injection. Around the 1950s, liquid silicone made its debut on the cosmetic market but was temporarily banned by the Federal Drug Administration (FDA) until several modifications were made to ensure its safety. In the early 1980s, bovine collagen was introduced in the United States. Although the aesthetic effects of this product only lasted approximately three to five months before re-injection was required for maintenance, bovine collagen remained the gold standard of fillers for many years. Hyaluronic acid (HA) products were introduced in the mid-1980s, and received FDA approval in 2003. Since then, a medley of injectable HA products has been developed and marketed. HA products were rapidly incorporated into cosmetic practices, and have become the most commonly used soft tissue filler products in the U.S. market.

As the desire for nonsurgical cosmetic procedures is on the increase, fillers have become an essential tool. In the year 2007 alone, approximately 1.5 million filler procedures were performed (1). The number of injectable procedures will continue to rapidly increase as new filler products are developed and patient demand continues to increase. With collagen and HA products paving the way, biomedical companies have strived to find an ideal filler that meets patients' cosmetic desires. Calcium hydroxylapatite, poly-L-lactic acid, porcine collagen, and polymethylmethacrylate have all been FDA approved for use as soft tissue fillers.

Given the development of all of these different fillers, it is only natural for our patients to wonder, "What is the best filler for me?." Each of these fillers has its utility as well as its limitations. In order to offer patients the best outcomes, cosmetic physicians should be familiar with all of the products and know when best to use each product. The goal of this chapter is to discuss the history of each filler, injection techniques,

procedural protocol, anatomical considerations, and the adverse event profiles of fillers used for augmentation of the nasolabial folds and for midface rejuvenation.

TYPES OF FILLERS

Fillers are generally classified as biodegradable or non-biodegradable. The aesthetic effects of biodegradable products are temporary and can last anywhere from 3 to 24 months, depending on the specific product. HAs, calcium hydroxylapatite, poly-L-lactic acid, bovine-based collagens, and porcine collagen are biodegradable fillers. Non-biodegradable fillers, on the other hand, are permanent; these include liquid silicone, polyacrylamide gels, polymethylmethacrylate, and synthetic derivatives. Table 2.5.1 shows the fillers currently approved for clinical use by the FDA; however, there are many other products currently approved outside the United States or that are currently under FDA approval.

BRIEF FACIAL ANATOMICAL OVERVIEW OF THE MIDFACE: CHEEKS AND NLFS

Before beginning with a comprehensive discussion of fillers for the cheeks and NLFs, it is important to understand the muscular and vascular anatomy of the midface (Fig. 2.5.1).

Vascular necrosis is a significant adverse event associated with the injection of soft tissue fillers. The risk of vascular necrosis is increased if knowledge of the facial vasculature anatomy is not adequately mastered. Vascular occlusion leading to necrosis can be caused by a direct intravascular injection of the filler or from an extravascular compression of too much filler adjacent to a blood vessel. A common reported site of vascular occlusion and skin necrosis is the glabella, which is in the vicinity of the supratrochlear artery and its branches. Another high-risk area is near the superior edge of the NLF, where the angular artery and vein, as well as their branches, lay in the immediate subdermal plane. Injection of the parotid

Table 2.5.1 Injectable Fillers for Augmentation of Cheeks and Nasolabial Folds

Classification	Filler	Products	Manufacturer	Whether FDA approved as an injectable filler
Biodegradable	Hyaluronic acids	Juvederm Ultra	Allergan	Yes
		Juvederm Ultra Plus	Allergan	Yes
		Prevelle Silk	Mentor	Yes
		Elevesse®	Anika (Woburn, Massachusetts, U.S.A.)	Yes
		Restylane	Medicis	Yes
		Perlane	Medicis	Yes
	Calcium Hydroxylapatite	Radiesse	Merz Pharmaceuticals	Yes
	Poly-L-lactic acid	Sculptra	Dermik Laboratories	Yes
Nonbiodegradable	Liquid silicone	Silikon-1000	Alcon Laboratories	For ophthalmic use only
		AdatoSil-5000	Bausch & Lomb	For ophthalmic use only
	Polymethylmethacrylate	Artefill®	Suneva Medical	Yes

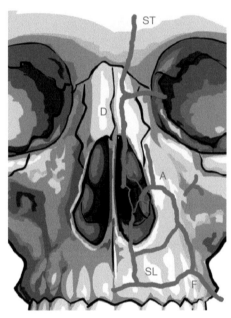

Figure 2.5.1 Vascular anatomy of the midface. The angular artery (a branch of the facial artery) anastomoses with the supratrochlear and dorsal nasal arteries (branches of the ophthalmic artery), joining the external carotid artery network with the internal carotid artery network. Occlusion or embolic events involving this network can lead to extensive tissue necrosis. *Abbreviations:* A, angular artery; D, dorsal nasal artery; F, facial artery; SF, superior labial artery; ST, supratrochlear artery.

duct, which overlies the buccinator muscle in the lateral cheek, should also be avoided. In addition to being cautious in these "high-risk" areas, it is also important to utilize the proper filler product; the risk of skin necrosis is increased if a robust, dense filler product is utilized in these areas. Calcium hydroxylapatite (Radiesse®, Merz Aesthetics, San Mateo, California, USA) is a robust filler that should be avoided in the glabellar area. In the author's experience (DJ), HA products such as Juvederm Ultra® (Allergan, Irvine, California, U.S.A) or Restylane® (Medicis Aesthetics, Scottsdale, Arizona, U.S.A.) are the most suitable fillers for the glabellar area, injected slowly and over multiple treatment sessions if needed (2).

In the case that vascular injection is suspected (manifested by a vascular watershed white blanching of tissue followed by a dusky blue-grey or maroon mottled appearance of surrounding soft tissue), topical nitroglycerin or a warm compress can be used to vasodilate the affected area. In the case of a HA product causing vascular compromise, the immediate injection of hyaluronidase may quickly reinstate vascular blood flow (3,4).

GENERAL CONSIDERATIONS: INJECTION TECHNIQUES

When assessing midface volume deficits, it is recommended to assess volume loss in the NLF as well as the superior malar and zygomatic areas. Thinning and drooping of the malar fat pad may accentuate nearby NLFs. Correction of cheek volume by filling the malar and infrazygomatic zones may optimize the appearance of NLFs by restoring the lost architecture to the midface.

The technique employed by a physician for the injection of fillers is dependent upon the nature of the volume deficit and the type of filler employed. There are several common injection techniques: serial puncture, linear threading, depot injection, fanning, and cross hatching. In order to avoid vascular injection, many seasoned physicians often use linear retrograde injection, where the needle is first inserted and advanced into the appropriate plane and the filler is injected linearly at a slow, even rate while withdrawing the needle. The fanning and cross-hatching techniques are variations on the linear threading technique. Both techniques employ retrograde injection. In cross hatching, multiple linear threads are injected at 90-degree angles to one another, creating a grid of threads, while fanning involves injecting several linear threads in a radial or fan-like fashion through a single injection site. A layered approach using linear threading, where successive threading is placed at various depths, can be used for the correction of more prominent wrinkles. With the serial puncture technique, very small aliquots are injected at regular intervals.

Depending on the specific type of filler, both linear threading and serial puncture techniques should be injected at the level of the immediate subdermal plane, subcutaneous fat, or supra-periosteal planes. Superficial intradermal injections should be avoided when volumizing, as dermal contour irregularities may result. It is important to note that there is an increased risk of bruising with multiple injections. However, this complication can be avoided with slower injection rates, fewer injection sites, and avoidance of anticoagulants for 7–10 days prior to treatment.

DISCUSSION OF SPECIFIC DERMAL FILLER PRODUCTS FOR CHEEKS AND NLFS

Biodegradable Fillers

Hyaluronic Acids

HA (hyaluron), a major component of the cutaneous extracellular matrix, is a glycosaminoglycan composed of repeating and alternating disaccharide units of sodium gluconorate and N-acetylglucosamine. HA is an important component of the body and exhibits a high turnover rate. It is involved in wound healing/tissue repair, joint lubrication, support of tissue architecture, cell motility and is a major component of the skin. HA's function in the skin is to bind and retain water, which is made possible through its hydrogen-binding capacity: 6 L of water can be bound with every gram of HA. HA is broken down by the tissue enzyme hyaluronidase and is later metabolized by the liver (5).

As a person ages, the amount of HA in the skin is reduced, which decreases the skin's water-binding capacity and tissue turgor, leading to visible wrinkles and drooping skin. The signs of aging are accelerated with sun exposure, specifically ultraviolet-B (UVB) radiation. A 2007 study reported that UVB radiation decreases the amount of HA in the dermis and upregulates the number of HA degradation products, including hyaluronidase (5). HA fillers are designed to restore a youthful appearance to the skin by replacing lost HA and binding water, thus reducing the appearance of sagging skin and skin folds.

Currently, there are several injectable HA products on the market. Injectable HAs are differentiated from one another by several variables (5): (*i*) molecular weight, (*ii*) concentration, (*iii*) method and degree of cross-linking, (*iv*) particle versus monophasic technology (*v*) avian versus bacterial origin, and (*vi*) presence or absence of lidocaine admixed as anesthesia. It is essential to understand all of these variables to intelligently understand the differences between products.

Molecular Weight

HA is composed of carbohydrate polymers (glycosaminoglycan chains) which are formed from repeating disaccharide monomer subunits, linked together like beads on a string. The longer the chain, the higher the molecular weight is. Lower molecular weight products, such as Voluma® (Corneal/Allergan, Irvine, California, U.S.A., not yet FDA approved), have a greater "lift" capacity and are intended for deep subcutaneous volumizing of the midface.

Concentration

HAs bind water avidly. At a certain point, HA binds a maximum amount of water and is fully saturated. Maximally saturated products tend to swell less upon injection and have relatively shorter tissue residence times (three months or less). Prevelle Silk® (Mentor Worldwide, Santa Barbara, California, U.S.A.) is in this category and has a HA concentration of 5.5 mg/cc and contains lidocaine. The Restylane/Perlane® (Medicis Aesthetics, Scottsdale, Arizona, U.S.A.) family of products contains 20 mg/cc of HA, while the Juvederm® family of products contains 24 mg/cc. The products of both the Restylane/Perlane and Juvederm (Allergan, Irvine, California, U.S.A.) families tend to persist longer, with up to a year or more of longevity after repeat injections. Because Restylane/Perlane and Juvederm are not maximally saturated and will absorb water following injection, overcorrection should be avoided.

Degree and Method of Cross-Linking

Un–cross-linked chains of HA are cleared from the skin within hours of injection. In order to increase tissue residence time, HA chains must be chemically cross linked. More heavily cross-linked products tend to be more robust and have a greater persistence in the skin.

Particle Vs. Monophasic Technology

After injectable HA is cross linked, it is a firm gel, much like a bowl of "Jell-O." It must be cut up to aid with injection. Restylane and Perlane products utilize particle technology. The gel is passed through a screen, which cuts and sizes the gel into identical, uniformly sized and shaped particles. The Juvederm family utilizes "Hylacross Technology" which cuts the gel into random sizes and shapes (analogous to putting the Jell-O in a blender); this appears to result in a more cohesive injectable product. Advocates of this technology posit that it results in a smoother, more even correction. These claims have yet to be established with controlled head-to-head clinical trials against particle technology products.

Avian Vs. Bacterial Origin

All available HA products on the market are of bacterial derivation, including Restylane/Perlane, Juvederm, and Prevelle Silk. Avian-derived products have a lower molecular weight but are no longer commercially available (Captique® and Hylaform®). It has not been proven that these products are more or less antigenic than bacterially derived HA.

Lidocaine

The inclusion of small amounts of lidocaine homogeneously mixed into certain HA products, including newer Juvederm-XC®, Restylane-L®, and Prevelle Silk products, represents a big advance in patient comfort, with greatly reduced pain on injection compared with products without lidocaine. The inclusion of lidocaine does not appear to alter the rheology or other characteristics of the HA product.

HAs meet many properties of an ideal filler in that they are noncarcinogenic, long-lasting, rarely allergenic, reversible, natural appearing, and smooth and supple to touch (Fig. 2.5.4). Prevelle Silk is seldom used as the persistence of correction appears to be very short (around three months) with this product (6). The Restylane/Perlane family and the Juvederm family (Juvederm Ultra and Juvederm Ultra Plus®), currently capture the largest share of the filler market. Perlane contains larger gel particle sizes compared to Restylane, while Juvederm Ultra Plus is more heavily cross linked than Juvederm Ultra. Perlane and Juvederm Ultra Plus are more robust fillers and are indicated for correction of deeper NLFs and mid cheek volume deficits. Restylane and Juvederm Ultra have been shown to be clinically superior to Zyplast® (Allergan) collagen for NLF correction in multicenter, double-masked, randomized, pivotal FDA studies in terms of 24-week persistence, as well as patient and investigator preference (6,7). In both trials, expected injection-related events included transient purpura, pain on injection, erythema, and edema. Restylane and Juvederm Ultra products achieve similar results with equivalent injection volumes and both products display increasing periods of longevity of up to a year or more after repeat injections (8,9). When treating NLFs, HAs should be injected in the immediate subdermal plane with a linear retrograde technique(Fig. 2.5.2). For midcheek volume

correction, (Fig. 2.5.3) the products should be injected deeply in the subdermal or epiperiosteal space deep to the muscle to avoid contour irregularities or the appearance of blue discoloration (Tyndall effect). Epiperiosteal injections should not be performed in the area of the infraorbital nerve which exits just inferior to the infraorbital rim in the mid-pupillary line.

A remarkable attribute of injectable hyaluronans is that they are reversible. They may be rapidly and safely degraded with the injection of hyaluronidase (3). Therefore, adverse events such as rare hypersensitivity reactions or misplacement of the product are treatable as long as the adverse event is properly identified or, in the case of vascular occlusion, promptly treated (4). It is recommended that the reader becomes thoroughly familiar with the use of hyaluronidase as reported in the literature. Juvederm products are more resistant to hyaluronidase than are

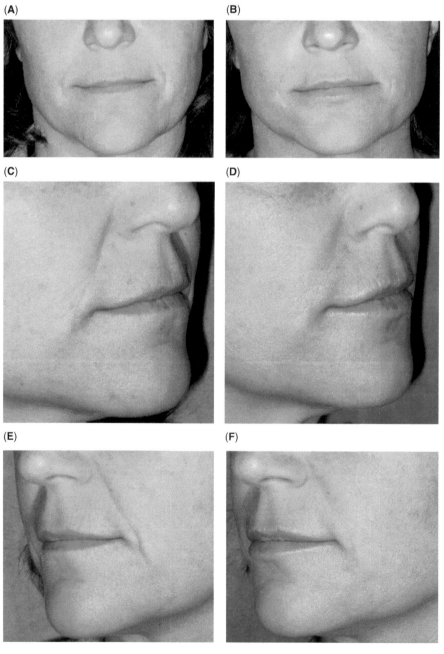

Figure 2.5.2 (**A,C,E**) Prior to treatment of the nasolabial folds (NLFs), oral commissures, and lips, prior to treatment with Juvederm Ultra. (**B,D,F**) Post treatment of the NLFs, oral commissures, and lips, after treatment with Juvederm Ultra.

Restylane products, but both are completely reversible with hyaluronidase (30). Although dose–response relationships need more evidence-based clarification, the authors recommend keeping Vitrase (hyaluronidase) immediately available and injecting about 5 units of product for each 0.1 cc of Restylane and 10 units for each 0.1 cc of Juvederm that the physician intends to dissolve(30).

Based on European experience, FDA safety and efficacy studies are underway for midface volumizing with more robust HA products such as Restylane Sub Q® (10) or Voluma® (11), which have a higher "lift" capacity compared with other hyaluronans. Restylane Sub Q shares the same properties as other Restylane products except that the gel particle sizes are larger compared with Perlane. Alternatively, Voluma, which is in the Juvederm family of products, is a monophasic 20 mg/cc HA product with a lower molecular weight and a higher cross-linking ratio which allows for retention of structure after deep injection. It is supplied in 2-cc syringes and is injected through larger bore needles into the subcutaneous or supraperiosteal plane. These products should not be injected into the dermis or the lips, as this may result in an uneven appearance.

Poly-L-Lactic Acid

Poly-L-lactic acid (PLLA) is a biodegradable synthetic polymer. PLLA is composed of alpha-hydroxy acid polymers and is molecularly similar to Vicryl® (Polyglactin 910, Ethicon, New Brunswick, New Jersey, U.S.A.) suture. The only FDA-approved injectable preparation of PLLA is Sculptra® (Dermik Laboratories, Bridgewater, New Jersey, U.S.A.), which is packaged as a sterile freeze-dried powder of 24.5% sodium carboxymethylcellulose (an emulsifier), 34.7% nonpyrogenic mannitol (provides osmosity), and 40.8% PLLA microparticles. The powder is reconstituted into a suspension with sterile water prior to injection.

When the product is injected into the subcutis, PLLA causes immediate and delayed volume restoration. Water suspension from the filler immediately causes edema, which resolves within a few days. A gradual foreign body tissue response is elicited, which leads to macrophage phagocytosis of PLLA, fibroblast proliferation, and subsequent neocollagenesis. This is believed to be the mechanism for the delayed volume reconstitution.

Sculptra was approved by the FDA in 2004 for human immunodeficiency virus (HIV)-associated lipoatrophy of the cheeks and temples. Of note, this product was granted fast-track approval for the unique needs of the HIV population with efficacy and safety based on published European data and small physician-sponsored investigational trails in the United States. It was not until 2009 that the FDA approved Sculptra Aesthetic® for the treatment of shallow to deep NLF contour deficiencies and other facial wrinkles in immune-competent patients. This approval was largely based on the results of a randomized, evaluator-blinded, parallel group, multicenter trial of 233 immunocompetent patients using a 5-cc dilution per vial of Sculptra, a 2-hour hydration time, and a deep dermal grid pattern injection technique to place product in the NLF in multiple treatment sessions (up to four in total) three weeks apart (12). Collagen (Cosmoplast®, Inamed Aesthetics, Irvine, California, U.S.A.) was used as the comparator in the contralateral NLF. Sculptra Aesthetic showed better improvement compared with the collagen control with a statistically significant improvement from baseline in the wrinkle assessment score at the 13-month follow-up and at all time points after week 3. Notably, a very large mean cumulative volume and a number of Sculptra treatments were required to reach optimal correction for one NLF: 11.7 cc (5-cc dilution per vial) over 3.2 treatment sessions. A large mean cumulative was also required with collagen: optimal correction for one NLF required 6.2 cc over 2.6 treatments. The results also show that Sculptra Aesthetic is associated with a gradual improvement of the NLF, with a time to peak correction of 192.7 days. During the extension phase study (19- and 25-month follow-up), the majority of Sculptra Aesthetic patients continued to demonstrate improvements in the wrinkle assessment score without retreatment. (Sculptra Aesthetic Package Insert, July 2009). Patients often reported redness, tenderness, swelling, and pain following the injections. Nodules (>5 mm) and papules

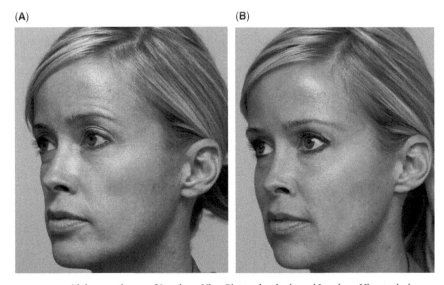

Figure 2.5.3 Pre- (**A**) and post treatment with larger volumes of Juvederm Ultra Plus to the cheeks and Juvederm Ultra to the brow area, nasolabial folds, and oral commissures in a patient with lean body mass (**B**).

(<5 mm) developed in 17.2% of PLLA patients, which was greater than the patients treated with collagen (12.8%). For Sculptra, the time to onset for nodules was a median of 160 days (mean 209 days); time to onset for papules was 55 days (mean 159 days). These papules and nodules typically resolve spontaneously, though one patient was treated with intralesional corticosteroids. The median duration of the papules was 110 days (mean 176 days) while the median duration of nodules was 100 days (mean 180 days). No serious adverse events were reported by the authors of the study.

In the author's experience (DJ), PLLA is usually not robust enough to obtain optimal correction of advanced cases of HIV facial lipoatrophy (stages 2–4). However, it is a good, albeit an expensive, option for those individuals with panfacial stage-1 facial lipoatrophy, which is often seen not only in cases of HIV but as a consequence of the normal aging process in otherwise healthy, lean individuals. In these individuals, repeated monthly injections of one to two vials strictly into the subcutis often achieves a subtle, yet significant, restoration of subcutaneous volume (Fig. 2.5.4). Patients should be aware that approximately three to six treatment sessions are needed to stimulate neocollagenesis. Optimal correction of subcutaneous fat loss with PLLA will gradually fade over 12–24 months, at which point patients often seek reinjection.

There have been several reports of nodule and papule development after the injection of PLLA (13,14). The risk of formation of these nodules can be greatly reduced if a careful injection technique is implemented. First, the product should be injected only into the subdermal space, and not intradermally. Intradermal injections have been associated with persistent granulomatous inflammatory dermal papules (14). We recommend a subcutaneous cross-hatched linear retrograde injection technique using a 2-inch 25-gauge needle (33). Smaller needles often become clogged. The needle entry site may be anesthetized with small intradermal injections of 1% lidocaine with epinephrine through a 30-gauge needle, and the resulting injections are quite tolerable. Intravascular injection and injection of the parotid duct should be avoided. Parotid duct occlusion has been reported with Sculptra (32). It is often advantageous to outline the treatment area before injection. The treated area must not extend above the inferior orbital rim. In the infraorbital area the product must be injected epiperiosteally in small amounts, deep into the muscle layer. Patients should also be made aware that the immediate post-treatment appearance will dissolve within two to four days. This instantaneous effect is due to fluid from the filler, which causes edema upon injection. Optimal augmentation will become apparent after multiple treatments at three- to four-week intervals, as new collagen is regenerated.

Subcutaneous lumps are also avoided if each vial is reconstituted with at least 5 cc or more of sterile water at least 24 hours prior to injection. Sculptra can be stored at room temperature before and after reconstitution. Although it is recommended to discard the reconstituted product 72 hours after it is reconstituted, anecdotal evidence suggests that the reconstituted product remains safe and viable for weeks. Unreconstituted product has a shelf life of two years. The reconstituted vial should be vigorously shaken immediately prior to transfer into the syringe as settling of the product in the syringe may lead to uneven application and contribute to nodule formation. Lastly, patients should be instructed to frequently massage the treated area in the days to weeks following the procedure to prevent the formation of uneven or lumpy fibroplasia. Some advocate the "rule of 5s" whereby the patient massages the area for 5 minutes, 5 times daily, for 5 days after the injection.

If nodules or papules do develop, several treatments are available. Early-onset nodules are best treated with sterile water injections or vigorous post-treatment massage. Later-onset nodules can be managed with injection of intralesional 5-fluorouracil or triamcinolone, followed by a daily dose of tetracycline (13,14).

Calcium Hydroxylapatite

Calcium hydroxylapatite is an organic salt found in human tissue that has been used for over a decade in reconstructive orthopedic surgery. It is a crystalline material composed of phosphate, calcium, and the main constituent of mature bone, hydroxide ions.

(A)   (B)

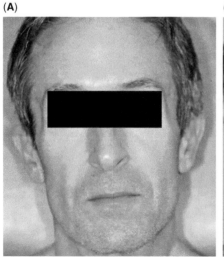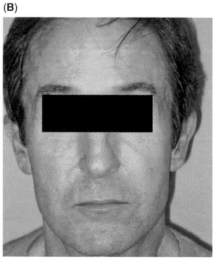

Figure 2.5.4 (**A**) Pre- and (**B**) 8-month post treatment of the cheeks and temples with 10 vials of Sculptra (5 treatments, 2 vials per treatment) over 4 months to correct facial fat loss associated with aging and lean body mass.

Radiesse is a semipermanent, biodegradable soft-tissue filler composed of calcium hydroxylapatite (CaHA) microspheres suspended in an aqueous gel carrier. The gel composed of sterile water, glycerin, and sodium carboxymethylcellulose is phagocytosed by macrophages upon injection, leaving only the CaHA microspheres behind. This process takes two to three months, during which time the CaHA microspheres act as a scaffold that promotes neocollagenesis. Fibroblasts anchor onto this scaffold and lay down a collagenous extracellular matrix, which becomes integrated into the surrounding soft tissue. Over a period of 9–18 months, the CaHA is gradually metabolized by the same metabolic pathways as bone debris into calcium and phosphate ions (15). Synthetic CaHA does not cause ossification when injected subdermally, and it does not require skin testing prior to injection in a patient. Although radiopaque, it does not confound or impede interpretation of x-rays. Its appearance on computed tomographic (CT) scans is distinct from surrounding bony tissues and does not interfere with normal analysis (16). CT scans of injected material prove that the material does not migrate and remains localized at the injection site.

Several studies have confirmed the safety and efficacy of CaHA. A recent multicenter two-year study evaluated the safety and perceived patient satisfaction of CaHA injections for the correction of NLFs. Seventy-five patients received one treatment injection while the remaining 38 patients had multiple sessions. Of the 113 patients, only seven reported minor complications that were resolved within four weeks. Ninety percent of patients reported very good or excellent results and were satisfied with the treatment (17). A separate randomized split-face study (the pivtol FDA study) showed that CaHA products offer significantly longer-lasting correction of NLFs compared with human collagen with fewer injections and less product volume (18).

Another multicenter randomized trial compared Radiesse with three different HAs. A total of 205 patients were injected with either CaHA or HA (Juvederm or Perlane), for correction of NLFs at week 0 and 4-month post-treatment. Patient surveys and measurements from the Global Aesthetic Improvement Scale (GAIS) revealed that CaHA-treated NLFs received significantly higher satisfaction scores and GAIS scores compared with the HAs (19).

In the author's (DJ) practice, Radiesse is recommended for patients with very deep NLFs, or significant midface lipoatrophy that requires a more robust filler with more lift capacity than the existing hyaluronans can offer (Fig. 2.5.5). Radiesse can be stored at room temperature for up to two years. The product is now supplied in two different sized syringes: 1.5 and 0.5 mL, with the smaller syringe intended for touch-up procedures. The addition of a small volume (0.1–0.15 cc) 2%

lidocaine to the syringe, mixed with a female to female adaptor, is now considered safe and is FDA approved, and has virtually eliminated the intense pain that was once common with Radiesse injections (20). For corrections of the zygomatic and malar regions of the face, a 27-gauge, 1.25 inch needle should be used for injection. The product should be injected in a linear retrograde fashion into the deep dermis or subcutaneous plane, using multiple small linear threads (0.05 mL per pass). For correction of HIV and non-HIV-associated midfacial lipoatrophy, a linear retrograde cross-hatched technique should be employed. For HIV facial lipoatrophy, significant volumes (>13 cc on an average) need to be injected subdermally to obtain an optimal correction (21).

CaHa is not recommended for use in lip or nasojugal groove (tear trough) augmentation. When injected into the lips, the pumping action of the orbicularis oris can cause the filler to clump and move toward the mucosa and vermillion sides. Treatment-related adverse events after injection of CaHA include ecchymosis, temporary edema, and short-duration pain. If the product is injected too superficially in the dermis, persistent nodules may form. Radiesse is a robust filler that can easily occlude the vascular lumen with intravascular injection or cause indirect vasoconstriction due to extravascular volumetric compression, both of which lead to tissue necrosis. The angular artery and vein and their branches lay in the immediate subdermal plane in the superior NLF and are particularly vulnerable. Slow injection technique and great care should be adopted when injecting in this area.

Cross-Linked Porcine Collagen

Evolence® (ColBar LifeScience, Herzliya, Israel) is a cross-linked porcine type I collagen gel, suspended in a phosphate-buffered saline solution and is supplied in a 1 mL (35 mg/cc) syringe. This porcine collagen is prepared using enzymatic digestion to remove immunogenic telopeptides, making the product nonimmunogenic in humans. The porcine collagen is then cross-linked with a sugar (ribose) metabolite (Glymatrix Technology), which gives the product a greater longevity (up to one year in animal models). Because the antigenic portions of the molecule are removed, hypersensitivity reactions should be minimal and there is no need for skin testing (22).

Narins et al. performed a randomized, multicenter study of 194 patients comparing Evolence with Restylane for NLF correction. It was found that both had similar safety profiles, efficacy, and patient satisfaction. The incidence of pain, swelling, and bruising was slightly higher with Restylane whereas incidence of induration was slightly increased with Evolence. Clinical evidence of immunologic reaction to Evolence was not seen (22).

(A) **(B)**

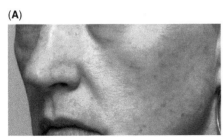 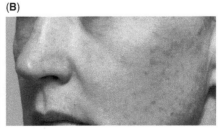

Figure 2.5.5 (**A**) Pre- and (**B**) post treatment of the midface with Radiesse in a patient with facial atrophy associated with aging and lean body mass.

Evolence was first licensed for use in Europe in 2004 and was later approved by the FDA in the United States in June 2008. It is indicated for the cosmetic correction of moderate to deep facial contour deformities, such as the NLFs. It should not be injected into the lips as there is potential for long-lasting nodules post injection and no reversing agent is available. Evolence Breeze®, which is approved for clinical use in Canada and Europe but not in the United States, can be used in fine lines and wrinkles of the face and may be a safer filler for the lips.

At the time of writing this chapter, manufacturing and distribution of Evolence has been discontinued due to an apparent lack of market demand.

NONBIODEGRADABLE FILLERS

Although biodegradable fillers are safe and reliable agents for facial augmentation, re-treatment is typically required within 3–12 months. Thus, nonbiodegradable fillers were developed with the intention of providing patients with permanent soft tissue augmentation. The two main nonbiodegradable fillers used for correction of NLFs and cheeks are discussed in detail next.

Liquid Injectable Silicone

Liquid injectable silicone (LIS) is composed of polydimethylsiloxane. Approved by the FDA as an injectable retinal tamponade for retinal detachment, LIS comes in two forms: Silikon®-1000 (Alcon Laboratories, Fort Worth, Texas, U.S.A.) and AdatoSil®-5000 (Bausch and Lomb, Rochester, New York, U.S.A.). The viscosity of silicone, which is reflected in the number at the end of the brand name, is expressed in centistokes (cS) units, with smaller values reflecting less viscous and increasing values reflecting more viscous products. Although it is not FDA approved for injectable soft tissue augmentation, Silikon-1000, due to its lower viscosity and ability to be injected through smaller gauge needles, is commonly used off-label for this purpose (23).

Liquid silicone was first used as injectable filler in the 1950s. It became more widely used in the 1970s–1980s, although there was no standardized FDA-approved product and many "medical grade" silicone oils of varying purity were injected often in large bolus form, leading to frequent product migration and foreign body inflammatory reactions (23). In the 1980s, mounting cases of adverse events led health authorities to investigate the cosmetic safety of this product. Several reports of ulceration, connective tissue disease, granulomas, and filler migration led to the legal banning of LIS for cosmetic indications in the early 1990s. After the FDA resolved safety issues regarding LIS, two important FDA provisions let LIS emerge on the market again in the mid to late 1990s after a brief hiatus. First, Silikon-1000 and AdatoSil-5000 were FDA approved for treating retinal detachment. A second concurrent event, the passage of the FDA Modernization Act, made it legal for FDA-approved injectable devices to be used off-label for other indications as long as such provisions were not openly advertised and physicians based their decision to use the device off-label on unique, individual patient needs (23).

Currently, opinion on liquid injectable silicone is polarized between opponents and advocates. Opponents advocate that despite use of proper technique and products, serious adverse events are common and unpredictable. Advocates rely on a wealth of anecdotal data to argue that liquid injectable silicone is safe and effective as long as three rules are employed: (*i*) use highly purified FDA-approved LIS; (*ii*) employ microdroplet serial puncture technique, defined as multiple injection of 0.01 cc into the subdermal plane or deeper at 3–5 mm intervals with no second pass, and (*iii*) use small volumes (0.5 cc for smaller defects and up to 2 cc for larger areas of atrophy) at each session with multiple sessions staged at monthly intervals or longer. Gradual fibroplasia ensues around each silicone microdroplet anchoring it in place and contributing to the ultimate result.

Recent reports have validated the safety of LIS in the treatment of HIV-associated facial lipoatrophy and acne scarring (Fig. 2.5.6). In a 2004 study from *Dermatologic Surgery*, 77 patients were treated with 1000-cS purified silicone oil for treatment of HIV-associated lipoatrophy using 2 cc of Silikon-1000 at monthly intervals with microdroplet technique until optimal correction was achieved (24). Results showed that facial contours were reliably reconstructed with an average of 6 cc (three treatments) for each stage of lipoatrophy severity. The mean volume was 12 cc (6 treatments), similar to the volume requirements of Radiesse for HIV facial lipoatrophy. It was concluded that 1000-cS purified silicone oil was safe and effective for treatment of lipoatrophy. A five-year follow-up has revealed no known serious adverse events, although four patients in a cohort of over 135 patients with greater than five-year follow-up developed mild to moderate subcutaneous firmness, which was responsive to intralesional cortisone or 5-FU injections (31). LIS also appears to be an exceptional filler for severe acne scarring (25).

(A)   **(B)**

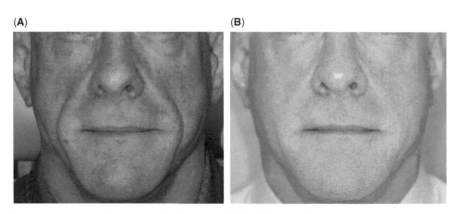

Figure 2.5.6 (**A**) Pre- and (**B**) post treatment with liquid injectable silicone for HIV facial lipoatrophy.

In a recent testimony, 35 skin biopsies obtained from target areas where LIS had been previously injected for correction of depressed facial scars were examined by light microscopy. The investigators found that LIS remained in the target areas in 100% of the cases biopsied without inducing any significant adverse complications. In several of the cases, LIS had been injected many years before the tissue was biopsied (26).

It is the author's opinion (DJ) that liquid injectable silicone should not be routinely employed for the average cosmetic patient until longer term studies with current products resolve some of the controversy regarding longer term safety and efficacy. However, for the unique and disfiguring defects associated with HIV facial lipoatrophy and serious acne scarring, patients and physicians should be aware of this excellent treatment modality which most frequently produces cosmetically superior and more durable results than currently available less permanent options.

Polymethylmethacrylate

Artefill® (Suneva Medical, San Diego, California, U.S.A.) is composed of 20% polymethylmethacrylate (PMMA) microspheres suspended in an 80% by volume bovine collagen gel matrix with 0.3% lidocaine. The product was approved in 2006 by the FDA for aesthetic correction of NLFs. The predecessor product of Artefill was Artecoll® (Rofil Medical, Breda, The Netherlands), which is a combination of PMMA and bovine collagen. Artecoll, which was never approved by the FDA, contained microspheres of varying sizes, including smaller nanoparticles less than 20 µm, which are easily engulfed by tissue macrophages and may contribute to granulomatous reactions. When redesigning the product to make Artefill, the surface of the particles was made smoother and particles less than 20 µm in size were removed. The newer product has been proven to cause fewer granulomatous foreign body reactions, presumably because of these changes.

One milliliter of Artefill contains approximately 6 million microspheres of PMMA. The microspheres stimulate tissue fibroblasts to encapsulate them, causing fibrous tissue formation in much the same way as LIS or PLLA induces tissue augmentation. However, unlike other fillers which are reabsorbed by the body after an extended period of time, PMMA stays permanent.

A recent study by Cohen et al. reported the five-year safety and efficacy of Artefill. This randomized controlled trial compared standardized photographs of NLFs injected with Artefill five years previously (n = 145) to baseline photographs before injection. Based on blinded observers' assessments of these photographs, subjects demonstrated a significant cosmetic improvement in the NLF five years following augmentation compared with baseline. Adverse events were noted at the following rates: 8.3% mild, 1.4% moderate, and 0.7% severe including lumpiness, persistent swelling, or redness; granuloma formation; or enlargement of the implant over time. This study confirms that Artefill demonstrates a continued correction of NLFs over a five-year period post injection with a serious adverse event rate of less than 1% at five years' follow-up (27).

Artefill can be used for aesthetic augmentation of NLFs, particularly deep NLFs that require a robust fill. Skin testing is required before treatment as the product contains bovine collagen. Before treatment, patients should be reminded that PMMA is a permanent treatment. Patients who have not previously been injected with temporary fillers for correction of NLFs should be encouraged to do so in order to visualize the aesthetic correction before committing to a permanent treatment option. The product should be stored in a refrigerator at 2–10 °C and warmed to room temperature before use. As it is a permanent filler, injection mistakes are hard to correct; therefore, small volumes of treatment should be injected over a period of time and overcorrection should be avoided. Since 0.3% lidocaine is already combined in the collagen matrix, an anesthetic is not necessarily required for small treatments. Topical anesthetic or nerve blocks may be used for larger treatments. A variety of injection methods can be used for deposition of this product, although many clinicians recommend the tunneling technique. Using a 26- or 27-gauge needle, the filler is layered in the deep dermis as the needle is passed back and forth. Superficial placement of product should be avoided as nodularity may occur. To reduce the risk of bruising and edema, the patient should be instructed to apply ice packs to the injection sites up to 24 hours post procedure. Minimal post-treatment edema and erythema may persist for a day or two.

A large number of European and Canadian studies have reported granulomatous reactions after injection with Artecoll (28). However, if granulomas do appear, they can be successfully treated with intralesional cortisone. It should be noted that in 2008 Artes Medical, the original manufacturer, went into chapter 7 bankruptcy; the product was temporarily unavailable, but is now being produced and distributed by Suneva Medical.

Hydrogel Polymers

Hydrogel polymers include the nonbiodegradable fillers Aquamid® (Contura International, Soeborg, Denmark) and Bio-Alcamid® (Polymekon, Milan, Italy). Aquamid is composed of 97% water and 3% polyacrylamide, while Bio-Alcimid is composed of 97% water and 3% alkylimide-amide groups. Both products are approved in other countries but not in the United States. The prostheses are highly biocompatible and nonabsorbable, yet can often be removed with incision and drainage if injected in bolus form. The implant is prepackaged in a syringe and is injected into the deep dermis/subcutis in the form of a bolus. Fibroplasia occurs around the periphery of the implant, thus creating an injectable, nonmigratory prosthesis. Although clinical trials have reported the efficacy of both products, adverse events, such as palpable subcutaneous lumps, delayed inflammatory reactions, migration, and late-appearing streptococcal bacterial abscesses have been common and may stall the approval of these products in the United States (29).

CONCLUSIONS

The current fillers on the market today provide patients with a variety of effective options that provide soft tissue augmentation for the NLFs and cheeks. Whether patients are interested in long-term or short-term correction, disease-related compatibility, or the comfort of reports of minimal risk, a product is available to fit their needs.

REFERENCES

1. American Society for Aesthetic Plastic Surgery. Cosmetic Procedures in 2007 [cited May 28, 2008].
2. Cohen J. Understanding, avoiding, and managing dermal filler complications. Dermatol Surg 2004; 34: S92–S9.
3. Brody HJ. Use of hyaluronidase in the treatment of granulomatous hyaluronic acid reactions or unwanted hyaluronic acid misplacement. Dermatol Surg 2005; 31 (8pt 1): 893–7.
4. Hirsch RJ, Cohen JL, Carruthers JD. Successful management of an unusual presentation of impending necrosis following a hyaluronic acid injection embolus and a proposed algorithm for management with hyaluronidase. Dermatol Surg 2007; 33: 357–60.
5. Tezel A, Fredrickson GH. The science of hyaluronic acid dermal fillers. J Cosmet Laser Ther 2008; 10: 35–42.
6. Carruthers A, Carey W, De Lorenzi C, et al. Randomized, double-blind comparison of the efficacy of two hyaluronic acid derivatives, estylane, erlane and ylaform, in the treatment of nasolabial folds. Dermatol Surg 2005; 31 (11pt 2): 1591–8; discussion 8.
7. Baumann LS, Shamban AT, Lupo MP, et al. Comparison of smooth-gel hyaluronic acid dermal fillers with cross-linked bovine collagen: a multicenter, double-masked, randomized, within-subject study. Dermatol Surg 2007; 33 (Suppl 1): S128–35.
8. Narins RS, Dayan SH, Brandt FS, Baldwin EK. Persistence and improvement of nasolabial fold correction with nonanimal-stabilized hyaluronic acid 100,000 gel particles/mL filler on two retreatment schedules: results up to 18 months on two retreatment schedules. Dermatol Surg 2008; 34 (Suppl 1): S2–8; discussion S8.
9. Smith S, Jones D. Poster Presentation: Efficacy and safety following repeat treatment for a new family of hyaluronic acid based fillers. American Academy of Dermatology Academy 2006 Meeting. San Diego, CA, 2006.
10. Lowe NJ, Grover R. Injectable hyaluronic acid implant for malar and mental enhancement. Dermatol Surg 2006; 32: 881–5; discussion 5.
11. Raspaldo H. Volumizing effect of a new hyaluronic acid sub-dermal filler: a retrospective analysis based on 102 cases. J Cosmet Laser Ther 2008; 10: 134–42.
12. Narins RS, Baumann L, Brandt FS, et al. A randomized study of the efficacy and safety of injectable poly-L-lactic acid versus human-based collagen implant in the treatment of nasolabial fold wrinkles. J Am Acad Dermatol 2010; 62: 448–62.
13. Stewart DB, Morganroth GS, Mooney MA, et al. Management of visible granulomas following periorbital injection of poly-L-lactic Acid. Ophthal Plast Reconstr Surg 2007; 23: 298–301.
14. Wildemore JK, Jones DH. Persistent granulomatous inflammatory response induced by injectable poly-L-lactic acid for HIV lipoatrophy. Dermatol Surg 2006; 32: 1407–9; discussion 9.
15. Goldberg D. Calcium hydroxlyapatite. Fillers in cosmetic dermatology. Informa UK Ltd: Abingdon, England, 2006.
16. Carruthers A, Liebeskind M, Carruthers J, Forster BB. Radiographic and computed tomographic studies of calcium hydroxylapatite for treatment of HIV-associated facial lipoatrophy and correction of nasolabial folds. Dermatol Surg 2008; 34 (Suppl 1): S78–84.
17. Sadick NS, Katz BE, Roy D. A multicenter, 47-month study of safety and efficacy of calcium hydroxylapatite for soft tissue augmentation of nasolabial folds and other areas of the face. Dermatol Surg 2007; 33 (Suppl 2): S122–6; discussion S6–7.
18. Smith S, Busso M, McClaren M, Bass LS. A randomized, bilateral, prospective comparison of calcium hydroxylapatite microspheres versus human-based collagen for the correction of nasolabial folds. Dermatol Surg 2007; 33 (Suppl 2): S112–21; discussion S21.
19. Moers-Carpi M, Vogt S, Santos BM, et al. A multicenter, randomized trial comparing calcium hydroxylapatite to two hyaluronic acids for treatment of nasolabial folds. Dermatol Surg 2007; 33 (Suppl 2): S144–51.
20. Busso M, Voigts R. An investigation of changes in physical properties of injectable calcium hydroxylapatite in a carrier gel when mixed with lidocaine and with lidocaine/epinephrine. Dermatol Surg 2008; 34 (Suppl 1): S16–23; discussion S4.
21. Carruthers A, Carruthers J. Evaluation of injectable calcium hydroxylapatite for the treatment of facial lipoatrophy associated with human immunodeficiency virus. Dermatol Surg 2008; 34: 1486–99.
22. Narins RS, Brandt FS, Lorenc PZ, et al. A randomized, multicenter study of the safety and efficacy of Dermicol-P35 and non-animal-stabilized hyaluronic acid gel for the correction of nasolabial folds. Dermatol Surg 2007; 33 (Suppl 2): S213–21.
23. Prather CL, Jones DH. Liquid injectable silicone for soft tissue augmentation. Dermatol Ther 2006; 19: 159–68.
24. Jones DH, Carruthers A, Orentreich D, et al. Highly purified 1000-cSt silicone oil for treatment of human immunodeficiency virus-associated facial lipoatrophy: an open pilot trial. Dermatol Surg 2004; 30: 1279–86.
25. Barnett JG, Barnett CR. Treatment of acne scars with liquid silicone injections: 30-year perspective. Dermatol Surg 2005; 31 (11pt 2): 1542–9.
26. Zappi E, Barnett JG, Zappi M, Barnett CR. The long-term host response to liquid silicone injected during soft tissue augmentation procedures: a microscopic appraisal. Dermatol Surg 2007; 33 (Suppl 2): S186–92; discussion S92.
27. Cohen SR, Berner CF, Busso M, et al. Five-year safety and efficacy of a novel polymethylmethacrylate aesthetic soft tissue filler for the correction of nasolabial folds. Dermatol Surg 2007; 33 (Suppl 2): S222–30.
28. Carruthers A, Carruthers JD. Polymethylmethacrylate microspheres/collagen as a tissue augmenting agent: personal experience over 5 years. Dermatol Surg 2005; 31 (11pt 2): 1561–4; discussion 5.
29. Jones DH, Carruthers A, Fitzgerald R, Sarantopoulos GP, Binder S. Late-appearing abscesses after injections of nonabsorbable hydrogel polymer for HIV-associated facial lipoatrophy. Dermatol Surg 2007; 33 (Suppl 2): S193–8.
30. Jones D, Tezel A, Borrell M. In vitro resistance to degradation of hyaluronic acid fillers by ovine testicular hyaluronidase. Dermatol Surg 2010; 36: 804–9.
31. Jones D. A report of 135 patients with 5 year and beyond follow up after treatment with highly purified Liquid Injectable Silicone (LIS) for HIV Associated Facial Lipoatrophy (HIV FLA). American Society for Dermatologic Surgery Annual Meeting. Chicago, IL, October 24, 2010.
32. Jones D. Commerntary: what lies beneath. Dermatol Surg 2011; 37: 387–8.
33. Jones D, Vleggaar D. Technique for injecting Poly-L-lactic acid. J Drugs Dermatol 2007; 6 (Suppl 2): S13–S17.

2.6 Perioral rejuvenation
*Frederick Beddingfield, Diane Murphy, Cherilyn Sheets,
Andrew Nelson, and Jenny Kim*

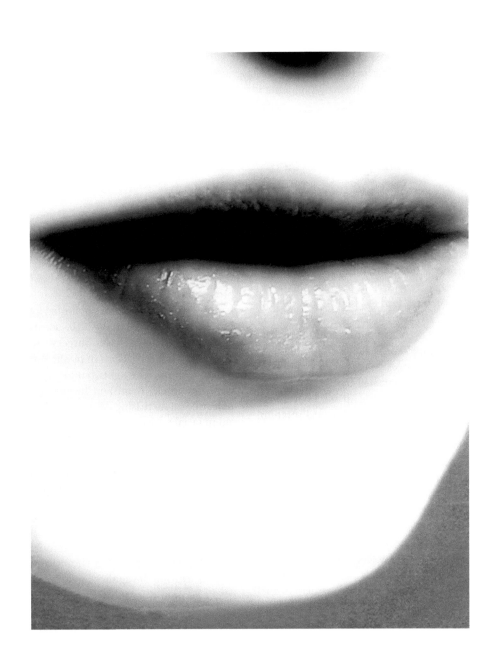

KEY POINTS

- Perioral aging is one of the great contributors to an overall aged appearance for patients
- Perioral aging results from the dynamic effects of muscle movement, an overall loss of volume, as well as the results of chronic photodamage
- Dermal soft tissue fillers can be used to improve the lost volume in the lips, as well as better define the appearance of the vermilion border. Soft tissue fillers can also be used to improve radiating perioral rhytides, and provide scaffolding support for the oral commissures
- Botulinum toxin is effective in improving the appearance of radiating perioral rhytides, melomental folds, mental creases, chin dimpling, as well as to alter a patient's smile. Caution should be exercised in treating these areas, as inappropriate treatment can result in loss of competence of the orbicularis oris muscles
- Skin resurfacing, via chemical peels or laser treatment, can significantly improve the appearance of mottled dyspigmentation, dyschromia, and lead to neocollagenesis as well
- Whenever discussing perioral rejuvenation, physicians should consider the impact of the appearance of the dentition, and involve a cosmetic dentist if necessary to achieve the best outcomes

INTRODUCTION

Facial aging is the result of several processes that arise from both intrinsic and extrinsic factors. With time, the loss of subcutaneous fat and skin elasticity, as well as the remodeling of bony and cartilaginous structures, lead to visible signs of aging in the face as a whole. Repetitive muscle activity can lead to the development of rhytides that deepen over time and ultimately remain apparent even when the face is at rest. Photodamage and smoking accelerate these changes. In the perioral region in particular (the section of face demarcated by the nasal base, cheeks, and chin), dentition changes, loss of lip fullness, resorption of mandibular and maxillary bone, and forward rotation and protrusion of the chin also contribute to the aging face. The primary goals of lower face rejuvenation are to restore volume, reduce mobility, and resurface when appropriate.

Historical solutions for the patient seeking a more youthful appearance were almost exclusively surgical interventions of varying degrees. A "facelift" can be quite expensive and requires that the patient have an extensive recovery time. The results provide dramatic and enduring changes in appearance; but, if they are not to the patient's liking, further surgical intervention is necessary. Additionally, it can result in a tell-tale unnatural "pulled-tight" appearance of the skin and corners of the mouth, as a facelift does not address volumetric losses associated with aging. With the more active lifestyles of today's aging population, the downtime from traditional plastic surgery has become less acceptable. Alternative treatments, including minimal downtime procedures such as dermal soft tissue fillers and botulinum toxin, have become much more popular in the last decade.

Because there are numerous factors that contribute to visible signs of aging, facial rejuvenation of the perioral area is most effectively achieved through combination treatment. Improving skin texture and fine lines as well as other signs of photoaging such as uneven pigmentation and redness is important.

Controlling muscle movement in addition to the restoration of volume is necessary (1). Treatment methods include the use of dermal fillers, botulinum toxin, laser treatments, chemical peels, cosmetics and cosmeceuticals, and surgical and dental procedures.

Nonsurgical procedures accounted for 83% of total cosmetic procedures conducted in 2010, according to the American Society for Aesthetic Plastic Surgery (ASAPS) annual survey of board-certified physicians in plastic surgery, dermatology, and otolaryngology. The top two nonsurgical cosmetic procedures were botulinum toxin and hyaluronic acid (HA) injections, reflecting an increasing demand for less invasive products that aid in facial rejuvenation (2).

Many of the treatment paradigms discussed herein represent off-label uses, but these practices have been used safely and successfully by practitioners under the advice of consensus recommendations and peer-reviewed literature.

CHARACTERISTICS OF THE AGING PERIORAL AREA

The aging rate and process for an individual is unique due to variables such as genetics, anatomy, environment, and lifestyle choices. During the aging process, collagen diminishes; elastic fibers become thin and fragmented; subcutaneous fat thins; and underlying facial muscles become weaker. These changes, in conjunction with gravity, result in an overall drooping of the face. Signs of perioral aging common across most individuals are the formation of rhytides, changes in lip shape or fullness, creation or deepening of the melomental crease and nasolabial folds (NLFs), and ptosis of the chin.

Rhytides

Rhytides (wrinkles) are formed due to the repeated contraction of the underlying circular orbicularis muscle in conjunction with slackening of the skin. In the perioral region, these fine lines radiate outward from the lips and are a common complaint of older women whose lipstick begins to "bleed" into these lines.

Lips

As aging proceeds, the upper lip becomes thin and elongated (3), and the lower lip thins and rolls inward. The result is a loss of show of the upper teeth and an increase in show of the lower teeth and sometimes gum. These effects also result in an overall reduction in the visible vermilion. There is a thickening of the epidermis, especially in the white roll of the upper lip. In addition, the Cupid's bow, the two high points of the upper vermilion, becomes flattened, and the philtral columns are not as prominent as we age.

Melomental Crease

Vertical lines at the oral commissures ("marionette lines") form and deepen due to hyperactivity of the depressor angularis oris (DAO) muscle and loss of skin structure and bony support inferiorly, resulting in a saddened or unhappy expression.

Nasolabial Folds (NLFs)

The nasolabial lines, from the corners of the nose to the corners of the mouth, become increasingly deep due to muscular activity and ptosis of the skin.

Chin

Over time, the chin loses its delineated look and begins to sag. The skin of the chin often becomes dimpled from the muscular contraction resulting in a so-called peau d'orange appearance.

Table 2.6.1 The Glogau Scale of Photoaging (51)

1. Early photoaging: mild pigmentary changes, no keratoses, minimal wrinkles
2. Early to moderate photoaging: early senile lentigines, no visible keratoses, wrinkles in motion
3. Advanced photoaging: dyschromia and telangiectasia, visible keratoses, wrinkles at rest
4. Severe photoaging: yellow-gray color skin, prior skin malignancies, wrinkled throughout—no normal skin, multiple actinic keratoses

Table 2.6.2 The Fitzpatrick Skin Phototype Classification Scale

I	White; very fair; red or blond hair; blue eyes; freckles	Always burns, never tans
II	White; fair; red or blond hair; blue, hazel, or green eyes	Usually burns, tans with difficulty
III	Cream white; fair with any eye or hair color; very common	Sometimes burns mildly, gradually tans
IV	Brown; typical Mediterranean Caucasian skin	Rarely burns, tans with ease
V	Dark brown; mid-eastern skin types	Very rarely burns, tans very easily
VI	Black	Never burns, tans very easily

Jowls often start to form from the sagging of the skin and loss of support, yielding an overall flattened look for the bottom of the face.

What Drives Treatment Decisions

Treatment of the perioral area differs from patient to patient, based on factors such as skin type, severity of photoaging, the individual patient's goals and expectations of treatment, and other factors such as recovery time. The Glogau Scale of photoaging (Table 2.6.1) and the Fitzpatrick Classification Scale for skin pigmentation (Table 2.6.2) are useful in the initial assessment of patients, and may help to direct treatment decisions. For example, patients with significant photodamage (i.e., higher categories on the Glogau Scale) will require more aggressive treatments to elicit satisfactory results, and patients with darker skin tones (i.e., Fitzpatrick skin type IV or higher) should be treated cautiously with certain types of chemical peels and laser treatments due to the higher risk of dyspigmentation in this population. The Wrinkle Severity Rating Scale (Table 2.6.3) and the Wrinkle Assessment Scale (Table 2.6.4) have often been used during clinical trials for NLFs (4,5), and another scale specific to lip size, the vermilion, and the vermilion border (CKC Scale, Table 2.6.5) may be useful when discussing lip treatment goals with patients (6).

The most critical step in developing a treatment plan is to understand the outcome sought by the patient—whether

Table 2.6.3 The Wrinkle Severity Rating Scale (52)

1 (absent)	No visible nasolabial fold (NLF); continuous skin line
2 (mild)	Shallow but visible NLF with a slight indentation; minor facial feature; implant is expected to produce a slight improvement in appearance
3 (moderate)	Moderately deep NLF; clear facial feature visible at normal appearance but not when stretched; excellent correction is expected from injectable implant
4 (severe)	Very long and deep NLF; prominent facial feature; <2-mm visible fold when stretched; significant improvement is expected from injectable implant
5 (extreme)	Extremely deep and long NLF; detrimental to facial appearance; 2–4 mm visible V-shaped fold when stretched; unlikely to have satisfactory correction with injectable implant alone

Table 2.6.4 The Wrinkle Assessment Scale for NLF Severity (4)

Score	Severity	Descriptions
0	None	No wrinkle
1	Mild	Shallow, just perceptible wrinkle
2	Moderate	Moderately deep wrinkle
3	Severe	Deep wrinkle, well-defined edges (but not overlapping)
4	Extreme	Very deep wrinkle, redundant fold (overlapping skin)

Table 2.6.5 The CKC lip evaluation scale (53)

Size

Score	Letter	Description	
−2	V	Very Thin	≤1:15
−1	T	Thin	1:15–1:10
0	M	Medium Sized	1:10–1:7
1	F	Full	1:7–1:4
2	E	Extremely Full	>1:4

Vermilion body

Score	Description
−1	Tight almost unlined
0	Rounded with natural lines
1	Less rounded with fine lines
2	Flattening with moderate wrinkles
3	Severe wrinkles

Vermilion border

Score	Description
−1	Protruding and/or creating peri oral shadow
0	Distinct and intact, with/without shadow from mid lower lip
1	Distinct but broken by fine lines, with/without shadow from mid lower lip
2	Indistinct and broken by moderate lines with/without shadow from mid lower lip
3	Indistinct and severely lined, with/without shadow from mid lower lip

enhancement or restoration. Younger patients typically seek enhancement, particularly of the lips, and older patients typically seek restoration. In both cases, a careful assessment of the overall face is necessary. Physicians need to treat the entire face by looking at how an area of the face relates to the whole (7).

For enhancement, it is important to determine the degree of enhancement sought by the patient. Is the patient satisfied with the existing shape but desiring fuller lips, or does the patient seek an entirely different look for his/her lips? Frequently, younger patients want to emulate the look of movie stars or public figures. A careful assessment of the appropriateness of that look in proportion to the rest of the patient's face is warranted. Volume enhancement not only increases the vertical height of the vermilion, but also increases lip volume circumferentially, potentially resulting in the undesirable "duck lip" appearance (8).

For restoration, it is important that the patient's specific concerns are determined first. Often, a single concern will necessitate treatment in multiple areas. Fixing a "lipstick bleed" may require treatment with dermal fillers in the lips as well as a laser treatment, or a chemical peel to remove very superficial lines. Conversely, sometimes treating one area, such as the oral commissures, can improve the overall appearance of the face. In general, though, it is best to view the face as a whole rather than as isolated regions. Treatments do not need to occur in a single session; especially for restoration, it is better to schedule multiple visits with gradual steps of treatment in order to better assess the effects of previous sessions on the overall restoration goal.

Finally, recovery time should be discussed with the patient. Botulinum toxin injections and most nonpermanent injectable fillers are usually touted as "lunchtime" procedures with very minimal recovery time. However, bruising is possible with any injection, and hydrophilic fillers such as HA fillers may result in temporary swelling following these "lunchtime"

procedures. Similarly, some laser procedures such as nonablative technologies can be performed with minimal downtime. However, ablative laser resurfacing, which often gives a considerable improvement in the appearance of perioral rhytides, may require several weeks of healing. Likewise, there are superficial, medium, and deep chemical peels; the deeper the peel, the longer the recovery time. The downtime the patient is willing to accept ultimately has a significant impact on the appropriate treatment options for perioral rejuvenation.

Finally, treatment decisions may be driven by cost. Surgical treatments, such as facelifts, cheek implants, and chin augmentation, while potentially longer lasting, cost significantly more upfront than nonsurgical treatments, such as dermal fillers or chemical peels. Even within dermal fillers there is a wide range of costs; autologous fat is more expensive than HA fillers after factoring in the costs to harvest and process; it has also been associated with variable duration and possible severe adverse events (9). In addition to determining the patient's treatment goals and describing the recovery time, the most cost-effective treatment should be presented to the patient for consideration.

DERMAL FILLERS FOR PERIORAL REJUVENATION

Soft tissue fillers are an effective and safe way to restore the lost volume in the perioral region of the face. They have been used effectively to reduce the appearance of NLFs and marionette lines, and to create fuller lips. An ideal filler will be one that is nonpermanent and reversible but long lasting, hypoallergenic, easy to use and inject, painless upon injection, with a quick onset, minimal side effect profile, cost-effective, and produces a natural appearance and feel. Although no single filler can provide all the solutions that patients may need to achieve their desired outcome, many dermal fillers are now available to meet an increasing demand. The U.S. dermal filler market is projected to continue increasing through 2011, due to the aging population, new and improved filler technologies, and increasing social acceptance of cosmetic procedures (10).

Dermal fillers are available in an array of biodegradable/nonpermanent and nonbiodegradable/permanent materials. Traditionally, fillers have been biodegradable, and they have a proven safety record in spite of the potential for hypersensitivity reactions. Biodegradable fillers, including collagen and HA-based fillers are temporary and generally last four to six months. One HA filler, Juvéderm® Ultra Plus (Allergan Inc, Irvine, California), has a labeled duration of 12 months (11). The disadvantage to biodegradable substances is that they have a relatively short duration of effect, in some cases necessitating injections every three months. Semipermanent fillers produce a longer effect but are associated with a higher incidence of granulomas, which are often of late-onset (i.e., one year or more after treatment). Permanent, nonbiodegradable fillers are available and are often used in patients with HIV lipoatrophy or stable morphea. They are associated with a higher incidence of granulomas and extrusion. However, filler duration in individual patients may vary due to external factors such as smoking or sun exposure. And, although permanent fillers are long lasting, the continual aging process may necessitate further treatments.

Table 2.6.6 lists some of the fillers available along with their approximate duration of effect. Treatment with dermal fillers generally falls into two different mechanistic actions: "stimulatory"

Table 2.6.6 Types of Dermal Fillers in the United States

Category	Material	Trade names	Approximate Duration of Effect
Temporary	Autologous fat	—	3–6 months (mo)
	Bovine collagen	Zyderm I Zyderm II Zyplast (no longer commercially available)	3–6 mo
	Human collagen	CosmoDerm I CosmoDerm II CosmoPlast (no longer commercially available)	3–6 mo
	Porcine collagen	Evolence (no longer commercially available)	6 mo
	Hyaluronic acid	Captique (Inamed Aesthetics, Santa Barbara, California) Elevess (Anika Therapeutics, Bedford, Massachusetts) Hylaform, Hylaform Plus (Genzyme, Ridgefield, New Jersey) Prevelle (Genzyme, Ridgefield, New Jersey) Juvéderm Ultra (with and without lidocaine); Juvéderm Ultra Plus (with and without lidocaine) (Allergan Inc, Irvine, California) Restylane, Perlane (Medicis Aesthetics, Scottsdale, Arizona)	Dependent on the viscosity of the product (3–18 mo)
Semipermanent	Calcium Hydroxylapatite	Radiesse (Merz Aesthetics, San Mateo, California)	9–12 mo
	Poly-L-lactic acid	Sculptra (Dermik Laboratories, Bridgewater, New Jersey)	18–24 mo
Permanent	Polymethylmethacrylate	ArteFill (Suneva Medical Inc, San Diego, California)	4–5 yrs
	Silicone oil	Adato Sil 5000 (Bausch & Lomb Inc, Rochester, New York) Silikon 1000 (Alcon Laboratories, Fort Worth, Texas)	

Table 2.6.7 Treatment Areas that Respond to Botox (Allergan Inc, Irvine, California)

Treatment For	Treated Muscle	Units	Placement of Injection
Perioral rhytides	Orbicularis oris of upper and lower lips	1–3 units in each lip quadrant	Superolateral to the oral commissure, at or approximately 3–5 mm above the vermilion border; 4–6 sites, 1 per lip quadrant; inject as needle is withdrawn
Oral commissure depression	Depressor anguli oris (DAO)	2–5 units per side	At mandibular insertion of the DAO; immediately above the angle of the mandible and 1 cm lateral to the lateral oral commissure; insert needle perpendicular to the skin
Chin dimpling	Mentalis	3–10 units	Into mentalis split between 1 and 2 sites; perpendicularly into the muscle; massage chin to diffuse the toxin
Prominence of mental crease	Mentalis	3–5 units	Into the bony mentum, perpendicularly into the muscle, split between 1 and 3 sites
Nasolabial folds	Lip elevators	1 unit per side	Into each lip elevator complex in the nasofacial groove

and "replacement." Stimulatory fillers stimulate endogenous tissue growth, such as collagen, and typically provide a delayed correction. Replacement fillers occupy the space left by the lost volume and provide a more immediate correction (12).

Temporary Fillers

Collagen, HA, and fat are normal constituents of the dermis and subcutaneous tissue and, as such, are less likely in general to cause hypersensitivity reactions than products utilizing nonnatural components (e.g. semipermanent, permanent, and synthetic fillers) (8).

Bovine Collagen

Zyderm®I, Zyderm®II, and Zyplast® were the first FDA-approved collagen fillers and were the most frequently used substances until 2003. They are now replaced by other fillers and are no longer marketed. Good results were obtained for depressed acne scars, NLFs, and lips. Since the source of the collagen is bovine, there is a high potential for allergic reactions, so two separate skin tests are required prior to use. Duration is limited, with an upper limit of ~6 months. In areas of greater mobility (e.g., the lips), it is rare for the effect to last

longer than three months. Patients with known connective tissue disorders (e.g., systemic lupus erythematosus) should not receive animal-based implants that can cause hypersensitivity reactions.

Human Collagen

Following on the heels of the bovine collagen fillers, Cosmo-Derm I, CosmoDerm II, and CosmoPlast use bioengineered human collagen. These, like bovine collagen, are no longer marketed. These did not require testing but had a short-duration effect like bovine collagen. These products were used in a number of sites because of their ease of injection and malleability. Collagen is often layered with other fillers such as HAs and can be used as a supporting framework to enhance the lips (8).

Porcine Collagen

The latest addition to the collagen filler group is Evolence™, a porcine-derived collagen. Because immunogenicity is low for porcine collagen, this product was touted as an improvement over bovine collagen and, like bioengineered human collagen, does not require a skin test (5). There is evidence that the longevity of correction from porcine collagen may exceed other collagen products. To date, it has failed to capture a large share of the market for fillers and is no longer marketed in many countries (13).

Hyaluronic Acid

All living organisms have naturally occurring HA as part of the extracellular matrix. First approved by the FDA in late 2003, HA fillers do not require allergy testing since HA is completely homologous in structure between species. Common sources of HA include bacterial cultures, rooster combs, and umbilical cords. The incidence of delayed hypersensitivity reactions is less than 1 out of 10,000. HA fillers initially provide correction by the volume from the hydrophilic injected material. They have been shown to stimulate fibroblasts to produce collagen which may help maintain the effects of treatment, but the exact clinical meaningfulness of any collagen stimulation is still uncertain (14). Cross-linking of the HA in the fillers results in larger, more stable molecules with longer duration than native HA (1), and this is critical because uncrosslinked HA would last less than a week (15). Cross-linking of the HA extends the longevity of correction to between 6 and 12 months. Excellent long-lasting results for lips, NLFs, marionette lines, and acne scars are observed (16), with duration being the key factor that has made HA fillers, particularly Restylane® and Juvéderm®, replace collagen as the gold standard wrinkle filler (17,18). Recently, HA products with lidocaine have been approved in Europe, the United States, and other countries; these products have rapidly replaced most of the HA without lidocaine products because of the substantial reduction in pain.

Autologous Fat

Autologous fat has been used since the late 19th century, but the technique has evolved dramatically over time. The possible mechanism of action is in stimulating an inflammatory response that is later replaced with fibrotic tissue. The advantages are that large volumes are utilized and it can be used for volume restoration anywhere on the face, specifically to NLFs, cheeks, and marionette lines. Due to its volume and viscosity, fine lines and small acne scars cannot be treated appropriately with autologous fat. It can be a cost-effective procedure when used in conjunction with liposuction as it requires extraction of the fat from a fat deposit. Because it is endogenous to the patient, there are no compatibility issues; however, due to reabsorption of the fat by the body, overcorrection of 30–50% is advised in order to achieve the best results. Multiple injections are often required to obtain a desirable result. Longevity is limited, and the irregular surface contours may not be optimal in mobile areas such as the lips (8).

Semipermanent Fillers

Calcium Hydroxylapatite

Calcium hydroxylapatite (CaHA) microspheres are suspended in a water-based carboxy methylcellulose gel carrier. The CaHA is identical in chemical composition to that found in bone and teeth, making it biocompatible and naturally degraded by the body. However, CaHA is not a normal constituent of the dermis and thus may rarely cause hypersensitivity reactions. The CaHA microspheres remain in the dermis after the carrier matrix degrades and serve as a "scaffold" for collagen deposits. The product should be injected in the subdermal plane as it may become visible if injected more superficially. This filler is used for NLFs, marionette lines, hollowing of cheeks, and substantial acne scars. The prejowl sulcus can be augmented. CaHA has also been used for "nonsurgical rhinoplasty." Formation of lumps and nodules, sometimes resulting in scarring, has been reported, especially if injected superficially or in mobile areas like the lips, so it is not recommended for lip augmentation (17,18).

Poly-L-lactic Acid

Poly-L-lactic acid is a biocompatible, biodegradable, synthetic polymer from the α-hydroxy-acid family. As this product is not a normal constituent of the dermis, hypersensitivity reactions may be more likely than with HA and collagen. The FDA has approved its use for lipoatrophy in people with HIV in 2004; cosmetic use of this product was recently approved in 2009. The filler should be injected into the subcutis, where it stimulates fibroplasia. Multiple treatment sessions are necessary (17), and results are not visible until collagen production has taken place (18). As with CaHA, nodules are a concern for poly-L-lactic acid (17).

Permanent Fillers

Polymethylmethacrylate Microspheres

Polymethylmethacrylate (PMMA) microspheres are formulated into a collagen carrier. After injection, the collagen suspension is slowly reabsorbed over one to three months, while the microspheres remain encapsulated in fibrous tissue. Correction is provided not only by the volume of injected material but also via fibrosis from the degraded collagen, resulting in further collagen production locally (19). Because the collagen carrier is from a bovine source, skin allergy tests are required. For full augmentation, successive treatments are required until the desired result is achieved, often requiring sequential treatment every two to three months (20). Because of its consistency and the reactivity potential of PMMA in the skin, this product (and its previous formulations) has led to reactions and nodules which can lead to lumpiness and unevenness in the lips (21). The company that originally developed this product filed for bankruptcy and the product was acquired by another company. This product does not constitute a large proportion of the filler market.

Silicone

Liquid injectable silicone has been in use for more than 40 years, but the cosmetic use of silicone oil products for lip augmentation is off-label in the United States and most other countries (22). Silicone as a filler has a longer lasting effect than other injectable fillers; however, a higher viscosity can lead to more bruising. There have been reports of granulomas, foreign-body reactions, migration, and extrusion, which may have been due to impurities or may be inherent to the reactivity of certain grades and formulations of silicone in the skin. The microdroplet technique has led to improved results (22) but silicone injections are still controversial, and the long-term risks are unknown (17).

Selecting the Proper Filler for Perioral Rejuvenation

Once the patient's treatment goals have been thoroughly vetted, the physician must choose the type of filler and the proper technique. No single filler is suitable for all areas in all situations (23). Skin type, severity of lines, and shaping versus filling must all be taken into consideration.

Skin type is a major determinant in the type of filler used. Thickness of skin tends to be different in men and women, and female skin tends to be more sensitive to irritants. Facial profiles vary among ethnic groups, and a patient's ethnicity may also impact the way they age. According to the ASAPS 2010 survey, Caucasians make up the majority of patients seeking cosmetic enhancements, followed by Hispanics, African-Americans, and people of Asian descent (2). Care must be taken not to apply Caucasian aesthetic ideals to other ethnic groups. Ethnic skin differs in the amount of pigmentation and how the skin reacts to minor trauma (such as hypertrophic scars and keloids) (1), although clinical studies have not shown an increased incidence of these reactions after HA-filler injections in skin of color (24). For a more complete discussion of injectable fillers in ethnic populations, please see the section of the book, "Beauty and Aging in Ethnic Skin."

Wrinkle severity also determines which type of filler is appropriate. In general, fillers with greater particle size or viscosity are injected deeper in order to correct more severe volume loss and wrinkle severity. Layering of fillers works well for deeper folds; larger particle fillers placed deeper provide a subdermal "bed" for finer particle materials injected into the middle and upper dermis. For superficial rhytides, a single-filler treatment may be sufficient. Sclafani provides a nice summary of which fillers to use where:

"Large particles placed too superficially can produce visible nodules, and … are most appropriately placed just below the dermis. Conversely, midsized particle substances … can be injected into the mid-dermis, and small particle injectables … can be used even more superficially. Any injectable filler should be placed as superficially as safely possible to maximize benefit" (19).

Injection Techniques for Dermal Fillers for Perioral Rejuvenation

For patients concerned with their lips, the type of filler chosen depends on the treatment goals. Shaping the lips requires different filler treatment than simply addressing rhytides. Assessments of the lips should include vertical height and bulk of the red lip, the horizontal vermilion arch, and the height of the white lip. Any lip asymmetry should be noted as well as the presence and severity of perioral wrinkles (20). The effect of aging on the lips is noted in an elongation of the upper lip and a drooping of the lower lip and lip corners. These changes are due to gravity and loss of skin elastosis and collagen, loss of dental and bony support of the mandible, and the effects of depressors of the lip corners such as the depressor anguli oris (DAO).

Published literature is plentiful regarding how to achieve optimal results with dermal fillers. Injection techniques include tunneling, serial puncture, threading, cross-hatching, and fanning (18). Some physicians provide recommendations as to which technique to use with which filler (25,26), but ultimately, the injection method is not as important as the location and quantity of the product injected (20).

It is critical to understand the underlying anatomy when deciding upon the treatment technique. One unique cadaver study demonstrated that there are distinct arteries and membranes that define and separate the philtral columns from the lateral lip compartments, which may affect how the philtral columns are addressed during treatment (27). In addition to understanding the anatomy, careful injection planning is important to deliver equal amounts to each side of the face to avoid asymmetries (1).

In general, injections in the lip vermilion produce volume, whereas injections in the rolled border produce definition (28). However, patients want individualized results that suit their specific lip goals. To achieve this, it can be useful to separate the lip into distinct zones for injection. These injection zones correspond to specific lip contouring or augmentation. The zones include the vermilion/white roll, subvermilion, peristomal, philtral column, and commissural. Within these major zones are lateral and medial sections, along with the Cupid's bow apex zone and philtral/central zone. The vermilion/white roll zones are injected to increase the size of the lip as well as to modify the curvature of the Cupid's bow. Injections into the subvermilion and peristomal zones both medially and laterally, can achieve fullness (29) (See Figs. 2.6.1A–C and 2.6.2A–C).

For perioral rhytides, degeneration of the collagen and elastic fibers around the mouth provides an easy potential space or passageway for small amounts of filler to travel (28). The commonly seen downturn of corners of the mouth with aging, which can create an unwanted sad look, can be addressed by a combination treatment of fillers injected inferiorly to provide a buttress and botulinum toxin injected into the DAO to reduce the dynamic downward pull of this muscle. (Figs. 2.6.3,2.6.4,2.6.5,2.6.6)

In 2007, a multidisciplinary group of experts in aesthetic treatments (the Facial Aesthetics Consensus Group) recommended using HA fillers and botulinum toxin type A (Botox) for facial rejuvenation. The excerpt below from the published consensus provides guidelines for the location and quantity:

"When treating the vermilion border with HA filler, approximately 80 percent of the faculty use Juvéderm® Ultra and the remaining use Restylane®. For volumizing the lips, Juvéderm® Ultra, Juvéderm® Ultra Plus, and Restylane® are preferred by 44 percent, 31 percent, and 25 percent of the faculty, respectively. For volume enhancement of the lips and shaping the vermilion border, 67 percent of the faculty use 1.0 mL of HA filler. The remaining 33 percent use 2.0 mL … It is important to think of shaping the lips, not simply adding volume … For marionette lines (melomental folds) and the prejowl sulcus, 56 percent of the faculty use one syringe of HA filler and the remaining 44 percent use two syringes" (1).

Adverse Events Associated with Dermal Fillers

Since many of the dermal fillers are used off-label for certain treatment areas, full elucidation of the common adverse events in clinical studies has not been performed. In general, dermal fillers have been demonstrated to be safe. Common adverse events are local to the injection site and include swelling, erythema, bruising, pain, and tenderness, and generally last less

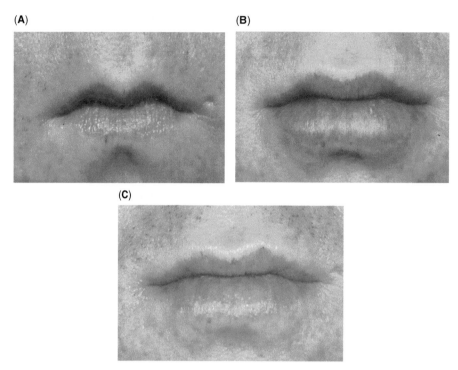

Figure 2.6.1 Patient before (**A**) and 2 weeks after (**B**) lip augmentation/rejuvenation with Juvederm Ultra hyaluronic acid filler injections. Note the enhanced volume of both the upper and lower lips, as well as the improved definition of the rolled border. After 48 weeks (**C**), the effect continues to persist.   *Source*: Photos courtesy of Allergan Inc, Irvine, California.

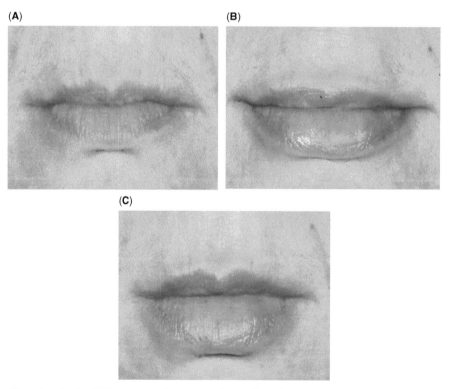

Figure 2.6.2 Patient before (**A**) and 2 weeks after (**B**) lip augmentation with Juvederm® Ultra hylauronic acid filler injections. Note the enhancement of the volume of both the upper and lower lip, as well as the reduction in the appearance of vertical rhytides in the lips themselves and the perioral rhytides. After 36 weeks (**C**), the effect continues to persist.   *Source*: Photos courtesy of Allergan Inc, Irvine, California.

(A)   (B)

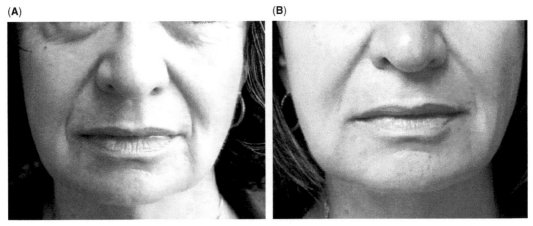

Figure 2.6.3 Patient before (**A**) and 4 weeks after (**B**) Juvederm Voluma® hyaluronic acid (HA) filler injections. HA filler was injected at the melomental fold and the lateral oral commissure to add volume, reduce static rhytides and buttress the corners of the lip.   *Source*: Photos courtesy of Drs. Jean and Alastair Carruthers.

(A)   (B)

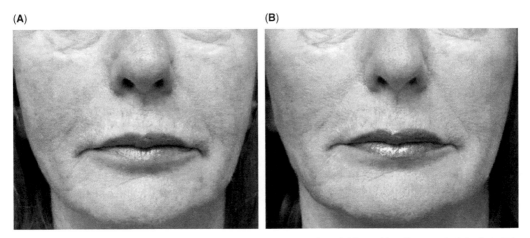

Figure 2.6.4 Patient before (**A**) and immediately after (**B**) Juvederm Voluma hyaluronic acid (HA) filler and botulinum toxin injections. HA was injected in the melomental fold and around the lateral oral commissure to reduce static rhytides and buttress the corners of the lip. Botulinum toxin (Botox) was injected into the depressor anguli oris (DAO) muscle to help elevate the corners of the mouth.   *Source*: Photos courtesy of Drs. Jean and Alastair Carruthers.

(A)   (B)

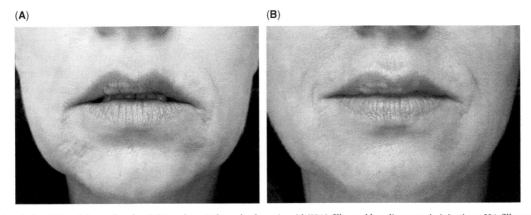

Figure 2.6.5 Patient before (**A**) and 6 months after (**B**) Juvederm Voluma hyaluronic acid (HA) filler and botulinum toxin injections. HA filler was injected in the melomental folds and around the lateral oral commissure to reduce static rhytides and buttress the corners of the lip. Botulinum toxin (Botox) was injected into the depressor anguli oris muscle to help elevate the corners of the mouth. Note the rejuvenated appearance, as the corners of the mouth are no longer downturned. *Source*: Photos courtesy of Drs. Jean and Alastair Carruthers.

(A)   (B)

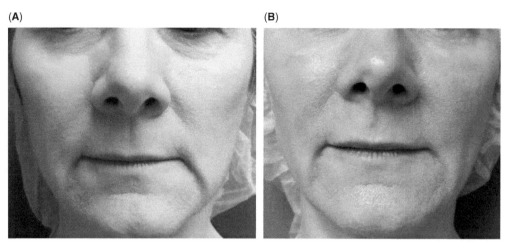

Figure 2.6.6 Patient before (**A**) and 2 weeks after (**B**) Juvederm Voluma hyaluronic acid (HA) filler and botulinum toxin injections. HA filler was injected around the lateral oral commissure as well as into the melomental fold to reduce static rhytides, buttress the corners of the lip, and improve the marionette lines. Botulinum toxin (Botox) was injected into the depressor anguli oris muscles. Note the marked reduction in the appearance of the melomental folds, as well as the improvement in the downturned corners of the mouth.   *Source*: Photos courtesy of Drs. Jean and Alastair Carruthers.

than seven days. Some of the fillers may cause transient lumps or mass formation which may last for several weeks or months. Local adverse events are primarily related to physician experience and injection technique (25). One study found that fanlike needle use, rapid injection and flow rates, and larger volumes may increase the incidence of local adverse events (30). Semipermanent and permanent fillers have been noted to generate nodules or granulomas, which may require corticosteroid injections to resolve (31,32). Some reactions such as nodules may be due to the formation of a biofilm. A biofilm is a microbiologic contamination which can form on any implanted medical device in the body including dermal fillers. It is possible that such biofilms contribute to reactions, especially those seen months after injection. Antibiotics which may treat the microbiologic component and the inflammatory reactions may be helpful when treating nodules and granulomas. To avoid allergic reactions, skin allergy tests must be conducted prior to using any filler that utilizes bovine collagen.

BOTOX® FOR PERIORAL REJUVENATION

Facial rhytides can occur from hyperactivity in certain facial muscles, which can negatively impact the aesthetic appearance of the face (33). This hyperkinetic state can be reduced through treatment with botulinum toxin. Botox (botulinum toxin type A) (Allergan, Inc., Irvine, California, U.S.A.) exerts its action by preventing the release of acetylcholine at the neuromuscular junction, inducing a flaccid paralysis of the treated area. Ongoing turnover of neuromuscular junctions allows a gradual return of function over a period of three to six months (34). The effects of Botox injections begin to appear within one to two days; the full effect of Botox treatment in facial line treatment is typically seen by day 14 and wears off gradually over three to four months; however, the duration is dose dependent with larger doses lasting longer and smaller doses lasting relatively less long (35). Historically, the application of botulinum toxin was primarily utilized for the upper third of the face, where its effects were well studied, well known, and predictable (33). While in the United States,

Botox Cosmetic is FDA-approved only for the treatment of glabellar lines in the upper face, in recent years, some physicians have utilized botulinum toxin in the lower two-thirds of the face to improve the appearance of perioral rhytides, "marionette lines" and the downturn of the oral commissures, chin dimpling, a prominent mental crease, and, in carefully selected patients, nasal contour and NLFs (33). These are however, considered off-label uses in the United States. Because the use of botulinum toxin in the lower face can result in functional loss as well as aesthetic issues, the lower face must be approached with more cautious doses and accurate delivery than the upper face (36). It is recommended that injection in the lower face only be attempted by physicians who are highly familiar with facial anatomy in order to avoid suboptimal outcomes (1). In addition, botulinum toxin can be used adjunctively in combination with dermal fillers to extend the life of the dermal fillers in areas of frequent muscle contraction/animation, such as the lips and melomental crease (36).

Contraindications to botulinum toxin treatment include neuromuscular disease such as myasthenia gravis or amyotrophic lateral sclerosis, infection at the injection site, or a known hypersensitivity to any of the contents of the product (35). Many authors consider pregnancy or lactation a contraindication as well (35,37,38). Ecchymosis and erythema at the injection site are the most common complications associated with botulinum toxin use. These effects can be minimized through the use of preserved saline diluent, topical anesthetics, and small-gauge needles, and by applying cold packs immediately after injection (39). Injection into muscles other than the targeted musculature can result in complications that may last as long as the duration of the effect. In the perioral area the targeted muscle and nontargeted muscles are often in close proximity and, thus, specificity of a technique and a lack of diffusion of the botulinum toxin utilized are critical. In particular with botulinum toxin treatment around the lips, localized muscular adverse effects could include inadequate sphincter closure of the mouth; inability to pucker or purse the lips; asymmetry; drooling; changes in the ability to articulate certain sounds;

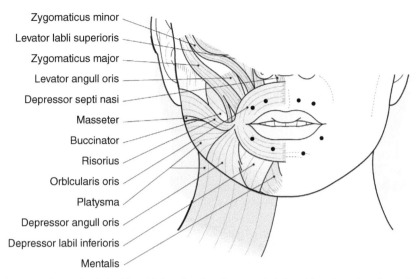

Figure 2.6.7 Injection points for improving perioral rhytides with low-dose botulinum toxin injected into the points shown. Botulinum toxin is injected into 2–4 injection points in the upper lip and 2–4 injection points in the lower lip, with 1–2 units of Botox administered in each injection point, for a total dose of 4–12 units of Botox. Botulinum toxin injections 3–5 mm superior to the vermilion border typically result in the effacement of fine perioral rhytides, while injection at the vermilion border is more likely to result in enhanced lip fullness.

involuntary biting of the lips, tongue, or inner cheek; biting, and lip paresthesias (1,33,40). The formation of neutralizing antibodies is very low and in general not a significant concern with Botox treatment (35).

Most clinicians use 1–3 mL of saline to reconstitute a vial of Botox Cosmetic. In general, higher doses of botulinum toxins delivered in smaller volumes keep the effects more localized with minimal diffusion, whereas smaller doses in larger volumes allow diffusion and cause more widespread effects (35). Once mixed, the vial should be stored under refrigeration (2–8ºC) and should be used within four hours (39). Additional botulinum toxins are being evaluated and studied and have been approved in some countries for cosmetic use including Dysport® (Medicis Aesthetics, Scottsdale, Arizona) and Xeomin® (Merz Aesthetics, Franksville, WI). It is important to remember that these are unique biologic products, and according to their package inserts they are not interchangeable and have important differences in doses and clinical effects. It is recommended that physicians who use a particular botulinum toxin be familiar and comfortable with its use in each clinical indication and the requirements for reconstitution, dilution, and storage.

Botulinum Toxin for Perioral Rhytides

Vertical perioral rhytides are a natural consequence of aging; they can also develop due to photodamage, smoking, or any repetitive contraction of the orbicularis oris muscle. These lines, known also as "smoker's lines" or "lipstick lines," can give the impression of disapproval or disappointment (33). These lines are most effectively treated through a multipronged approach, combining dermal filler injections, facial skin resurfacing by laser, chemical peels, surgery, and injection of botulinum toxin. The use of botulinum toxins in conjunction with dermal fillers is particularly useful, since reduced muscle contraction of the lips may serve to prolong the effect of the filler. Dynamic wrinkles of the lips, such as those produced by pursing the lips, can be diminished by

treatment with botulinum toxin, though small doses should be used by experienced injectors for best results. Static wrinkling, usually produced by photodamage or age, is generally not as readily impacted by treatment with botulinum toxin (33). Because of the complexity of the orbicularis oris and the differences between patients in terms of the appearance of perioral rhytides, each patient should be evaluated and treated individually. Botulinum toxin should not be injected according to standardized injection points; rather, it should be injected into the area with maximal muscle contraction. In the orbicularis oris, the injections should be placed into each pars peripheralis of the upper and lower lips at the level of the lower dermis. Injection points can be either at the vermilion border or 3–5 mm superior to the vermilion border. The decision of how much to inject and the precise location of each injection point is largely based on the patient's treatment history (41). It has been recommended that Botox be administered symmetrically and, for most patients, at doses no higher than 2 U per site (3–5 U per lip) (33,42), though the doses in each quadrant of the lips can vary depending on the number and depth of rhytides. A common pattern used with Botox Cosmetic is 2–4 injections in the upper lip and 2–4 injections in the lower lip, with 1–2 units of Botox administered in each injection point, for a total dose of 4–12 units of Botox (Fig. 2.6.7). For patients who have had repeated treatments, 3 to 4 U of Botox per site are sometimes used; in general, high total doses above 10–12 units total should not be used commonly for most patients (40). The corners and midline of the lip should be avoided to prevent loss of function and flattening of the Cupid's bow (33). Injection of Botox 3–5 mm superior to the vermilion border is more likely to result in the effacement of fine perioral rhytides, while injection at the vermilion border is more likely to result in enhanced lip fullness (43).

Botulinum toxin injection in the perioral region can also be successfully used to improve the effects of resurfacing treatments and to lengthen the duration of effect of dermal fillers.

Botulinum Toxin for Melomental Folds

Melomental folds, also known as "marionette lines," are the vertical lines that extend from the oral commissures to the mandible and give the impression of sadness or disapproval. These lines can be effaced using dermal fillers, skin resurfacing procedures, and surgical procedures; however, the addition of botulinum toxin injections can improve the results seen with other methods. Melomental folds are produced by the hyperkinetic activity of the DAO muscle, which pulls on the lateral oral commissures. This muscle activity, combined with age in some individuals, can contribute to produce a subtle or pronounced "sad" appearance. By weakening the DAO, the action of the zygomatic muscles is unopposed, resulting in an elevation of the corners of the mouth and a more pleasant-seeming countenance (33). The appearance of these lines can be improved by injecting 2 to 5 U of Botox at the mandible at a point inferior to an imaginary vertical line that passes through the nasolabial sulcus. The muscle can be located by having the patient forcibly turn down the corners of the mouth. Treatment in this area relaxes the DAO to allow the unopposed elevation of the corners of the mouth, thus giving a more youthful, relaxed, and pleasant appearance (40).

Botulinum Toxin for Mental Crease and Chin Dimpling

Botulinum toxin has also been used successfully to lessen the appearance of a deep mental crease created by a hyperkinetic mentalis muscle and to reduce chin puckering, or "peau d'orange" appearance, during animation. To correct a deep mental crease in patients with a broad or square chin, Botox 3–5 can be injected subcutaneously or intramuscularly at one point on both sides of the midline at the apex of the mentum, above the lower edge of the mandible (Fig. 2.6.8). For patients with a narrower chin, 4–8 U of Botox can be injected into one point in the center of the mentum at the apex of the chin close to the inferior border of the body of the mandible. It may be advisable to inject a low dose first and use a second injection if needed, because an overtreatment in this area can lead to oral incompetence (44). This treatment relaxes the mentalis and reduces or eliminates chin puckering and helps efface a deep mental crease. For cases in which the mental crease is resistant to Botox treatment, injection with dermal fillers is an alternative treatment (40).

The use of lower doses of botulinum toxin (i.e., "baby Botox") than those used originally to induce total chemodenervation prevents functional loss and allows for a more consistent, sustained result. By sustaining the result with lower doses of botulinum toxin, a notable remodeling of the skin has been seen (e.g., deep rhytides fade over time) (34). Of course, from clinical experience and dose–response curves, it is known that lower doses do not have as sustained a duration as higher doses; this duration also varies depending on the individual muscles injected.

Botulinum Toxin for NLFs

The NLF extends from the alae nasi to the lateral aspect of the lips. It can result from the loss of subcutaneous tissue due to aging or lipoatrophy, and is further produced by four muscles: levator anguli oris, levator anguli superioris alaeque nasi, zygomaticus major, and zygomaticus minor (36,42). The most common treatment for NLFs has been dermal fillers and laser resurfacing. Botulinum toxin injections directly into the area of the fold can result in an asymmetric smile and upper lip ptosis. Treatment in the lip elevator muscles and zygomaticus and risorius muscles flattens the midface and elongates the upper lip (35). Some patients with a shorter upper lip may benefit from treatment with very small doses (1 U of Botox) to each lip elevator complex; however, due to the elongation of the upper lip, patients should be carefully selected (35). This treatment can also be used to improve the appearance of a "gummy smile" due to the shortening of the upper lip by overactivity of the lip elevator muscles.

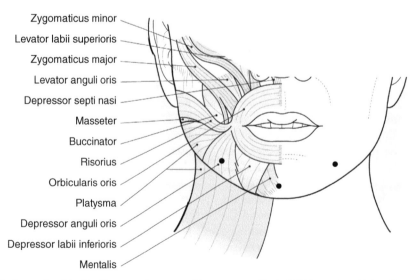

Zygomaticus minor
Levator labii superioris
Zygomaticus major
Levator anguli oris
Depressor septi nasi
Masseter
Buccinator
Risorius
Orbicularis oris
Platysma
Depressor anguli oris
Depressor labii inferioris
Mentalis

Figure 2.6.8 Injection points for improving chin dimpling, mental crease, and depressor anguli oris (DAO) muscles with botulinum toxin. The DAO is targeted by injecting botulinum toxin at the angle of the mandible, as shown by the black circles. The mentalis muscle is targeted by injecting in a single point at the midpoint of the chin, shown by the gray circle. Alternatively, the dose can be divided into haves and injected on both sides of the midline at the apex of the mentum.

All modalities of skin resurfacing treat photodamaged skin by the administration of a controlled wound to the epidermis or dermis in order to promote the growth of new skin with improved surface characteristics (39). The depth of this wound can be superficial, medium, or deep. Superficial wounds go to the depth of the stratum corneum trough and the papillary dermis. Medium-depth wounds go to the upper reticular dermis. Deep wounds go to the mid-reticular dermis. The three most common modalities for resurfacing are chemical peeling, laser resurfacing, and dermabrasion. Dermabrasion has largely been replaced by laser for the treatment of facial rhytides, acne scarring, and pigmentary alterations (45). Generally, the degree of photodamage and other skin surface irregularities is proportional to the depth of the wound required to treat it. The Glogau classification system is a useful tool to aid in the selection of the appropriate resurfacing treatment (39). The patient's Fitzpatrick skin class is important in aiding patient selection, as darker skin types have a higher risk for hyper and hypopigmentation with resurfacing treatments (42).

Chemical Peels for Perioral Resurfacing

Chemical peels are a method for improving skin texture, pigmentation, and the underlying collagen matrix. Chemical peels induce collagen remodeling through the induction of a controlled wound to all or part of the epidermis and part of the dermis depending on the depth of the peel (46). Depending upon the depth of the wound created by the peel, chemical peels are divided into three categories: superficial, medium, or deep. Patients with mild photoaging (Glogau I and II) can benefit from superficial peels, though a series of peels, as repeated treatments are often needed in order to obtain the best results (39). Medium-depth peels are required for the treatment of moderate photoaging (Glogau II or III). Patients in Glogau categories III and IV will benefit from deep peels. In general, superficial peels address acne and certain types of abnormalities of pigmentation or texture, whereas deeper peels address deep rhytides or severe photoaging (47). Lighter peels are associated with shorter healing times and fewer risks, but, unfortunately, slower and milder results compared with deeper peels. Deeper peels may result in more dramatic results, but are also associated with longer healing times and the possibility of serious complications (such as hypopigmentation, scarring, and systemic toxicity). As peels become deeper, the risk for permanent changes in pigmentation increases.

Superficial peels penetrate the epidermis only and can be subcategorized into "very light" and "light." Very light peels create a wound to the level of the stratum spinosum and include solutions of 10–15% trichloroacetic acid (TCA), alpha hydroxy acid, and beta-hydroxy acids (e.g., salicylic acid, tretinoin, and Jessner's solution). Very light peels tend to be safe and appropriate for all skin types. A single treatment with a very light peel induces exfoliation, but a series of very light peels may be necessary in order to achieve additional benefit. Very light peels can also be used prior to initiating topical 5-fluorouracil (5-FU) therapy for actinic keratoses, in order to increase penetration and effectiveness of 5-FU. Glycolic acid, alpha hydroxy acid, and salicylic acid peels are useful in the treatment of acne vulgaris.

Salicylic acid, in particular, is helpful for acne because it is lipophilic and penetrates the sebaceous units. Scaling, erythema, and postinflammatory hyperpigmentation (PIH) are possible side effects but are temporary and usually resolve with no long-term effects. For Fitzpatrick skin types IV–VI, salicylic acid as a very light peel seems to result in a lower incidence of PIH. With increasing depths of peels, caution must be exercised in patients with darker skin (i.e., Fitzpatrick types IV and VI).

Light peels penetrate the entire epidermis and include solutions of 20–35% TCA, 70% glycolic acid, and Jessner's solution. Light chemical peels are more effective than very light peels for the treatment of actinic keratoses, solar lentigines, and epidermal growths such as thin seborrheic keratoses. Erythema and scaling are common postoperatively; however, healing time is faster if patients are pretreated with topical tretinoin for two weeks prior to the peel.

Medium-depth peels penetrate the entire epidermis and wound to the level of the upper reticular dermis and include 35–40% TCA and 88% phenol (if left unoccluded) (46). Combination treatment is commonly used to achieve medium to deep peels, such as solid CO_2 plus TCA, Jessner's solution plus TCA, or 70% glycolic acid plus TCA. These combination peels are more effective than 50% TCA for the treatment of actinic keratoses, rhytides, melasma, seborrheic keratoses, and solar lentigines; they also result in greater improvement in skin texture compared with superficial peels. As patients with a darker skin are at a higher risk for PIH with deeper peels, Fitzpatrick types I–III are generally most appropriate for these medium-depth peels. With medium-depth peels, patients with Fitzpatrick skin types IV–VI are at a significant risk of PIH, which may be long term. Hydroquinone or kojic acid used either before or after the peel may be effective in preventing or treating PIH. Erythema and desquamation result from a medium peel and may last 8 to 10 days postoperatively. Patients with acne or rosacea may not benefit from a medium-depth peel.

Deep peels penetrate to the level of the mid-reticular dermis and are comparable to CO_2 laser resurfacing. A Baker–Gordon peel (croton oil, phenol, and septisol soap) is one example of a deep chemical peel. Due to the risk of PIH, this type of peel is usually appropriate only for patients with light skin, such as Fitzpatrick types I and II. A deep peel can dramatically improve deep rhytides, acne scarring, and skin laxity. Scaling and crusting last for up to 14 days postoperatively. Erythema may last for weeks or months. Patients may develop temporary or permanent PIH or hypopigmentation following these deep peels. Given the potential cardiotoxicity of phenol peels, these peels should only be performed by experienced practitioners in a setting where close patient monitoring is available. Additionally, patients must be aware of and prepared for the significant healing time and wound care associated with these deep peels.

Pretreatment recommendations vary according to the individual needs of the patient and the type of peel. Light peels may occasionally trigger herpetic infections or interactions with photosensitizing drugs, but medium and deep peels have a greater risk of these complications. Antiviral medications may be used as prophylaxis. Herpetic activation is more common with medium and deep peels; therefore, most patients should receive prophylaxis with an antiviral medication such as valacyclovir 500 mg twice daily for up to two weeks (47).

Other pretreatment options include 100% acetone applied evenly immediately prior to the peel to remove the outer layer of oil and the stratum corneum or an additional primer of Jessner's solution applied prior to TCA peels (34). Pretreatment with Botox (reconstituted with 2 mL of saline, 1.5 U injected into each quadrant of the lip) has been shown to result in a greater long-term effect of chemical peels in the perioral region (48).

Post-treatment recommendations also vary according to the individual needs of the patient and the type of peel. Immediately following the application of a medium or deep peeling agent, pain relieving methods can be employed such as the application of an ice pack, the use of a patient-held fan, or application of hydrogel wound dressings. Following a deep peel, pain medications and sleep aids should be offered to the patient (47). Pruritus is a common part of the healing process, especially after medium and deep peels. Recommendations for treatment of pruritus include aspirin, topical corticosteroids, oral antihistamines, or mild moisturizers (47).

Common complications due to TCA peels include prolonged erythema, dyspigmentation, and lines of demarcation between treated and untreated areas (46). Lighter peels are typically associated with hyperpigmentation while deeper peels cause hypopigmentation (47).

Considerations for patient selection for chemical peels include history of herpes simplex virus (treat prophylactically with antivirals), HIV (poor candidate due to prolonged healing time and possibility of infection following chemical peels), history of keloid formation, previous x-ray therapy of the skin (which can cause delayed re-epithelialization), smoking status (nicotine decreases blood supply to skin and delays wound healing), oral isotretinoin use (should wait 6–12 months post completion of treatment for optimal wound healing), and history of a facelift or a brow lift (wait 6–12 months before undergoing a medium or deep peel). Patients' skin type and degree of photoaging also impact patient selection. Patients categorized as Glogau type I will benefit from superficial peels, whereas patients categorized as Glogau type IV will benefit more from deeper peels. Patients categorized as Fitzpatrick types I and II are less likely to experience hyperpigmentation reactions from chemical peels, whereas care must be taken with patients categorized as Fitzpatrick types III–VI. On the other hand, all Fitzpatrick skin types are at risk for hypopigmentation. Patients with sebaceous skin may require preparatory degreasing of the skin prior to the peel in order to achieve the same level of penetration. Patients with underlying inflammatory skin conditions (e.g., seborrheic dermatitis or psoriasis) are at risk for increased absorption of the peel and may inadvertently sustain a deeper peel than intended. Hypersensitivity reactions are also a risk for this population. Patients with psoriasis may exhibit a Koebner phenomenon after a peel.

Laser Treatments for Perioral Resurfacing

Laser resurfacing was first introduced in the 1980s with ablative continuous wave (CW) CO_2 lasers to resurface photodamaged or scarred skin (49). Since then, progressive advancement has taken place in laser resurfacing technology, resulting in a wide variety of choices, including ablative, nonablative, and fractional modalities. Laser treatments are indicated for the improvement of the appearance of acne scars and various signs of photodamage, including dyspigmentation, lentigines, rhytides, and actinic keratoses. Patients with Glogau III photodamage are usually candidates for laser resurfacing. Different types of laser treatments produce different results based on the intensity of the treatment, which is controlled by selection of the laser itself, the length of time the laser is permitted to dwell on the skin, and the continuous or pulsed nature of the laser application. By controlling these various factors, the physician can control the depth of the wound and the percentage of the treated area that is wounded. Aesthetic results from laser resurfacing are comparable to those seen with chemical peeling; however, the benefit of laser treatments over chemical peels is the greater precision and control of the wound.

Ablative Laser Treatments

Ablative resurfacing is carried out by the controlled destruction of the whole epidermis, leading to remodeling of collagen and regeneration of a healthy epidermis (50). Perioral rhytides, photoaging, and scarring respond well to ablative treatment. Examples of ablative lasers include the 10,600-nm wavelength CO_2 laser, either pulsed or scanned, and the 2940-nm wavelength erbium-doped yttrium aluminum garnet (Er:YAG) laser.

The 10,600-nm CO_2 laser is strongly absorbed by water; thus, the penetration depth is dependent upon the water content of the skin. Due to risks of desiccation, charring, and deep thermal damage with CW CO_2 lasers, high-pulsed or scanned lasers have evolved in order to more precisely control the depth of thermal damage during treatment. With less than 1 msec of exposure (either pulsed or scanned), CO_2 lasers can penetrate 20–30 μm into tissue. By comparison, Er:YAG lasers have a penetration depth of 1–3 μm, allowing for more precise control. Because they cause less thermal damage, Er:YAG lasers have reduced side effects of discomfort, erythema, and edema compared with the CO_2 laser; however, the Er:YAG lasers are associated with less tissue tightening, more bleeding, and slightly less effect on rhytides compared with CO_2 lasers. Both treatments result in neocollagenesis approximately six weeks postoperatively. Skin resurfacing with "nitrogen plasma" (created by passing radiofrequency through nitrogen gas) causes limited tissue ablation and minimal unwanted thermal damage, and results in epidermal regeneration after 7 days and neocollagenesis by 90 days. Results of this method of treatment have been reported to be similar to gentle resurfacing with CO_2 or Er:YAG (49).

With ablative laser treatments, the entire epidermis is removed from the treated area. Thus, anesthesia is generally required, especially if CO_2 lasers are used. For localized treatment of just one area of the face, topical anesthetic creams can be used with or without an additional nerve block. For whole face treatment, regimens typically include a combination of intramuscular sedation, nerve blocks, topical and/or injectable anesthetics, inhalation anesthetics, and total intravenous anesthesia including propofol, an anxiolytic narcotic such as fentanyl, and a laryngeal mask adapter. Depending on the exact regimen used, an anesthesiologist may be required to sedate the patient. Post-treatment, edema, exudation, and sloughing of collagen occur during the first one to three days. Edema can be treated with ice packs, head elevation, and corticosteroids. Cool compresses are applied and wet debridement is performed through the first week. Bio-occlusive dressings during the first 24–72 hours can speed up re-epithelialization and improve patient comfort. Re-epithelialization typically occurs over three to 10 days, depending on the number of passes of the laser; this process occurs more rapidly after treatment with Er:YAG lasers than with CO_2 lasers. Use of petrolatum ointments, especially if utilized for more than two to three days, can be associated with acneiform eruptions. Postlaser erythema can last for weeks to months in some cases. Antivirals, analgesics, and gram-positive antibiotics are given after ablative resurfacing for antiviral and antibacterial prophylaxis. Oral antihistamines and topical corticosteroids may also be given in order to control the pruritus associated with healing. Mild topical steroids applied during the first few days post procedure may be helpful in our experience.

Nonablative Laser Treatments

While ablative CO_2 and Er:YAG lasers are the gold standard for rejuvenating photodamaged or scarred skin, they are associated with a significant risk of side effects and a prolonged and unpleasant postoperative recovery period. Nonablative laser systems stimulate neocollagenesis by delivering laser energy selectively to the dermis while sparing the epidermis. This modality is appropriate for the effacement of fine lines and nondynamic rhytides. Nonablative laser treatments are associated with shorter healing times, less discomfort, and less risk of short-term or permanent side effects. No anesthesia or wound care other than standard sunscreen and moisturizers are generally required before or after treatment. Nonablative lasers are classified into three main categories: mid-infrared lasers, visible lasers, and intense pulsed light (IPL).

Mid-Infrared lasers

The prototype of nonablative rejuvenation is the infrared 1320-nm Nd:YAG laser with a pulse duration of 200 msec and, more recently, the diode laser at 1450 nm, and the erbium:glass laser at 1540 nm. Clinical studies have demonstrated mild but reproducible improvement in the appearance of rhytides and scars. A new infrared device at 1100–1800 nm wavelengths has been used for the treatment of skin laxity. Because infrared lasers target the dermis rather than the epidermis, these devices have limited benefit for patients with epidermal damage such as photoaging. Infrared laser treatments are administered every two to four weeks for a total of five to six treatments; one to three passes may be administered per treatment depending on the device used. To protect the epidermis, a cryogen spray is applied to the skin milliseconds before the laser.

Visible Lasers

Visible lasers are used to improve the appearance of photoaged skin, hypertrophic scars, striae distensae, acne scars, and mild to severe rhytides. Examples of visible lasers include the 595-nm pulsed dye laser (PDL), the pulsed 532-nm potassium titanyl phosphatase (KTP) laser, and the 1064-nm neodymium yttrium aluminum garnet (Nd:YAG) laser. The long-pulsed PDL has enhanced efficacy in the treatment of photoaging when the precursor photosensitizer aminolevulinic acid (ALA) is applied prior to treatment. Redness associated with photoaging or rosacea is effectively and safely treated with the PDL. In order to achieve the desired results, a total of five treatments are typically required, with each treatment three to four weeks apart.

Intense Pulsed Light

IPL has the advantage of targeting both melanin and hemoglobin, resulting in global improvement of dyspigmentation and vascularity. Its effects on rhytide effacement are more modest. IPL devices require the application of cold aqueous gels prior to treatment. A series of five to six treatments with IPL are typically used in order to achieve the desired effect.

Nonablative laser rejuvenation can be effective for patients with mild, moderate, and severe rhytides and photodamage. They are an option for patients who are willing to accept minimal efficacy in exchange for minimal risk and faster recovery time. Post-treatment pigmentary alterations are a risk of nonablative laser resurfacing. Pregnant women should postpone treatment until after delivery and breastfeeding due to the pain associated with the procedure as well as the increased risk for hyperpigmentation. Patients who have been treated with oral isotretinoin should wait at least six months after stopping this treatment before the first treatment session due to the possibility of impaired wound healing.

For pulsed dye, KTP, and IPL treatments, general anesthesia is not required. A topical anesthetic cream, such as lidocaine and prilocaine cream (EMLA) or 4–5% lidocaine (LMX, LMX-5), is applied one hour prior to treatment, and cold packs applied immediately after resurfacing can further increase comfort. Postoperative care beyond sunscreen and a good moisturizer is typically not necessary with nonablative resurfacing; mild erythema and edema usually resolve within several hours. A majority of patients can return to normal life immediately after treatment. In patients with a history of rosacea or flushing, vesiculation may occur more frequently; premedication with antihistamines can prevent this occurrence. If vesiculation does occur, the patient is advised to apply a petrolatum-based ointment twice daily until healed.

Fractional Laser Treatments for Perioral Rejuvenation

The newest laser technology is fractional resurfacing, a technique in which thermal wounds are produced to columns of tissue within only a fraction of the total treatment area, leaving intervening areas untouched. The 1550-nm erbium-doped mid-infrared fiber laser creates 2000 microscopic, cylindrical wounds per square centimeter. The zones that are treated directly by the laser are 70–150 μm in width and 400–700 μm deep, penetrating to the dermis. These zones comprise approximately 15–25% of the skin surface area per treatment session. Treatment with fractional lasers results in faster recovery and fewer side effects than other laser treatments. Typically, erythema and edema will resolve within a few days. However, while these devices appear to be safer than traditional ablative devices and the results have been reported as quite impressive, in general, improvement in rhytides and photodamage is not as impressive as that seen with ablative resurfacing. Additionally, while these devices appear safe, there are rare reports of hypo and hyperpigmentation, as well as scarring. To achieve the desired effect, five to 6 sessions are required, spaced at one- to four-week intervals. Pigmentation issues related to photodamage improve more rapidly, while rhytides require more treatments.

For fractional laser resurfacing, topical anesthesia is required and cold air cooling is used during the treatment in order to minimize discomfort. To prevent and treat edema caused by fractional laser treatment, some advocate a three-day course of oral prednisone 30 mg starting the day of the procedure. Mild topical steroids for one to three days as needed, a nonirritating sunscreen and a good moisturizing cream are helpful in our experience during the postprocedure period.

DENTAL PROCEDURES FOR PERIORAL REJUVENATION

Introduction

The impact of the dentition and the oral facial supportive structures on facial beauty can be easily overlooked. As one evaluates the face for aesthetic appeal, the role that a patient's dentition plays in the overall appearance must also be considered. The power of an aesthetic smile and the overall effect on facial beauty is easy to recognize. As the lips separate to expose the underlying teeth during a smile or a speech, an image of the patient is revealed that may indicate youth or age, harmony or disharmony, and beauty or a compromised aesthetic appearance. Additionally, the teeth and their supporting bony housing form the soft tissue drape for the facial tissues, which can be both a help and a hindrance in achieving conservative facial aesthetic enhancements. The role of the dermatologist in identifying some simple dental aesthetic problems is critical in creating the most idealized appearance for the patient. This section of the chapter will focus on the various elements that are associated with an aesthetically pleasing dental facial complex.

The Ideal Dentition

A complete aesthetic dental analysis of the face requires an evaluation of three key oral-facial areas: the overall facial balance, the lip profile, and the aesthetic appeal of the teeth. These aspects of the patient's facial appearance will impact the lower third of the face and should be evaluated in both the frontal and lateral views.

Overall Facial Balance

In an aging face, the worn dentition will have implications far beyond the loss of chewing efficiency. The loss of height of the teeth also creates a reduced vertical support of the lower third of the face. The resultant loss of soft tissue scaffolding potentially creates a reversed smile line, an exaggerated rotation of the chin to a forward position, formation of rhytides, and exaggerated labial soft tissue folds. Therefore, an aging mouth reflects an aging face and needs to be addressed in conjunction with the face for a more complete reversal of the signs of aging. By increasing the occlusal vertical height through orthodontics, restorations, oral surgery or a combination of these treatments, a correction of the height of the lower third of the face can be accomplished (Figs. 2.6.9 and 2.6.10).

The Lip Profile

Certainly lip anatomy is critical to an aesthetic face. The underlying oral environment can either enhance or detract from the overall effect of the mouth. The teeth and its supporting alveolus should create an idealized functional scaffold for the lips during smiling and speech. Compromises in support typically result in severe tooth crowding, heavily worn dentition, missing teeth, and/or skeletal compromises that create a deficient underlying foundation making the lips appear thinned or collapsed (Figs. 2.6.11 and 2.6.12).

Soft tissue support or lip support can be recreated by either moving the biological components (surgically or orthodontically), or creating artificially support through augmentative restorative options, or a combination of both. Even minor changes in the position of the teeth can change the facial appearance, both positively and negatively.

The Aesthetic Appeal of the Teeth

The overall aesthetic appeal of the teeth is a result of the combination of tooth arrangement, tooth color, and tooth contours. Ideally, each of these elements must be in harmony to create an aesthetic result for the patient.

Tooth Arrangement: If the teeth do not have sufficient space to be aligned correctly in the mouth, crowding and malalignment will occur, resulting in an unaesthetic smile and diminished soft tissue support. Developing a harmonious positional relationship between the teeth can be accomplished through orthodontic treatment or, in more severe cases, orthognathic surgery where a combined orthodontic/surgical approach is

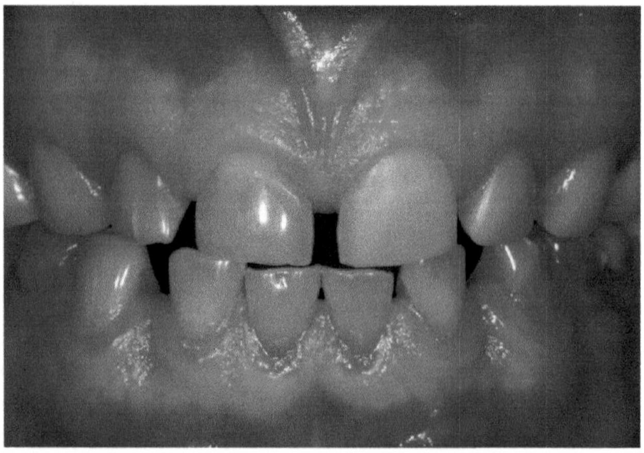

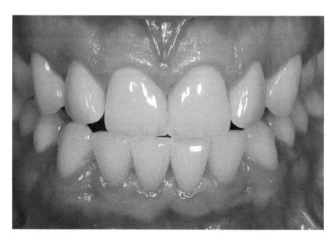

Figure 2.6.9 Patient with severely worn dentition. Note the reduced lower third facial height, discoloration, and decreased chewing efficacy.

Figure 2.6.10 Patient status post dental reconstruction. Porcelain veneers and crowns were used to restore the correct occlusal vertical dimension, improve the discoloration, and rejuvenate the mouth.

required. If crowding/malalignment is more minor, it can be masked through a restorative treatment alone. Porcelain bonded restorations are often used to accomplish this goal in appropriate situations (Figs. 2.6.13,2.6.14,2.6.15).

For example, the maxillary teeth provide support for the upper lip. If the arch is not broad enough, the maxillary lip appears longer, vertical lines appear deeper, and the lip vermilion is thinner. The patient shown in Figures 2.6.16 and 2.6.17 illustrates the difference in the anatomy of the lip as the arrangement of the patient's teeth is altered. Even isolated malalignment of teeth can trigger lip asymmetries, which can be more exaggerated during speech.

Tooth Color: The most easily recognized aspect of a dentition is the color of the teeth. A lot of emphasis is placed on the lightness or brightness of the teeth as this factor is associated with youthfulness. Tooth whitening procedures today are universally

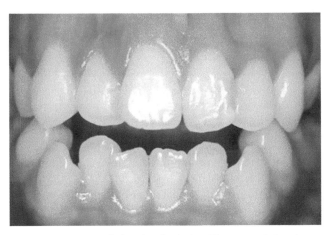

Figure 2.6.11 Patient with inadequate lip support: deficient teeth position resulting in a thinned or collapsed lip appearance.

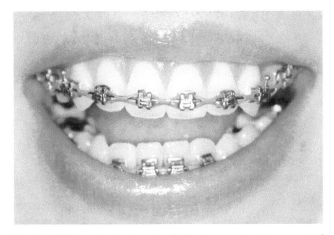

Figure 2.6.12 Note the improved lip support. All ceramic crowns were used to reposition teeth for increased soft tissue support.

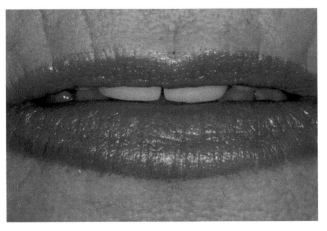

Figure 2.6.13 Patient with dental malocclusion. The retracted view shows a compromised tooth arrangement.

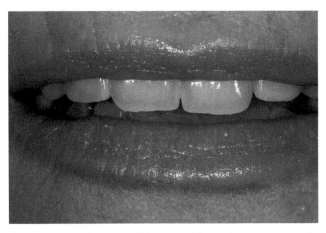

Figure 2.6.14 The patient underwent orthodontic correction to improve tooth malalignment (no orthognathic surgery was performed).

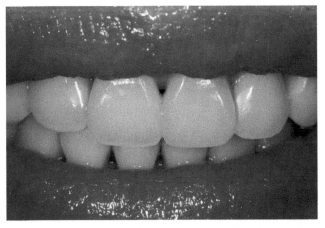

Figure 2.6.15 The patient has achieved a harmonious lip support with her orthodontic correction. Not the corrected tooth positioning and lip symmetry.

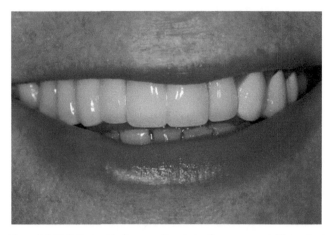

Figure 2.6.16 Patient with disproportionate tooth arrangement. The patient has incorrect tooth contours and proportions resulting in an aged and unnatural "denture-like" appearance.

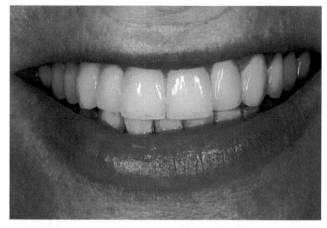

Figure 2.6.17 The patient has undergone full mouth dental reconstruction, resulting in corrected tooth contours, proportions and positioning to create an aesthetic tooth display.

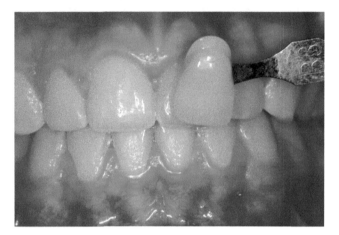

Figure 2.6.18 Patient with accumulated superficial staining of the teeth resulting in an aged appearance.

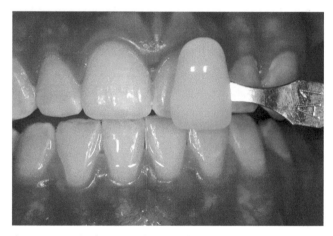

Figure 2.6.19 Patient's improved tooth color after 1 hour of in-office vital bleaching, utilizing 25% hydrogen peroxide ("zoom") to improve the superficial staining.

practiced and accepted as a conservative and safe treatment option. Extensive research has been devoted to establishing the efficacy and reliability of this protocol. Certainly, if color is the primary issue, vital tooth bleaching is a simple and dramatic solution. As we age, our teeth accumulate stain and also darken due to internal calcification of the underlying dentin. Lifestyle also plays a large role in the color of patients' teeth. People who use staining items in their daily life such as tobacco, coffee, tea, soy sauce, and highly colored liquids will have darker teeth than a person who does not consume these items. Certain drugs cause a discoloration of the internal dentin and can create a dark gray opalescence to the color of the teeth (tetracycline and minocycline are two of the most damaging). No matter what the cause is, the conservative technique of tooth bleaching can often make a dramatic improvement to the color in a cost-effective manner. The patient illustrated in Figures 2.6.18 and 2.6.19 shows the dramatic change that simple tooth bleaching can achieve.

If the color cannot be sufficiently corrected through bleaching, porcelain bonded restorations or full-coverage ceramic/metal ceramic restorations may be considered. Lifelike ceramic porcelain systems available today can replicate the natural light reflective properties of the natural dentition restoring the youthful vitality that often gets lost through time and damage. Obtaining symmetry, ideal proportions, correct

aerial inclination, and appropriate smile line significantly impacts oral facial balance (Figs. 2.6.20, 2.6.21).

Tooth contours: If the actual shape of the tooth is inharmonious due to wear, irregular restorations, angulation or congenital malformation, it can be changed through aesthetic reshaping, bonding, porcelain bonded restorations or other restorative options (Figs. 2.6.22, 2.6.23).

Conclusions Regarding Dental Restoration

It is possible to enhance conservative dermatological procedures by synergistically combining them with conservative dental procedures to create a more dramatic aesthetic change for the patient. Aesthetic dentistry is able to reverse the signs of aging as well as simply enhance the patient's current appearance. Significantly, very conservative dental treatment options can provide dramatic results in the oral-facial zone, especially when used in combination with additional perioral rejuvenation procedures.

CONCLUSIONS AND THE BENEFITS OF COMBINATION TREATMENTS

Our experience is that patients benefit from having an aesthetic evaluation and consultation of their full face. All patients are

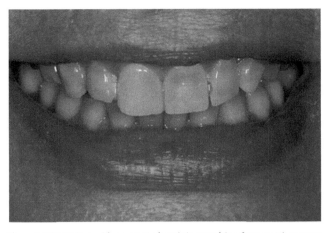

Figure 2.6.20 Patient with severe teeth staining resulting from previous tetracycline usage. Unfortunately, this staining was/is not treatable with vital bleaching alone.

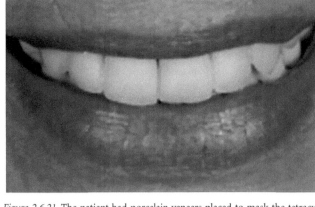

Figure 2.6.21 The patient had porcelain veneers placed to mask the tetracycline discoloration, resulting in a significant improvement of the tooth color.

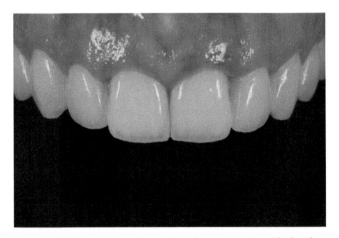

Figure 2.6.22 The patient underwent dental reconstruction with the placement of porcelain veneers and crowns to correct tooth contour and color.

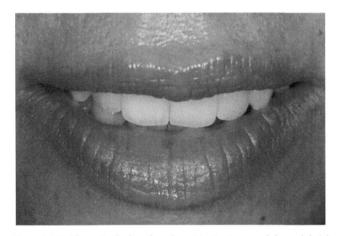

Figure 2.6.23 The patient's altered tooth positioning improved the oral-facial balance and resulted in an enhanced smile and rejuvenated lower third of the face.

started on a home care regimen that preferably involves the use of a topical retinoid, and, if tolerated, glycolic acid, as well as a sunscreen and good moisturizer. Once these basic guidelines are followed, we then discuss specific recommendations for treating the remaining underlying cosmetic issues. The emerging treatment paradigm for perioral rejuvenation is to combine different treatment modalities to achieve optimal results.

Dynamic rhytides, including perioral vertical rhytides are best treated with botulinum toxin. Dermal fillers, such as HA fillers and collagens, correct fine lines and deeper rhytides, restructure and volumize the lips, soften the NLFs and marionette lines, and support the buttresses of the oral commissures. Lasers and peels are utilized to reduce the redness and pigmentary effects of photoaging, as well as stimulate collagen remodeling. Dental care can help correct underlying anatomical abnormalities and enhance the aesthetic appearance of the teeth and in turn the smile.

While it is generally accepted that combination regimens help achieve greater cosmetic improvements in patients, the preferred sequence and ideal timing for the treatments are not clearly defined. One recommendation is to pretreat perioral rhytides with Botox before filler placement, with a rationale that the longevity of the filler will be increased with reduced muscular activity (34). However, 87% of the Facial

Aesthetics Consensus Group treated their patients with dermal fillers prior to Botox treatment (1). Ultimately, it is up to the individual practitioner to decide the exact timing and sequence of these multimodality approaches. Conservative treatments, followed by re-evaluation, and multiple treatments (or retreatments) are the norm to achieve the best results. By combining these treatment modalities, proceduralists can help their patients to achieve their aesthetic goals, reduce the aging process, and significantly rejuvenate the perioral area.

REFERENCES

1. Carruthers J, Glogau R, Blitzer A; and the Facial Aesthetics Consensus Group Faculty. Advances in Facial Rejuvenation: Botulinum Toxin Type A, Hyaluronic Acid Dermal Fillers, and Combination Therapies – Consensus Recommendations. Plast Reconstr Surg 2008; 121: 5S–30S.
2. Cosmetic Surgery National Data Bank Statistics 2010, American Society for Aesthetic Plastic Surgery. [Available from: http://www.surgery.org/sites/default/files/Stats2010_1.pdf]. (Accessed 6/22/11).
3. Ibher N, Kloepper J, Penna V, Bartholomae JP, Stark GB. Changes in the aging upper lip – a photomorphic and MRI-based study (on a quest to find the right rejuvenation approach). J Plast Reconstr Aesthet Surg 2008; 61: 1170–6.
4. Baumann LS, Shamban AT, Lupo MP, et al. Comparison of smooth-gel hyaluronic acid dermal fillers with cross-linked bovine collagen: a multicenter, double-masked, randomized, within-subject study. Dermatol Surg 2007; 33: S128–35.

5. Narins R, Brandt F, Lorenc P, et al. A randomized, multicenter study of the safety and efficacy of Dermicol-P35 and non–animal-stabilized hyaluronic acid gel for the correction of nasolabial folds. Dermatol Surg 2007; 33: S213–21.

6. Downie J, Mao Z, Lo TWR, et al. A double-blind, clinical evaluation of facial augmentation treatments: a comparison of PRI 1, PRI 2, Zyplast® and Perlane®. J Plast Reconstr Aesthet Surg 2009; 62: 1636–43.

7. Werschler W. Treating the aging face: a multidisciplinary approach with calcium hydroxylapatite and other fillers, Part 2. Cosmet Dermatol 2007; 20: 791–6.

8. Ali M, Ende K, Maas C. Perioral rejuvenation and lip augmentation. Facial Plast Surg Clin North Am 2007; 15: 491–500.

9. Kaufman MR, Miller TA, Huang C, et al. Autologous fat transfer for facial recontouring: is there science behind the art? Plast Reconstr Surg 2007; 119: 2287–96.

10. Executive summary global market for dermal fillers 2005–2011. Medical Insight, Inc. 2006.

11. Werschler WP, Kane M. Optimal use of facial filing agents: understanding the products. Cosmet Dermatol 2007; 20: S2–7.

12. Narins R, Brandt F, Lorenc P, et al. Twelve-month persistency of a novel ribose–cross-linked collagen dermal filler. Dermatol Surg 2008; 34: S31–9.

13. Wang F, Garza LA, Kang S, et al. In vivo stimulation of de novo collagen production caused by cross-linked hyaluronic acid dermal filler injections in photodamaged human skin. Arch Dermatol 2007; 143: 155–63.

14. Tezel A, Fredrickson G. The science of hyaluronic acid dermal fillers. J Cosmet Laser Ther 2008; 10: 35–42.

15. Perkins NW, Smith SP Jr, Williams EF 3rd. Perioral rejuvenation: complementary techniques and procedures. Facial Plast Surg Clin North Am 2007; 15: 423–32.

16. Dayan SH, Bassichis BA. Facial dermal fillers: selection of appropriate products and techniques. Aesthet Surg J 2008; 28: 335–47.

17. Alam M, Gladstone H, Kramer EM, et al.; with the Guidelines Task Force. ASDS guidelines of care: injectable fillers. Dermatol Surg 2008; 34: S115–S48.

18. Scalfani AP. Soft tissue fillers for management of the aging perioral complex. Facial Plast Surg 2005; 21: 74–8.

19. Segall L, Ellis DA. Therapeutic options for lip augmentation. Facial Plast Surg Clin North Am 2007; 15: 485–90.

20. ArteFill instructions for use. [Available from: http://www.fda.gov/cdrh/pdf2/P020012c.pdf]. (Accessed 12/9/08).

21. Barnett JG, Barnett CR. Silicone augmentation of the lip. Facial Plast Surg Clin N Am 2007; 15: 501–12.

22. Werschler W. Combining advanced injection techniques: integrating new therapies into clinical practice. Cosmet Dermatol 2008; 21 (2 Suppl 1): 3–6.

23. Grimes PE, Thomas JA, Murphy DK. Safety and effectiveness of hyaluronic acid fillers in skin of color. J Cosmet Dermatol 2009; 8: 162–8.

24. Vedamurthy M; IADVL Dematosurgery Task Force. Standard guidelines for the use of dermal fillers. Indian J Dermatol Venereol Leprol 2008; 74: S23–7.

25. Kelly PE. Injectable success: from fillers to botox. Facial Plast Surg 2007; 23: 7–18.

26. Garcia de Mitchell CA, Pessa JE, Schaverien MV, Rohrich RJ. The philtrum: anatomical observations from a new perspective. Plast Reconstr Surg 2008; 122: 1756–60.

27. Beer KR. Rejuvenation of the lip with injectables. Skin Therapy Lett 2007; 12: 5–7.

28. Jacono AA. A new classification of lip zones to customize injectable lip augmentation. Arch Facial Plast Surg 2008; 10: 25–9.

29. Juvéderm® package insert. [Available from: http://www.juvederm.com/content/pdf/juvederm_dfu.pdf]. (Accessed 23 May 2011).

30. Glogau RG, Kane MA. Effect of injection techniques on the rate of local adverse events in patients implanted with nonanimal hyaluronic acid gel dermal fillers. Dermatol Surg 2008; 34: S105–9.

31. Broder KW, Cohen SR. An overview of permanent and semipermanent fillers. Plast Reconstr Surg 2006; 118: 7S–14S.

32. Lowe NJ, Maxwell CA, Patnaik R. Adverse reactions to dermal fillers: review. Dermatol Surg 2005; 31 (11 Pt 2): 1616–25.

33. Kaplan SE, Sherris DA, Gassner HG, Friedman O. The use of botulinum toxin A in perioral rejuvenation. Facial Plast Surg Clin North Am 2007; 15: 415–21.

34. Perkins NW, Smith SP, Williams EF. Perioral rejuvenation: complimentary techniques and procedures. Facial Plast Surg Clin North Am 2007; 15: 423–32.

35. Carruthers J, Carruthers A. Botulinum toxin A in the mid and lower face and neck. Dermatol Clin 2004; 22: 151–8.

36. Lowe NJ, Yamauchi P. Cosmetic uses of Botulinum toxins for lower aspects of the face and neck. Clin Dermatol 2004; 22: 18–22.

37. Wynn R, Bentsianov BL, Blitzer A. Botulinum toxin injection for the lower face and neck. Oper Tech Otolaryngol Head Neck Surg 2004; 15: 139–42.

38. Beer K, Yohn M, Closter J. A double-blinded placebo-controlled study of Botox for the treatment of subjects with chin rhytids. J Drugs Dermatol 2005; 4: 417–22.

39. Hegedus F, Diecidue R, Taub D, Nyirady J. Non-surgical treatment modalities of facial photodamage: practical knowledge for the oral and maxillofacial professional. Int J Oral Maxillofac Surg 2006; 35: 389–98.

40. Benedetto AV. Cosmetic uses of botulinum toxin A in the lower face, neck, and upper chest. In: Benedetto AV, ed. Botulinum Toxin in Clinical Dermatology. Oxfordshire, UK: Taylor & Francis, 2006: 163–205.

41. Semchyshyn N, Sengelmann RD. Botulinum toxin A treatment of perioral rhytides. Dermatol Surg 2003; 29: 490–5.

42. Suryadevara AC. Update on perioral cosmetic enhancement. Curr Opin Otolaryngol Head Neck Surg 2008; 16: 347–51.

43. Atamoros FP. Botulinum toxin in the lower one third of the face. Clin Dermatol 2003; 21: 505–12.

44. Kane MA. The functional anatomy of the lower face as it applies to rejuvenation via chemodenervation. Facial Plast Surg 2005; 21: 55–64.

45. Niamtu J. Cosmetic oral and maxillofacial surgery options. J Am Dent Assoc 2000; 131: 756–64.

46. Tse Y. Choosing the correct peel for the appropriate person. In: Rubin MG, ed. Chemical Peels. Philadelphia, PA: Elsevier, Inc, 2006: 13–20.

47. Duffy DM. Avoiding complications. In: Rubin MG, ed. Chemical Peels. Philadelphia, PA: Elsevier, Inc., 2006: 137–69.

48. Kadunc BV, Trindade DE Almeida AR, Vanti AA, DI Chiacchio N. Botulinum toxin A adjunctive use in manual chemabrasion: controlled long-term study for treatment of upper perioral vertical wrinkles. Dermatol Surg 2007; 33: 1066–72.

49. Alexiades-Armenakas MR, Dover JS, Arndt KA. The spectrum of laser skin resurfaing: Nonablative, fractional, and ablative laser resurfacing. J Am Acad Dermatol 2008; 58: 719–37.

50. Shook BA, Hruza GJ. Periorbital ablative and nonablative resurfacing. Facial Plast Surg Clin N Am 2005; 13: 571–82.

51. Glogau RG. Aesthetic and anatomic analysis of the aging skin. Semin Cutan Med Surg 1996; 15: 134–8.

52. Day DJ, Littler CM, Swift RW, Gottleib S. The wrinkle severity rating scale a validation study. Am J Clin Dermatol 2004; 5: 49–52.

53. Downie J, Mao Z, Rachel Lo TW, et al. A double-blind, clinical evaluation of facial augmentation treatments: a comparison of PRI 1, PRI 2, Zyplast and Perlane. J Plast Reconstr Aesthet Surg 2009; 62: 1636–43.

2.7 Surgical interventions for the aging face: Rhytidectomy (facelift)
Tom S. Liu and Andrew L. DaLio

KEY POINTS

- While there are many temporary measures to improve facial aging, a facelift offers the most long-lasting results
- Prior to the procedure, a full pre-operative evaluation should be performed including a complete history and physical, evaluation for any cutaneous contraindications, and a screen for body dysmorphic disorder
- There are multiple facelift techniques, including a skin-subcutaneous lift, skin-SMAS (superficial musculoaponeurotic system) lift, subperiosteal, and suspension sutures
- Depending on the facelift technique used, a variety of anesthesia techniques can be adopted including full general anesthesia and local infiltration
- Complications of facelifts include hematoma, facial nerve injury, infection, skin necrosis, scars, and alopecia
- In order to obtain the best results, facelifts can be combined with injectable fillers and Botox

---

In the year 2000, approximately one out of six Americans was 60 years old or more (1). One consequence of our increased lifespan and healthier lifestyle choices is that our golden years have a better quality of life than those of our forebears. Most of us don't feel our age and few of us wish to look it. While there are many treatment techniques such as Botox (Allergan Inc, Irvine, California), chemical peels, lasers, and soft tissue fillers to reduce the appearance of aging, they are temporary. The only real way to achieve long-term facial rejuvenation is through a facelift.

The term "facelift" encompasses a wide variety of techniques, but they all have the same underlying approach: a circumferential excision extending from the temporal hairline in front of the ear around the lobule and behind the ear and then into the posterior hairline. The face is then dissected away from the underlying anatomy, elevated as a flap, and then redraped over the facial skeleton. Since the face loses some of its underlying fat (and therefore volume) as it ages, it takes less skin to cover the surface area of the face and the excess skin can be trimmed away. Though the external incisions are virtually the same for all facelifts, treatment of the underlying fascial layers vary tremendously among plastic surgeons. Facial scars heal quickly and since the incision follows the hairline, when done correctly, the scarring that results from a facelift should be nearly invisible. The end result is a more youthful, rejuvenated face (Fig. 2.7.1).

PREOPERATIVE ANALYSIS

Even in our youth-obsessed culture, cosmetic surgery is always elective. Facial rejuvenation may improve a patient's quality of life, but there is no such thing as a life-saving facelift. So it is important that anyone considering facial rejuvenation (or any other cosmetic procedure, for that matter) undergo a complete medical evaluation that includes a thorough medical history and physical examination. This evaluation should focus on the patient's cardiopulmonary health to determine whether they are fit enough to undergo an extended operation under anesthesia. The type of anesthesia will vary according to the scope of the procedure (see the section, "Anesthesia"), and the length of the surgery will depend upon the type of procedure (or procedures, if the patient elects to combine multiple cosmetic procedures into a single operation) and the skill of the surgeon. Some of the "better" plastic surgeons may take twice the time to perform the same procedure, whereas others may achieve a "better" outcome in half the time—there is no proven correlation between operative time and the quality of outcome. Each surgeon will have his/her own norm, but the expected length of the procedure should play into the preoperative evaluation. Similarly, a patient's hematologic/coagulation axis (including renal and liver diseases) and blood pressure control can have an impact on the outcome of facial surgery (see the section, "Complications") and should be carefully evaluated prior to surgery.

There are certain genetic skin conditions that, although rare, should be checked for prior to surgery, and some patients with these conditions should not be cleared for surgical cervicofacial procedures.

Cutis Laxa (Elastolysis)

This is a rare, acquired or inherited skin disorder characterized by degenerative changes in the skin's elastic fibers. The result is a loose and pendulous skin. Patients with this condition can benefit from facelift procedures, as long as the surgeon is aware of the condition and incorporates it into the operative plan.

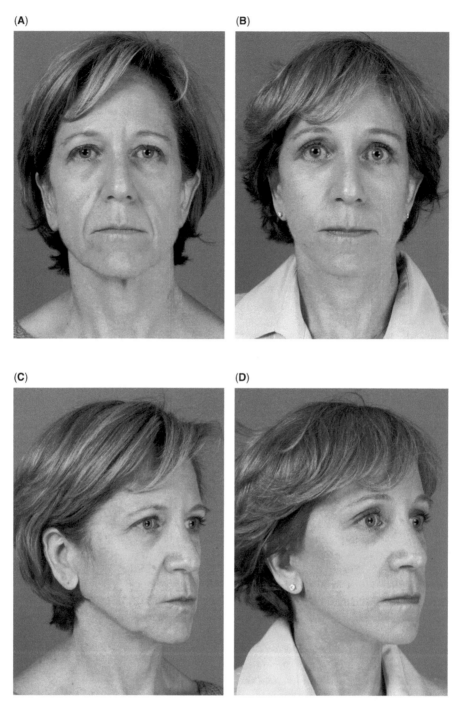

Figure 2.7.1 (**A**) A 55-year-old woman requested facial rejuvenation of the entire face to improve significant facial skin laxity; frontal view. (**B**) Preoperative presentation; oblique view, (**C**) One-year postoperative result following a standard facial rhytidectomy with a pre-parotid superficial musculoaponeurotic system flap, coronal browlift, and transconjunctival lower blepharoplasties; frontal view. (**D**) Postoperative result; oblique view.

Ehlers–Danlos Syndrome

This is an inherited skin disorder characterized by defects in collagen and connective tissue. In addition to its effects on the skin, the condition impacts other tissue, such as joints (hypermobility) and blood vessels (predisposition to aneurysmal changes). Facelift surgery is contraindicated in patients with Ehlers–Danlos syndrome and should not be performed.

Pseudoxanthoma Elasticum

This is a rare, inherited skin disorder characterized by progressive calcification and fragmentation of the skin's elastic fibers.

Pseudoxanthoma elasticum can also affect other tissue like the retina (progressive retinal hemorrhage) and the cardiovascular system (peripheral vascular disease and mitral valve prolapsed). Facelift surgery is contraindicated for patients with this condition and should not be performed.

Werner's Syndrome (Adult Progenies)

This is a rare, inherited skin disorder caused by a mutation in the WS gene, which affects connective tissue throughout the body. This disorder is characterized by premature aging, and may not manifest itself until a patient is in his or her late teens (with some cases not manifesting themselves until patients are in their early 30s). Facelift surgery is contraindicated for patients with this condition and should not be performed.

After an appropriate medical examination, evaluation of the face should proceed in detail. The skin quality should be carefully noted. Advanced photoaging (dermatoheliosis, or sun damaged skin resulting from chronic ultraviolet exposure) cannot be corrected with a facelift procedure, and facelifts can sometimes deepen or distort pre-existing rhytides (2). Patients with thick skin or "heavy faces" are often poor candidates for facelifts, and the correction a facelift can offer such patients is often minimal and short lived. The hair pattern along the temporal region and occiput should also be evaluated for alopecia (thinning hair or baldness), and patients with alopecia or who wear their hair up or have short hair should be counseled regarding the postoperative visibility of the facelift's scar and the potential for hairline distortion. Male patients should also be counseled that the rotation of skin from the cheeks and neck will also impact their facial hair (hair follicles travel with the skin). Finally, facial contour asymmetries, facial nerve activity and symmetry, and prior facial cosmetic surgery scars should be carefully noted and incorporated into the surgical plan.

PREOPERATIVE PSYCHOLOGY

While plastic surgeons are not psychologists (nor should cosmetic surgery be viewed as an antidote to psychological issues) it is important that they are cognizant of the external and internal factors that motivate a patient's desire to seek facial rejuvenation through elective cosmetic surgery. Patients will commonly cite reasons such as a change in relationship status (typically a recent breakup or the desire to begin dating again), the desire for social or job advancement (cosmetic procedures are often seen as a way to circumvent the ageism prevalent in corporate America), and the desire to improve their own self-confidence. On the surface, all of those factors sound reasonable and healthy enough, but patients with unrealistic expectations who espouse a desire to have their youth completely restored, or expect cosmetic surgery to immediately solve all their relationship problems, or believe a facelift will make them professionally successful will always be disappointed and should be counseled against having surgery.

It is important to emphasize that cosmetic procedures, both surgical and nonsurgical, have real risks associated with them and the decision to undergo surgery should not be made lightly. However, a well-informed patient, whose face shows objective signs of aging, who has taken the time to weigh the risks and benefits of surgical facial rejuvenation, and who elects to undergo surgery based on internal motivating factors with a realistic expectation of its outcome will likely benefit from a cosmetic procedure.

ANESTHESIA

The choice of which anesthesia should be used during cervicofacial contouring procedures is a decision best left to the experience of the cosmetic surgeon. The term "facelift" encompasses a broad range of procedures, both surgical and nonsurgical. And the type and depth of anesthesia used during a facelift will vary according to the level of dissection involved in the procedure (see the section, "Techniques").

Local anesthesia with or without sedation is often used by plastic surgeons when performing minimal surgical procedures (such as scar revision or minimal access and superficial dissections). Simple "liquid" or "filler" injection facelifts can be achieved with only a topical or local anesthesia. However, most plastic surgeons will choose to use general anesthesia with local anesthesia infiltration of the dissection planes for additional patient analgesia and more importantly, hemostasis. General anesthesia allows for a complete control of the patient's physiology and allows the surgeon to focus completely on the task at hand.

Regardless of the type of anesthesia used, the surgeon must take special care to monitor and control their patient's blood pressure, as blood pressure impacts hematoma formation and hematoma formation remains the most common complication following facelift surgery. The preoperative optimization of blood pressure is therefore critical to achieving an optimal outcome, and patients with uncontrolled or occult (hidden) hypertensive conditions should undergo an additional medical workup in order to optimize their blood pressure prior to surgery. Hypertensive patients who achieve normotension prior to surgery should continue taking their anti-hypertensive medication on the morning of surgery and through the postoperative period, and their medication may be supplemented with additional antihypertensives for breakthrough control.

All patients who undergo general anesthesia—and especially those with labile blood pressure—should be observed overnight in a hospital or a recovery facility capable of monitoring their blood pressure and administering both oral and intravenous medications as needed.

In addition to a patient's blood pressure, special attention should be paid to postoperative nausea. When nauseated patients retch, the act of retching will invariably elevate their blood pressure and their elevated blood pressure will predispose them to hematoma formation. The potential for postoperative nausea can be diminished by avoiding narcotics and certain inhaled anesthesia agents and through the aggressive use of chemoprophylaxis. The use of antiemetic medication should be a standard part of the facelift patient's postoperative treatment (3).

FACELIFT ANATOMY

The pivotal works of Skoog and then Mitz, and Peyronie in the 1970s highlight the importance of understanding the anatomy of the facial layers and the role they play in facial rejuvenation (4,5). Together, they describe a superficial facial fascia layer that interconnects the platysma muscle with the mimetic muscles of the face, now commonly known as SMAS, that is, superficial musculoaponeurotic system. Understanding the anatomy of these facial layers and the pathways of the facial nerve is critical to any surgical cervicofacial rejuvenation procedures.

Facial Layers

The head and neck can be divided into three main aesthetic regions: the scalp and brow, the face, and the neck. Throughout the head and neck, there are five main layers with analogous parts across the three regions (Table 2.7.1).

Table 2.7.1 Comparison of Anatomic Layers of Head and Neck

Layers	Scalp/Brow	Face	Neck
Skin	Skin	Skin	Skin
Subcutaneous	Subcutaneous	Subcutaneous	Subcutaneous
Muscular-aponeurotic layer (Superficial fascia)	Temporoparietal fascia Galeal Frontalis	SMAS-mimetic muscle	Platysma
Subareolar (Loose) Connective Layer			
Deep fascia	Innominate fascia Deep temporal fascia	Parotid-masseteric fascia	Deep cervical fascia
Periosteum	Pericranium	Periosteum	Periosteum

Abbreviation: SMAS, superficial musculoaponeurotic system.

Main Layers (Superficial to Deep)

1. Skin (epidermis and dermis)
2. Subcutaneous tissue
3. Muscular-aponeurotic layer (superficial fascia)

Subareolar (Loose) Connective Layers

4. Deep fascia
5. Periosteum

It should be noted that the loose areolar layer readily seen in the scalp becomes variable in thickness in the face and neck (6).

Facial Nerve

The facial nerve (cranial nerve VII) is solely responsible for the innervations of the facial mimetic muscles, which provide both facial animation, as well as sphincteric support of ocular, nasal, and oral orifices. The facial nerve makes its extracranial exit from the stylomastoid foramen and then follows a predictive pattern of arborization into five main branches: frontal-temporal, zygomatic, buccal, (marginal) mandibular, and cervical. Innervation of the facial mimetic muscles occurs at the undersurface of the muscles, with the exception of the buccinator, levator anguli oris, and mentalis muscles. Therefore, dissection superficial to the SMAS-mimetic musculature layer (with the exception of the three muscles mentioned earlier) can typically be made without injury to the facial nerve. In large series studies, less than 1% of patients experienced any complications related to damage to the facial nerve; however, damage to the facial nerve can result in weakened or paralyzed facial musculature. It is a stressful complication for both the patient and surgeon and should serve as a reminder of the risks associated with facial surgery. Most surgeons, therefore, commonly avoid any sub-SMAS dissection in order to minimize the risk of facial nerve injury.

Injuries to the zygomatic and buccal branches of the facial nerve are far more common and often go unrecognized. These branches of the facial nerve possess multiple cross-innervations (70%), resulting in non-clinical manifestations if an accessory branch is injured. The frontal and mandibular branches of the facial nerve, however, are terminal 85% of the time, and injury to either can result in a noticeable clinical defect. Injury to the frontal branch of the facial nerve can result in a ptotic and/or a frozen brow, and injury to the mandibular branch of the facial nerve can result in an asymmetric smile (6). And patients who receive platysma contribution to their smile may develop smile asymmetry in the context of cervical branch palsy, despite an intact mandibular nerve—the so-called "pseudo-mandibular" nerve palsy (7).

Facial Sensation

Somatic sensation is supplied by the three branches of the trigeminal nerve (CN V): supraorbital (V1), infraorbital (V2), and mental (V3). These nerves exit the craniofacial structure along a deep to superficial, medial to lateral pathway and are rarely encountered or injured during a majority of facelift procedures (the exception to this rule occurs during the subperiosteal technique).

The distal nerve endings, which supply cutaneous sensation, are invariably affected during any facial surgery, and patients can expect to experience transient postoperative anesthesia (numbness) in the areas undermined during the procedure. Over the time, this feeling of numbness will fade as the cutaneous regions are reinnervated by end nerve fibers.

The great auricular nerve, which provides sensation to the inferior lobular portion of the ear, must be approached with caution. It is a branch of the cervical nerve C2-C3 located 6 cm below the tragus at the anterior margin of the sternocleidomastoid and 9.5 cm below the tragus at the posterior margin of the sternocleidomastoid. And as a consequence of its location, the great auricular nerve is vulnerable to injury during the neck dissection that occurs during a facelift (8).

Retaining Ligaments

The facial retaining ligaments can be divided into two categories: osteocutaneous and fasciocutaneous. Furnas described the two main osteocutaneous ligaments in the malar region (the zygomatic retaining ligaments or "McGregor's Patch") and the mandibular region (9). The fixed osteocutaneous retaining ligaments form a predictable line of aging, manifested as a deepened nasolabial fold and jowling that occurs as the soft tissues of the mid face and lower face progressively descend. Stuzin, Baker, and Gordon described two additional areas of retaining ligaments that originated from a fascial layer of fixed facial structures rather than from the bone. These are the parotid-cutaneous and masseteric-cutaneous ligaments (10). Together, these ligaments provide the underlying tension that allows the face to maintain its shape, and they can be repositioned and/or tightened during surgery to correct specific defects in the structure or shape of the face (11).

FACELIFT TECHNIQUES

The origin of the modern facelift can be traced back to skin-tightening procedures developed in the early years of the twentieth century. The techniques evolved along with our understanding of facial anatomy and the planes or layers of the face. In the 1970s, the pivotal work of Skoog and then Mitz and Peyronie documented the importance of the SMAS layer (4,5). Most of the techniques used in modern facelift procedures represent some variation of Skoog's SMAS manipulation.

Due to the inherent bias of surgical techniques and patient selection, it is impossible to document which facelift technique provides the best and longest lasting results. One study with two different types of facelifts (limited SMAS vs. extended SMAS) performed by the same surgeon on opposite sides of patients' faces showed no difference at 6 and 12 months (12). However, the authors cautioned against the "riskier" extended-SMAS techniques, which in their experience offered no benefit when compared with simpler and "safer" limited-SMAS techniques. Another study involved eight sets of identical twins where different facelift techniques were performed on each twin. The authors compared the results and found no discernable difference between the outcomes obtained from the skin only, SMAS plication, and SMASectomy techniques (13). Another twin study divided the pairs between four notable plastic surgeons (Baker, Hamra, Owsley and Ramirez); each one utilized his preferred technique, and at the 10-year mark, each surgeon noted good results in terms of appearance when compared with his patients' preoperative photos taken a decade earlier (14).

Which is all to say that there is no proven, ideal facelift technique and rather than chasing after the technique that is currently in vogue, a patient considering a facelift should look through a surgeon's before and after photos. All surgeons have their own preferred technique, and whatever that technique is, it's usually the one they are most proficient with and the one with which they are able to give their best results to their patients. Patients considering a facelift may have to consult with several surgeons and look through several photo books before they find the right surgeon whose preferred technique will give them the result they are looking for. And however long the process takes, it will prove to be time well spent in the end.

Skin-Subcutaneous Facelift

The modern facelift, as noted above, traces its origins to skin tightening procedures developed in the early 1900s. Surgeons would elevate the skin flap, redrape it over the face (often pulled as taut as possible to efface the facial wrinkles), excise the excess skin and suture it into place. Up until the 1960s, these subcutaneous facelifts were the only facelifts performed. Surgeons would vary the incisions, flap thickness, and scope of dissection; however, their reliance on the skin envelope as the sole agent to address the ptotic soft facial tissue did not address the underlying anatomic derangement and often resulted in an unfavorable, overly taut, "pulled" look.

The skin-subcutaneous facelift's limited ability to address the jowls and platysmal bands led surgeons to develop various forms of SMAS imbricating (layering) and suture suspension, which have improved the technique's aesthetic results. This combination of skin-subcutaneous and SMAS imbrication facelifts accounts for one-third of facelifts performed by plastic surgeons today (15).

Skin and SMAS Facelift

In 1974, Skoog described a facelift technique that suspended the skin and the underlying SMAS as a single unit (4). The pivotal work by Mitz and Peyronie in 1976 also brought attention to the existence and importance of the SMAS (5). However, Skoog's technique yielded poor results at the nasolabial fold and the anterior neck (submental laxity), and over the next two decades, multiple variations of the skin-SMAS facelift techniques were developed in order to improve upon Skoog's results (16).

Hamra popularized a composite facelift technique, which elevates the cheek fat pad along with the skin flap, lower orbicularis oculi muscle and, platysma (17,18). Barton extended the concept of the deep plane facelift with a fixation of the SMAS flap to the deep temporal fascia for a more elevated purchase (19). Owsley developed a SMAS-platysma flap undermined in the sub-SMAS and sub-platysmal plane from the zygomatic arch and pretragal region down to the mid face and neck as a single unit (16,20). The SMAS flap is then elevated in the vertical vector and the platysma flap in the vertical-lateral vector with profound and lasting correction of the nasolabial fold depth, submental laxity, and cervicomental obliquity.

Minimal SMAS dissection techniques were developed in order to minimize the risk of injuring the facial nerve during deep plane dissection. These alternative SMAS techniques include limited dissection over the parotid with subsequent SMAS suspension and suture fixation. This allows the surgeon to resuspend the elevated SMAS to an elevated fixed position, such as the deep temporal fascia.

The lateral SMASectomy popularized by Baker offers an alternative to formal SMAS dissection (21). In this approach, a 2-cm strip of SMAS parallel to the nasolabial fold is excised along the anterior border of the parotid. The ends of the resulting SMAS defect are then sutured to itself creating a vector of elevation. The ease of this technique reduces the operative time and minimizes the risk of injury to the facial nerve.

Subperiosteal Facelift

Tessier first described a technique for the dissection of the subperiosteal plane in the 1980s; this technique was further modified, extended (in its dissection), and popularized by Ramirez (22–24).This approach relies on fixation sutures to resuspend the face and secure its newly lifted position. Care must be taken to avoid the frontal branch of the facial nerve during the temporal dissection (25). Of all the techniques utilized by plastic surgeons, the subperiosteal facelift remains the least commonly performed (26).

Suspension Suture

The minimally invasive facelift has seen a resurgence in its popularity in recent years, due to its ability to offer patients a relatively shorter recovery period and less dramatic changes to the overall appearance of the face. The contemporary approach was first described by Saylan in 1999. He utilized an S-lift with permanent sutures to resuspend ptotic tissue (27). Tonnard and Verpaele modified this technique and termed it the MACS lift (minimal access cranial suspension) and published their results in 2002 (28). The rising popularity of "barbed" sutures now allows surgeons to apply more creative touches to their facial and neck rejuvenations (26).

BASIC SURGICAL FACELIFT TECHNIQUE

After selecting the appropriate anesthesia, the incisions are marked and local anesthesia is infiltrated along the marked incisions and planes of dissection. The incision—either pretragal or retro-/intertragal—begins along (or within) the temporal hairline and the anterior contour of the ear. When operating on male patients, most surgeons will typically select a pretragal incision in order to minimize the distortion of external anatomy, namely facial hair. The incision continues around the lobule, behind the retroauricular sulcus, crosses over the mastoid region, and, depending on the degree of laxity of neck skin, into or along the posterior occipital hairline. The flaps are then elevated in the subcutaneous plane and then continued in the same or deeper plane, depending on the type of facelift technique being utilized. The SMAS is left alone, imbricated, plicated, or undermined and resuspended. The skin is redraped and trimmed to fit. The use of closed suction drains and dressings are surgeon dependent.

Submental liposuction can be performed simultaneously to remove submental fat deposits and redrape the neck skin. The submental incision can then be extended to allow for an anterior dissection of the platysma to medially plicate the platysma as a corset platysmaplasty (29). Lateral platysma suspension and placation can also be performed through the posterior exposure of the facelift incision.

COMPLICATIONS

Like all surgical procedures, facelifts carry a certain amount of risk. Patients should be thoroughly counseled about the complications inherent in the procedure and the potential for an adverse event or a negative outcome.

Hematoma

A hematoma is the most common complication resulting from a facelift surgery. In its simplest terms, a hematoma is a swelling of clotted blood underneath the skin flaps elevated during the procedure. The majority (87%) of hematomas occurs in the first 24 hours after surgery and 58% of them occur unilaterally (30). In most cases, the consequences of a hematoma are minor; however, it can lead to skin flap necrosis, edema, skin coloration changes, puckering, subcutaneous thickening, and masses, and may require reoperation to drain or to correct otherwise.

A recent survey of 570 members of the American Society of Plastic Surgeons found that hematomas occur in 5.7% of female patients and 11.1% of male patients (Table 2.7.2) (15,31–35). Blood pressure plays a key role in hematoma formation, and exercising control over preoperative, intraoperative, and postoperative blood pressure has decreased the frequency of hematoma formation. Surgeons typically use hypertension medication with additional anti-emetic and sedative qualities (such as clonidine and thorazine) in order to regulate patients' blood pressure during the course of their surgical care (36–38). Additionally, surgeons may use closed suction drains, dressings, and fibrin glue to minimize the risk of hematoma formation, even though there is no clinical evidence that conclusively proves these techniques have any effect (39,40,15). Lastly, anti-platelet medication (aspirin, plavix, etc.) should be discontinued 10–14 days prior to surgery and not resumed for 7 days postoperatively. If the patient is on anticoagulation (warfarin, lovenox, etc.) and/or antiplatelet medication and cannot medically discontinue them, the surgeon should reconsider whether they are an appropriate candidate for cosmetic surgery.

Facial Nerve Injury

A study of 12,192 facelifts found that facial nerve injury occurred in 2.1% cases, and in less than 0.1% the nerve injuries were permanent (15). Most of the injuries were to the frontal and mandibular branches of the facial nerve, and the permanent injuries (those persistent after one year) were present in the frontal, mandibular, and cervical branches. Since there is no proven way to prevent nerve injuries, it is paramount that the surgeon fully understands the anatomy of the facial nerve in order to avoid damaging, especially when performing SMAS and sub-SMAS dissections. A recent publication by Owsley and Agarwal illustrates how to safely navigate the facial nerve planes during a facelift surgery (41).

Infection

As with any surgical procedure, there is always an inherent risk of infection. Infections after facelift surgery are rare, but they do occur. Perioperative antibiotics with first-generation cephalosporin are administered as a prophylaxis, but continuation of antibiotics beyond the perioperative period has never been shown to reduce the incidence of surgical site infections for clean surgical procedures. If an infection occurs, it may require additional postoperative care and, potentially, reoperation to clean the infected area.

Skin Necrosis

Skin slough can occur due to the random nature of perfusion to the skin flaps. The robust vascularity of the face often results in the preservation of skin flaps, despite wide undermining. However, an excessive thinning of the skin flaps, tension on the skin closure, and smoking increase the risk of skin sloughing. Smoking should be discontinued four weeks prior to surgery in order to reverse its vasoconstrictive and toxic effects. Active smoking up to the day of surgery increases the risk of complications and in such cases it will be wise to cancel surgery.

Scars

Scars on the face heal tremendously well. The hidden nature of the facelift incision, combined with the improved healing of the face, results in a concealed scar. However, excessive tension and skin slough can result in unfavorable scarring and can potentially distort key facial elements (e.g., the tragus, ear, and hairline).

Table 2.7.2 Complications of Face Lifts

	Baker and Gordon(35)	Conway(32)	Leist(31)	Matarasso(15)	McDowell(33)	McGregor(34)
Alopecia	-	-	8.4	1.7	0	2.5
Hematoma	4.2	6.6	3.3	4.4	2.8	8.1
Infection	1	-	-	-	-	-
Nerve Injury	0.5	0.7	0.8	2.1	1.9	2.5
Numbness	-	5	-	1.8	-	-
Scarring	-	-	11.8	2.3	-	-
Skin Slough	1.1	0.3	-	1.5	0.9	3

Table 2.7.3 Comparisons of Various Fillers

Product	Trade Name (Concentration of HA mg/ml)	Approved Use	Estimated Duration	Level of Injection
Hyaluronic acid (HA)	Restylane® (20) Perlane® (20) [Medicis Aesthetics, Scottsdale, Arizona]; Juvaderm Ultra® (24) [Allergan Inc, Irvine, California]; Juvaderm Ultra Plus® (24) [Allergan inc, Irvine, California]; Hydrelle™ (28) [Anika Therapeutics, Bedford, Massachusetts]; Prevelle® [Genzyme, Ridgefield, New Jersey]	Nasolabial folds	6–12 mo	Mid dermis to deep dermis
Hydroxylapatite microspheres	Radiesse® [Merz Aesthetics, San Mateo, California]	Nasolabial folds HIV facial lipoatrophy	12–24 mo	Subcutaneous
Poly-L-lactic acid	Sculptra® [Dermik Laboratories, Bridgewater, New Jersey]	Nasolabial folds HIV facial lipoatrophy	12–24 mo	Subcutaneous

Alopecia

Alopecia (baldness) is often iatrogenic (caused by the procedure) due to incisions made within the hairline (with resultant damage to the hair follicles) rather than along it, and excessive resection of the skin flaps resulting in excision of the hair. This results in a superior-posterior shift of the temporal and occipital hairline. And once such a complication occurs, there is really no way to correct it, other than to wear hats.

A list and incidence of complications from published series is summarized in Table 2.7.2.

FACIAL SOFT TISSUE AUGMENTATION

The advent of soft tissue fillers (or simply "fillers") provides a number of options for increasing facial volume (lost during the natural aging process) in order to improve its overall aesthetic appearance. Fillers can be used to replace lost facial volume, soften some of the face's hollows, and mask the effects of gravitational ptosis. And for patients who are in need of mild or modest facial correction, fillers can provide a short-term, low-cost alternative to a facelift procedure.

Hyaluronic acid (HA) remains the most widely used facial filler due to its ease of use, availability, consistent results, and favorable side-effect profile. Other classes (such as hydroxylapatite spheres and poly-L-lactic acid) can offer relatively longer lasting results and can also be used to restore lost facial volume. Collagen can be used for similar purposes, but due to its significant risk for allergic reaction (requiring testing at 72 hours and 4 weeks), it has fallen out of favor with most plastic surgeons. Autologous structural fat grafting has also emerged as a popular method of soft tissue augmentation (42). With any of these fillers, the depth of injection begins at the mid dermis and progresses deeper, down to the subcutaneous layer or even the peri- or subperiosteal layer. The depth varies according to the filler particle size and its longevity. The "finer" and "short-term" fillers are injected more superficially (Table 2.7.3).

This method of treating facial aging does have its limitations, most notably, the results are short lived. HA fillers last anywhere from six to 12 months, depending on the site of injection and the concentration of HA in the product. Hydroxylapatite microspheres and poly-L-lactic acid fillers can last anywhere from 12 to 24 months. Fat injections produce variable and unpredictable results. While fillers offer a low-cost alternative to a facelift procedure, the cumulative cost of the repeat injections necessary to sustain the result make it cost prohibitive as a long-term solution. And no filler can match the longevity of a well-done facelift.

CONCLUSIONS

The things we enjoy in life, most notably the sun and the outdoors, take a considerable toll on the health of our skin. And as the population continues to age, in our youth-obsessed culture, there will be an ever-increasing demand for cosmetic procedures that can let us continue to look as young as we feel. Lasers, creams, and peels offer a number of superficial treatments that can minimize the effects that sun damage and time have on our skin. Soft tissue fillers offer an alternative to surgical correction, but the most aesthetically appealing and long lasting results come from a facelift. The techniques used today achieve far better—more natural, more subtle, less stretched, and windblown—aesthetic results than those used a generation ago.

REFERENCES

1. US Census.
2. James WD, Berger T, Elston D. Andrews' Diseases of the Skin: clinical Dermatology. Saunders Elsevier, 2006.
3. Owsley JQ. Aesthetic Facial Surgery. Philadelphia: WB Saunders, 1994.
4. Skoog T. Plastic Surgery: New Methods and Refinements. Philadelphia: WB Saunders, 1975.
5. Mitz V, Peyronie M. The superficial musculoaponeurotic system (SMAS) in the parotid and cheek area. Plast Reconstr Surg 1976; 58: 80.
6. Greer SE, Benhaim P, Lorenz HP, et al. Handbook of Plastic Surgery. New York: Marcel Dekker, 2004.
7. Daane SP, Owsley JQ. Incidence of cervical branch injury with "marginal mandibular nerve pseudo-paralysis" in patients undergoing facelift. Plast Reconstr Surg 2003; 111: 2414.
8. McKinney P, Katrana DJ. Prevention of injury to the great auricular nerve during rhytidectomy. Plast Reconstr Surg 1980; 66: 675.
9. Furnas D. The retaining ligaments of the cheek. Plast Reconstr Surg 1989; 83: 11.
10. Stuzin J, Baker T, Gordon H. The relationship of the superficial and deep facial fascias: relevance to rhytidectomy and aging. Plast Reconstr Surg 1992; 89: 441.
11. Hirohiko K, Simon N, Geva M, et al. Oculoplastic surgery for lower eyelid reconstruction after periocular cutaneous carcinoma. Int Ophthalmol Clin Fall 2009; 49: 143–55.
12. Ivy EJ, Paul LZ, Ashton SJ. Is there a difference? A prospective study comparing lateral and standard SMAS face lifts with extended SMAS and composite rhytidectomies. Plast Reconstr Surg 1996; 98: 1135.
13. Antell DE, Orseck MJ. A comparison of face lift techniques in eight consecutive sets of identical twins. Plast Reconstr Surg 2007; 120: 1667.
14. Alpert BS, Baker DC, Hamra ST, et al. Identical face lifts with differing techniques: a 10-year follow-up. Plast Reconstr Surg 2009; 123: 1025.
15. Matarasso A, Elkwood A, Rankin M, et al. National plastic surgery survey: facelift techniques and complications. Plast Reconstr Surg 2000; 106: 1185.
16. Owsley JQ. Plastyma-fascial rhytidectomy: a preliminary report. Plast Reconstr Surg 1977; 60: 843.
17. Hamra ST. The deep-plane rhytidectomy. Plast Reconstr Surg 1990; 86: 53.
18. Hamra ST. Composite rhytidectomy. Plast Reconstr Surg 1992; 90: 1.
19. Barton FE. Rhytidectomy and the nasolabial fold. Plast Reconstr Surg 1992; 90: 601.
20. Owsley JQ. SMAS-plastyma face lift. Plast Reconstr Surg 1983; 71: 573.
21. Baker DC. Lateral SMASectomy. Plast Reconstr Surg 1997; 100: 509.
22. Tessier P. Lifing facial sous-perioste. Ann Chir Plast Esthet 1989; 34: 193.
23. Ramirez OM, Maillard GF, Musolas A. The extended subperiosteal face lift: a definitive soft-tissue remodeling for facial rejuvenation. Plast Reconstr Surg 1991; 88: 227.
24. Ramirez OM. The subperiosteal rhytidectomy: the thirdgeneration face-lift. Ann Plast Surg 1992; 28: 218.
25. Stuzin JM, Wagstrom L, Kawamoto HK, et al. Anatomy of the frontal branch of the facial nerve: The significance of the temporal fat pad. Plast Reconstr Surg 1989; 83: 265.
26. Villa MT, White LE, Alam M, et al. Barbed sutures: a review of the literature. Plast Reconstr Surg 2008; 121: 102.
27. Saylan Z. The S-lift: Less is more. Aesthetic Surg J 1999; 19: 406.
28. Tonnard P, Verpaele A, Monstrey S, et al. Minimal access cranial suspension lift: a modified S-lift. Plast Reconstr Surg 2002; 109: 2074–86.
29. Feldman JJ. Corset platysmaplasty. Plast Reconstr Surg 1990; 85: 333.
30. Baker DC, Stefani WA, Chiu ES. Reducing the incidence of hematoma requiring surgical evacuation following male rhytidectomy: a 30-year review of 985 cases. Plast Reconstr Surg 2005; 116: 1973.
31. Leist FD, Masson JK, Erich JB. A review of 324 rhytidectomies, emphasizing complications and patient dissatisfaction. Plast Reconstr Surg 1977; 59: 525.
32. Conway H. Analysis of 25 consecutive rhytidectomies. NY J Med 1967; 67: 790.
33. McDowell A. Effective practical steps to avoid complications in facelifting. Plast Reconstr Surg 1972; 50: 563.
34. McGregor M, et al. Complications of facelifting. In Symposium of Aesthetic Surgery of the Face, Eyelid and Breast, Vol. 4 St. Louis, Mosby, 1972.
35. Baker TJ, Gordon HL. Complications of rhytidectomy. Plast Reconstr Surg 1967; 40: 31.
36. Man D. Premedication with oral clonidine for facial rhytidectomy. Plast Reconstr Surg 1994; 94: 214.
37. Beninger FG, Pritchard SJ. Clonidine in the management of blood pressure during rhytidectomy. Aesthetic Surg J 1999; 18: 89.
38. Berner RE, Morain WD, Noe JM. Postoperative hypertension as an etiological factor in hematoma after rhytidectomy: prevention with chlorpromazine. Plast Reconstr Surg 1976; 57: 314.
39. Oliver DW, Hamilton SA, Figle AA, et al. A prospective, randomized, double-blind trial of the use of fibrin sealant for facelifts. Plast Reconstr Surg 2001; 108: 2101.
40. Fezza JP, Cartwright M, Mack W. The use of aerosolized fibrin glue in face-lift surgery. Plast Reconstr Surg 2002; 110: 658.
41. Owsley JQ, Agarwal CA. Safely navigating around the facial nerve in three dimensions. Clin Plast Surg 2009; 35: 469.
42. Coleman SR. Structural fat grafting: more than a permanent filler. Plast Reconstr Surg 2006; 118: 108S.

3.1 Introduction to hair
Jamie Zussman

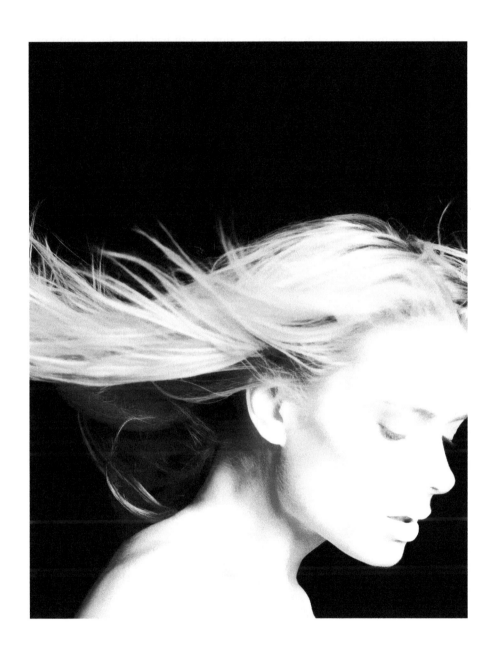

Like the eponymous mammary glands, hair is one of the defining features of mammals. It is a remarkable substance: light, flexible, and resilient. A single strand of human hair is capable of supporting 50–100 g, meaning that the total tensile strength of a normal head of hair could support over 12 metric tons (1). Hair first appeared in nature over 200 million years ago (2) and conventional wisdom is that hair originated as a part of the development of endothermy, or warm-bloodedness, to assist with insulation (3). New research however suggests that hair emerged during the complex process of skin evolution that took place during the transition of the mammalian species from aqueous to terrestrial environments (2). Although the precise evolutionary path remains unclear, the important role that hair plays in nature and society is undisputed.

Hair's functions include offering protection from the elements, camouflaging from predators, providing specialized sensory mechanisms, and acting as an important form of ornamentation. In each of these cases, the characteristics of hair are specifically adapted to fit its needed role.

For humans, hair is an important part of body image; it is one of the few parts of the body that can be easily modified, and it is on display daily for the world to see. Within the norms of a given society, hair has the ability to make statements about politics, identity, and style (4). A healthy head of hair can contribute to feelings of self-esteem and attractiveness as well.

Hair distribution not only plays a role in how individuals view themselves, but also in how they are viewed by others. The true value that our culture places on hairstyle is reflected in the massive amount of money spent on hair care products every year.

Until recently, hair care and hair styling were almost entirely the domain of the cosmetologist, with medical concern for hair limited to changes reflective of a disease. However, with medicine's increasing ability to address hair-related concerns through surgery, laser treatments, and pharmacology, it has become commonplace for patients to turn to their physicians for advice. The goal of this section is to familiarize the practitioner with hair physiology and to provide clinically relevant information about existing hair care modalities. We will discuss the structure and biology of hair, existing environmental and innate impediments to maintaining healthy hair, aesthetic hair care, hair removal, and transplantation techniques.

REFERENCES

1. Franbourg A, Leroy F. Hair structure, function, and physiochemical properties. In: Bouillon C, ed. The Science of Hair Care. 2nd edn. Boca Raton, Taylor & Francis: 2005: 1–66.
2. Maderson PF. Mammalian skin evolution: a reevaluation. Exp Dermatol 2003; 12: 233–6.
3. Wong K. What's the difference between hair and fur? Sci Am 2001; 284.
4. Synnott A. Shame and glory: a sociology of hair. Br J Sociol 1987; 38: 381–413.

3.2 Structure and function of hair
Gurpreet Ahluwalia

KEY POINTS

- Hair has evolved from a functional appendage to a largely cosmetic aspect of human life
- There are three main types of hair on the human body: vellus, intermediate, and terminal
- They are distributed to varying degrees depending on the anatomical site
- The most cosmetically visible terminal hairs are coarse, thick, and pigmented; they are composed of a medulla at the center of the fiber, which is surrounded by the cortex and the outermost layer of fully keratinized, hardened cuticular cells. Vellus hairs, which are unpigmented fine hair, are present on most of the body surface
- Hair seen above the skin surface originates from the hair follicle present 3–6 mm deep in the dermal layer of the skin, and its formation and character are closely regulated by many molecular signals
- A unique feature of human hair growth is the "hair cycle," whereby hair undergoes periods of growth (anagen), transition (catagen), rest (telogen), shedding (exogen), and regrowth. For a given body area, the maximum hair length achieved is dependent on the anagen duration of the hair cycle and the growth rate
- Hair growth can be hormone dependent or hormone independent, for example, androgen-dependent male beard growth and male pattern scalp hair loss (androgenic alopecia); hormone-independent growth of eyebrows and eyelashes
- Human hair growth is an asynchronous process, whereby each hair follicle cycles independent of the neighboring follicles so that the hair shedding is scattered with no significant day-to-day change in the global appearance of hair on a person's body. Many molecular signals closely regulate this process
- As we age, hair naturally changes colors and becomes more brittle, dry, and less dense

---

THE ORIGIN AND EVOLUTION OF HAIR

While evolutionary biologists have not yet been able to identify precisely when hair first appeared, it is clear that it evolved at least 200 million years ago (1). Because the most obvious benefit of hair in the wilderness was insulation, conventional wisdom has been that hair originated as a part of the development of endothermy or warm-bloodedness (2). Although not without controversy, accumulating scientific data now suggest that the development of hair was a part of a more complex process of skin evolution that took place during the transition of mammalian ancestors from aqueous to terrestrial environments. During this transition, glands were internalized as the skin became less mucogenic, and the evolution of keratins and lamellar bodies reduced cutaneous water loss, allowing for survival in a dry environment (1). Simultaneously, genetic changes led to the proliferation of epidermal appendages whose initial function was as mechanosensory organs, and whose most direct descendents are vibrissae (1,3). These appendages provided an additional benefit of mechanical protection, but as primitive mammals moved out of aqueous environments and became endothermic, the insulating

capacity of the proto-hairs became increasingly vital (4). Subsequent genetic changes in the keratins and the keratin-associated proteins (KRTAPs) over time led to the current morphology of hair, and provided an adaptive advantage that played a critical role in the ascendance of mammals (5).

While its protective and insulating function provided a major selective advantage for its evolution, hair has since taken on a vast array of other functions. In contemporary mammals, hair growth happens in three cyclic stages and shares the same fundamental structure of cuticle, cortex, and cell membrane complexes (6). Despite these fundamental similarities in architecture and growth, hair serves in a variety of important roles in differing species, as reflected by substantial hair polymorphism, including downy hair, bristles, vibrissae, and spines, to name just a few (3). Hair has many functions; it protects the body from the elements and provides camouflage from predators. It helps in specialized sensation and acts as an important form of ornamentation. In each of these cases, the characteristics of the hair is specifically adapted to fit its needed role, from the highly insulating and camouflaged hairs of the polar bear to the stiff whiskers and richly innervated hair follicles of the rat, which are optimized to detect mechanical stimuli. Hair has even been adapted for use as a weapon—the quills of a porcupine are actually specialized hairs. Hair length and distribution also play an important role in sexual dimorphism, helping to establish the difference in appearance between males and females of the same species.

In humans, hair no longer fulfills its major evolutionary role of thermal insulation and mechanical protection, and we are the only primates that lack insulating fur (7). Indeed, it is clear that there has been a significant evolutionary trend among humans toward less body hair. Interestingly, humans have the same density of hair follicles as other primates, meaning that it is the quality of the hair that has changed rather than the much more ancient trait of hair distribution (5). Many theories have been put forward to explain this trend, including man's ability to clothe himself, the need to cool a more active body, and even a proposed period of time in which humans were aquatic (8–10). Probably the best current theory invokes diminished hair as an adaptation against fur-dwelling parasites (7). In this model, humans began to have less hair at approximately the same time as humans began to band together in more permanent settlements, which is associated with an increased parasite burden. Sociobiologists believe that sexual selection further reinforced the trend. While it is generally well established that men tend to prefer women with less body hair, this theory suggests that there is a practical reason behind this preference.

HAIR AND SOCIETY

While hair's functional role in insulation and protection in humans has diminished, it has taken on an increasingly important role in social interaction, especially eyelashes, eyebrows, and scalp hair. While it is true that the eyelashes provide some protection for the eye, a $3.7-billion global market for mascara and the recent marketing of prostaglandin analogs to stimulate eyelash growth suggest that the cosmetic appearance of eyelashes is substantially more important than any protective function (11). Similarly, eyebrows play a small role in shunting sweat away from the eyes, but research has shown that eyebrows play an important role in facial recognition, emotional expression, and attractiveness (12). And while the hair on top of our heads provides some measure of heat retention and padding, by far the most important role it plays is as a social signal and a marker of our identity.

As far back in history as we can look, humanity has been preoccupied with its hair. In social interactions, our physical appearance is the most impactful and obvious characteristic. Hair is a unique feature of our bodies with its ability to be cut and styled at will. Within the norms of a given society, hair also has the ability to make statements about politics, identity, and individuality (13). The punk rocker's rebellious Mohawk or the defiantly boyish look of the Jazz Age flapper's bob cut serves as a visual symbol of the wearer's social values and his social identity. In the same manner, institutions that emphasize conformity, such as the military or the prison system, may require recruits or prisoners to symbolically give up part of their individual identity by shaving their heads. The relatively recent phenomenon of women removing their body hair in the United States, only dating back to the first half of the 20th century, has come to be a symbol of femininity. In one study, over 80% of women removed their body hair, with the groups least likely to do so being feminists and lesbians who were consciously rejecting social norms (14).

With all of the significance that we place on our hair, it comes as little surprise that the appearance of hair plays a large role in our conception of beauty—both in others and in ourselves. But research is beginning to show that beauty is more than just an artificial social construct. Rather, certain aspects of what we find beautiful have been hard-wired into our aesthetic sensibilities over eons of evolution. Archetypes of beauty for both men and women have been molded by their roles in reproduction, with men being drawn to women's attractiveness as a sign of youth and reproductive health. Desirable physical traits in men, on the other hand, tend to represent their health and ability to be a provider. Unwanted changes in hair (whether gain, loss, or graying) play an important role in our social interactions, and can have significant psychological and emotional effects. Researchers have found that, on an average, people who are considered more beautiful tend to make more money and their résumés are looked at more favorably (15,16). The importance that we place on the way that our hair appears is reflected in the massive amounts of money spent on hair care products—retail sales of these products in the United States alone were over $6 billion in the year 2000 and have continued to grow.

For women, the social role of hair is heavily associated with their sexuality. When women flirt, they toss and flip their hair (17). Some evolutionary psychologists have hypothesized, and begun to substantiate, that hair is a visible sign of female health and availability for reproduction (18). In fact, studies have even suggested that women are more attentive to grooming and choose more revealing clothing during ovulation (19). Underlying all of this is the general principle that women are not reproductively limited by the number of men that are willing to reproduce, but rather the quality and quantity of resources available to them and the quality of their suitor's genetic material. In other words, woman can be choosy, and so it behooves them to have a wide range of men from which to choose. Men, on the other hand, tend to compete over women, and their relationship with their hair is not quite as straightforward. A wider range of hair patterns on men are attractive to women, both on the body and on the head. Despite this, men are just as sensitive to changes in their hair—particularly when it comes to baldness. Researchers have shown that male pattern baldness may lead to less favorable initial impressions, lower ratings of physical attractiveness, and less desirable judgment of personal and interpersonal characteristics (20). Consistent with the theory that women are choosy and men are competitive, the anxieties associated with hair loss are about the loss of power and virility—a narrative encoded in the biblical story of Samson whose strength was lost when his hair was cut.

HAIR-FOLLICLE STRUCTURE AND HAIR FORMATION

The visible hair fiber above the skin surface is a flexible tube of high tensile strength made of dead, fully keratinized epithelial cells. Hair fibers vary in color, length, thickness and cross-sectional shape between individuals, ethnic groups, and also between different body regions in the same individual.

Morphologically, the superficial hair in humans can be characterized into three different types: vellus, intermediate, and terminal. Vellus hairs lack a medulla and are generally short, soft, and non-pigmented. They are approximately 0.03 mm or less in diameter and generally less than 1 cm in length. They are present on all skin surfaces with the exception of plantar skin (palms and soles). The intermediate hair, also referred to as vellus-like, similarly lacks a medulla and is fine and thin; however, these intermediate hairs are pigmented. In contrast, terminal hairs contain a medulla and are coarser and pigmented. Their thickness is greater than 0.03 mm (average 0.05 mm) and the length is usually greater than 2 cm. Hair found on the scalp, axilla, pubic region, lower limbs, eyelashes, eyebrows, and the male face are all examples of terminal hair.

Anatomically, the hair follicle extends 3–6 mm into the dermis and subcutaneous fat. At birth, the human body is covered with approximately 5 million hair follicles and no new additional follicles are formed after birth (21). The character of hair fibers formed by these follicles however does change throughout life under the influence of various hormones and growth factors. The hair follicle can be divided into four major regions: the infundibulum, the sebaceous gland region, the isthmus, and the hair bulb (22). The infundibulum, which is contiguous with the skin surface, extends to the opening of the sebaceous gland. The sebaceous gland region is composed of a lobular gland that secretes lipid-rich sebum into the infundibulum. The isthmus is the middle portion of the follicle that extends from the sebaceous gland to the bulge area near the insertion of the arrector pili muscle. The bulb is the center of metabolic activity and hair fiber formation. It contains epithelial and germinative matrix cells that envelop the mesenchyme-derived dermal papilla (Fig. 3.2.1).

Hair fiber formation starts at the base of the hair follicle in the hair bulb. The bulb region contains an undifferentiated germinative epithelial cell population as well as pigment producing melanocytes in the hair matrix. They surround the dermal papilla and are separated by a basement membrane (23). The proliferation and differentiation of matrix cells are controlled by the dermal papilla composed of highly specialized fibroblast cells (21). The matrix cells display a very high rate of metabolic activity with a proliferation rate that is among the highest of any body tissue (24). This is the reason why aggressive chemotherapy severely affects hair growth.

The suprabulbar region is also referred to as the keratinization zone (25). This area is rich in enzymatic activity responsible for the post-translational modification of proteins and synthesis of specific keratin proteins, including low- and high-molecular-weight sulfur-rich keratins. The matrix cells differentiate into the outer root sheath, the three layers of the inner root sheath, and the hair shaft.

A fully formed terminal hair is composed of the medulla at the center of the fiber, the surrounding cortex (composed of longitudinally arranged microfibers), and the outermost layer of fully keratinized, hardened cuticular cells (Fig. 3.2.2). The central medulla becomes more prominent in thicker hairs such as the male beard. The cuticular cells are arranged as overlapping scales, with their free ends directed toward the outside of the body giving a hair fiber its strength, rigidity, and flexibility as well as a unique character and appearance. The cuticular scales are interlocked with scales of the opposite direction in the inner root sheath allowing the layers to move together during hair growth. These interlocked layers with overlapping

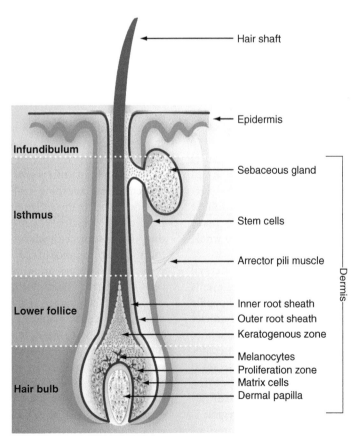

Figure 3.2.1 Structure of a hair follicle.   *Source*: Photo courtesy of Allergan Inc.

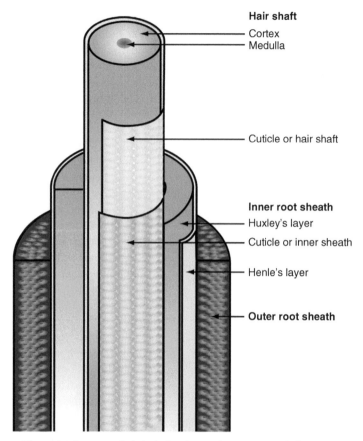

Figure 3.2.2 Structure of a hair shaft.   *Source:* Photo courtesy of Allergan Inc.

cuticle cells, together with Huxley's and the Henley's layers, make up the inner root sheath. The inner root sheath supports and molds the hair fiber and guides its upward movement. As the fiber emerges from the skin surface it sheds its inner root sheath covering, leaving the fiber cuticle to be its outmost layer.

The outer root sheath, composed of concentric multilayer epithelial cells that line the outer surface of the hair follicle, forms a contiguous extension of the epithelial cell lining of the epidermis. Just below the sebaceous gland region, the outer root sheath forms a distinct bulge that houses the hair follicle stem cell population, which is characterized by an extremely low proliferation rate and the capacity to form several cell types (26). These pluripotent cells are responsible for regenerating the hair follicle at each cycle. Separating the hair follicle from the dermal fibroblasts is a fibrous connective tissue sheath composed of collagen bundles that envelop the whole follicle structure.

Hair fiber formation is tightly regulated by the dermal papilla cells which control molecular and biochemical events critical for hair growth and melanogenesis. The dermal papilla is believed to control both the rate of growth and the character of hair, including color, length, thickness, and coarseness. Molecular signals such as keratinocyte growth factor, hepatocyte growth factor, and insulin-like growth factor are secreted by dermal papilla cells to regulate various growth and cycling functions of the hair follicle. In humans, the growing hair follicle descends to the hypodermis so that the bulb region is highly vascularized and immersed in adipose tissue, presumably to meet the high energy demand of the growing follicle.

The pigment in hair fibers comes from a specialized population of cells, melanocytes, located at the apex of the dermal papilla region. The melanocytes are responsible for the formation of melanin pigment, and have a well-developed dendritic system for transferring the synthesized melanin to the differentiating keratinocytes.

HAIR CYCLE

In contrast to the continuous production of the stratum corneum by epidermal skin cells, hair growth follows a cyclic pattern with periods of growth and rest. This hair cycle is also asynchronous, meaning each hair follicle possesses its own genetic individuality and maintains a cycle independent of the neighboring follicles (27). Asynchronicity results in hair shedding that is scattered with no significant day-to-day change in the global appearance of hair on a person's body.

Dramatic changes are observed in the microanatomy and cellular activity of hair follicles during the three distinct phases of the hair cycle: anagen or growth phase, catagen or transition phase, and telogen or resting phase (28,29). In the active anagen growth phase, multiple factors promoting proliferation, differentiation, and survival predominate; in the regressive catagen phase, molecular signals characteristic of apoptosis are most active (30–32). The anagen phase is characterized by the active and continuous formation of the hair fiber. In response to signals from the dermal papilla cells, the matrix cells undergo tightly regulated proliferation and differentiation resulting in the formation of new hair fibers (26).

Molecular signals from dermal papilla are essential for both induction and maintenance of hair growth (33).

Once a hair reaches its genetically predetermined length a short apoptosis-driven involution phase follows. Apoptosis is a process by which hair follicle cells undergo a "programmed cell death" to achieve a hibernating state (telogen phase). This transitional catagen phase is characterized by well-coordinated programmed cell death occurring in the proximal part of the hair follicle resulting in its disintegration. The follicular apoptosis is regulated by a delicate balance between molecules that inhibit or prevent apoptosis, such as *surviving, Bcl-2,* and *c-kit* and those that induce apoptosis such as *p53* and *TNF*-α (34). The majority of the epithelial keratinocytes are susceptible to apoptosis, while the fibroblast cells of dermal papilla show resistance (35,36). As the catagen phase progresses, proliferation, differentiation, and melanogenesis decrease dramatically and the production of new hair shaft is halted. The dermal papilla and matrix cells become separated and disengaged; the regressing follicle shortens in length by as much as 70% during this process.

Telogen, the resting phase of the hair cycle, represents a quiescent hair follicle with little or no metabolic activity or demonstrable cell proliferation. Histologically, the telogen follicles lack an inner root sheath and lack pigment-producing melanocytes. Though hair growth stops in telogen, it can be activated by applying certain mechanical or chemical stimuli. For instance, epilating hair in telogen can initiate new hair growth (37).

The duration of the hair cycle can vary considerably not only between individuals but also from one body region to the other. The relative duration of each cycle varies with the age of the individual. For example, scalp hair can stay in the anagen growth phase for as long as two to six years, which gives its characteristic long length, whereas the anagen phase of hair on eyelashes, eyebrows, and axilla is in the order of 30–90 days (29). The length of a given terminal hair is most influenced by the duration of its anagen phase. An additional factor that contributes to length is the growth rate of hair, which in most body areas ranges between 0.15 and 0.35 mm per day (38,39). The duration of the catagen phase is approximately two weeks for most hair types, and the telogen phase generally varies between two and six months (29,38). Dermal papillae regulate the length and character of hair by controlling the time period a follicle spends in each phase of the cycle, the proliferation rate of matrix cells, the differentiation processes, and melanogenesis (21).

The melanogenic activity of hair follicles is mostly associated with the anagen growth phase (40,41). Melanocytes located in the lower hair bulb produce and transport melanin to the differentiating keratinocytes. The biochemical pathways involved in the melanogenesis process have been well studied. Two types of melanin are found in hair, brown/black pigment known as eumelanin and red pigment known as pheomelanin (42). The synthesis of these two forms of melanin is controlled by several enzymes uniquely expressed in melanocytes. The key rate-limiting enzyme is tyrosinase. The rate of melanin formation, as well as the proliferation, differentiation, and dendricity of melanocytes is further regulated by the hormone α-*MSH*. Differences in these pathways result in the multitude of possible hair colors.

THE AGING PROCESS OF HAIR

As we age, hair undergoes a number of normal, but often undesirable, changes. The most common of these is graying or whitening (canities), the prevalence of which has been described by a "rule of 50s": 50% of the population will have 50% gray hair by the age of 50 (43). While the mechanisms underlying the graying of hair aren't completely understood, recent research has begun to identify genetic changes that may predispose melanocytic stem cells to undergo premature apoptosis and thus hair graying (44).

Along with color changes, both men and women experience changes in hair density as they age. The most obvious example is that of alopecia, which disproportionately affects men; however, both men and women experience an overall thinning of the hair as they age. Long-term photographic studies of scalps have shown that this thinning is the result of a decline in the activity of the follicles, resulting in a reduction in the diameter of the individual hair strands, a shorter growth cycle, and a protracted interval between growth cycles (45).

Finally, there are reductions in the scalp's sebum production that accompany aging, particularly in women (6). This decline in oil production leads to dryness of both the hair and the scalp. There is also evidence that the lipid composition of the sebum changes as we age, although the consequences of this change are not as well understood (46).

CONCLUSIONS

Hair is a complex organ that is thought to have initially developed to serve a thermoregulatory function; in humans, however, hair has largely evolved to serve a cosmetic purpose in our lives. The structure of hair is specially suited to serve its multiple functions. In order to understand the effects of the aging process and the damage that hair undergoes, it is important to understand its structure. Finally, with a solid understanding of the structure of hair and biochemical mechanisms that regulate its growth, it is possible to discuss treatment options for excess hair or loss of hair.

REFERENCES

1. Maderson PF. Mammalian skin evolution: a reevaluation. Exp Dermatol 2003; 12: 233–6.
2. Wong K. What's the difference between hair and fur? Sci Am 2001; 284.
3. Chernova O. Evolutionary aspects of hair polymorphism. Biol Bull 2006; 33: 43–52.
4. Ruben JA, Jones TD. Selective factors associated with the origin of fur and feathers. Am Zool 2000; 40: 585–96.
5. Wu DD, Irwin DM, Zhang YP. Molecular evolution of the keratin associated protein gene family in mammals, role in the evolution of mammalian hair. BMC Evol Biol 2008; 8: 241.
6. Robbins CR. Chemical and physical behavior of human hair. 4th edn. New York: Springer, 2002.
7. Rantala MJ. Evolution of nakedness in homo sapiens. J Zool 2007; 273: 1–7.
8. Glass B. Evolution of hairlessness in man. Science 1966; 152: 294.
9. Hardy A. Was man more aquatic in the past? New Sci 1960; 7: 642–5.
10. Morris D. The naked ape; a zoologist's study of the human animal. London: Cape, 1967.
11. Cohen JL. Enhancing the growth of natural eyelashes: the mechanism of bimatoprost-induced eyelash growth. Dermatol Surg 2010; 36: 1361–71.
12. Sadr J, Jarudi I, Sinha P. The role of eyebrows in face recognition. Perception 2003; 32: 285–93.

13. Synnott A. Shame and glory: a sociology of hair. Br J Sociol 1987; 38: 381–413.
14. Basow SA. Women and their body hair. Psychol Women Q 1991; 15: 83–96.
15. Hamermesh DS, Biddle JE. Beauty and the labor market. Am Econ Rev 1994; 84: 1174–94.
16. Cash T, Kilcullen R. The aye of the beholder: susceptibility to sexism and Beautyism in the evaluation of managerial applicants. J Appl Soc Psychol 1985; 15: 591–605.
17. Moore MM. Nonverbal courtship patterns in women: context and consequences. Ethol Sociobiol 1985; 6: 237–47.
18. Hinsz VB, Matz DC, Patience RA. Does women's hair signal reproductive potential? J Exp Soc Psychol 2001; 37: 166–72.
19. Haselton MG, Mortezaie M, Pillsworth EG, Bleske-Rechek A, Frederick DA. Ovulatory shifts in human. Female ornamentation: near ovulation, women dress to impress. Horm Behav 2007; 51: 40–5.
20. Cash T. Losing hair, losing points?: the effects of male pattern baldness on social impression formation. J Appl Soc Psychol 1990; 20: 154–67.
21. Paus R, Cotsarelis G. The biology of hair follicles. N Engl J Med 1999; 341: 491–7.
22. Abell E. Embryology and anatomy of the hair follicle. Disorders of hair growth: diagnosis and treatment. In: Olsen E, ed. McGraw-Hill, 1994.
23. Nutbrown M, Randall VA. Differences between connective tissue-epithelial junctions in human skin and the anagen hair follicle. J Invest Dermatol 1995; 104: 90–4.
24. Moschella SL, Hurley HJ. Dermatology. 3rd edn. Philadelphia: WB Saunders Co., 1992.
25. Langbein L, Schweizer J. Keratins of the human hair follicle. Int Rev Cytol 2005; 243: 1–78.
26. Cotsarelis G, Sun TT, Lavker RM. Label-retaining cells reside in the bulge area of pilosebaceous unit: implications for follicular stem cells, hair cycle, and skin carcinogenesis. Cell 1990; 61: 1329–37.
27. Danforth CH. Physiology of human hair. Physiol Rev 1939; 19: 94
28. Stenn KS, Combates NJ, Eilertsen KJ, et al. Hair follicle growth controls. Dermatol Clin 1996; 14: 543–58.
29. Saitoh M, Uzuka M, Sakamoto M. Human hair cycle. J Invest Dermatol 1970; 54: 65–81.
30. Kligman AM. The human hair cycle. J Invest Dermatol 1959; 33: 307–16.
31. Botchkarev VA, Kishimoto J. Molecular control of epithelial-mesenchymal interactions during hair follicle cycling. J Invest Dermatol Symp Proc 2003; 8: 46–55.
32. Botchkareva NV, Ahluwalia G, Shander D. Apoptosis in the hair follicle. J Invest Dermatol 2006; 126: 258–64.
33. Weinberg WC, Goodman LV, George C, et al. Reconstitution of hair follicle development in-vivo: determination of follicle formation, hair growth and hair quality by dermal cells. J Invest Dermatol 1993; 100: 229–36.
34. Randall VA, Botchkareva NV. The biology of hair growth. In: Ahluwalia GS, ed. Cosmetic Applications of Laser and Light-Based Systems. New York: William Andrew, Inc., 2009: 3–35.
35. Lindner G, Botchkarev VA, Botchkareva NV, et al. Analysis of apoptosis during hair follicle regression (catagen). Am J Pathol 1997; 151: 1601–17.
36. Seiberg M, Marthinuss J, Stenn KS. Changes in expression of apoptosis-associated genes in skin mark early catagen. J Invest Dermatol 1995; 104: 7882.
37. Muller_Rover S, Handjiski B, van_der_Veen C, et al. A comprehensive guide for the accurate classification of murine hair follicles in distinct hair cycle stages. J Invest Dermatol 2001; 117: 3–15.
38. Braun-Falco O, Heilgemeir GP. The trichogram: structural and functional basis, performance, and interpretation. Semin Dermatol 1985; 4: 40–52.
39. Faber EM, Lobitz WC. The physiology of the skin. Annu Rev Physiol 1952; 14: 519–34.
40. Slominski A, Paus R, Costantino R. Differential expression and activity of melanogenesis-related proteins during induced hair growth in mice. J Invest Dermatol 1991; 96: 172–9.
41. Tobin DJ, Slominski A, Botchkarev V, Paus R. The fate of hair follicle melanocytes during the hair growth cycle. J Invest Dermatol 1999; 4: 323–32.
42. Lin JY, Fisher DE. Melanocyte biology and skin pigmentation. Nature 2007; 445: 843–50.
43. Trueb RM. Aging of hair. J Cosmet Dermatol 2005; 4: 60–72.
44. Steingrimsson E, Copeland NG, Jenkins NA. Melanocyte stem cell maintenance and hair graying. Cell 2005; 121: 9–12.
45. Courtois M, Loussouarn G, Hourseau C, Grollier JF. Ageing and hair cycles. Br J Dermatol 1995; 132: 86–93.
46. Pochi PE, Strauss JS, Downing DT. Age-related changes in sebaceous gland activity. J Investig Dermatol 1979; 73: 108–11.

3.3 What factors play a role in unhealthy hair?
Jamie Zussman

KEY POINTS

- Many synergistic factors contribute to damaged hair
- Ultraviolet light exposure causes hair to become dry, brittle, and discolored. These damages are accentuated by high or low levels of humidity
- Chemical alterations including relaxing solutions, permanent waves, bleaching, and hair dyes all cause significant permanent damage to hair by disrupting the cuticle and the cortex of the hair follicle
- Mechanical insults from blow-drying, hair extensions, and irons for curling and straightening hair cause further damage
- Finally, innate insults including hormonal changes as we age, substance abuse, and systemic disease cause systemic damage to hair
- Simple steps such as leave-in conditioners, moisturizing products, and minimizing exposure to damaging chemicals and mechanical insults can all lead to healthy hair

Environmental, iatrogenic, and innate insults can all play a role in hair shaft damage. Certain factors, such as chronological aging and the accompanying hormonal changes, are unavoidable. However, voluntary manipulation of the normal structure of the hair shaft with the use of chemicals and various styling techniques is epidemic. The permanent effects of these mistreatments may be minimized with a proper understanding of the mechanisms by which they inflict harm and an awareness of available protective strategies. This section provides a summary of the various acquired causes of unhealthy hair and advises on how to minimize their detrimental effects.

ULTRAVIOLET DAMAGE

Thankfully, in contrast to the neoplastic transformation that ultraviolet (UV) radiation may cause in the skin, the deleterious effects of UV exposure on hair are solely a cosmetic concern. UV wavelengths of 254–400 nm cause hair protein degradation, clinically manifested by sun-exposed hair that becomes dry, brittle, and dull; in addition, photodamaged hair loses its strength and changes color. Research into the mechanisms by which this photodamage occurs and finding ways for protecting hair is minimal, but some basic conclusions can be drawn.

Hair has intrinsic photoprotection in the form of melanin granules located within the cortex. Two types of melanin exist naturally in hair and are responsible for hair color, eumelanin (brown-black), and pheomelanin (red). Melanins provide protection by absorbing and filtering UV radiation and by neutralizing free radicals formed by the radiation. However, in performing their protective functions, melanin granules degrade gradually, leading to the hair lightening seen after continuous sun exposure (1). Melanin granules exist only in the cortex of the hair shaft, leaving the cuticle susceptible to photodamage as it is the outermost layer. UV radiation induces changes in the amino acids throughout the cuticle and can cause rupture and detachment of the outermost layers creating "split ends" (1). After both the melanin granules and the cuticle have incurred sufficient insult, the proteins within the cortex become susceptible to degradation. Specifically, cystine disulfide bonds, which are essential to the hair shaft's strength and survival, are targeted and undergo increased destruction (1,2).

In the laboratory, the susceptibility of hair to UV damage changes with alterations in humidity. At both very high and very low levels of humidity, UV exposure induces more changes in hair's mechanical properties than at moderate 30% relative humidity (1). These findings can translate into research-based clinical advice: patients should avoid sun exposure with wet hair and in very dry, desert-like climates. In a dry climate it may be beneficial to gently hydrate the hair with a styling product if the sun exposure cannot be avoided.

In general, the most effective strategy to avoid UV-induced hair damage is to avoid sun exposure when possible and to use physical protection such as hats and scarves when necessary. In addition, many products on the market claim to help protect the hair from UV-induced damage. When recommending these products, several factors should be considered. (1) What is the likely distribution of the product; will it cover all aspects of the hair shaft and follicle and remain in place? Leave-in conditioners, gels, and mousses may accomplish this more effectively than sprays and shampoos. (2) What are the cosmetic results of product application; does it leave hair greasy and weighed-down? (3) What published evidence exists to support the use of this product for sun protection?

CHEMICAL DAMAGE

Hair care products that alter the texture, color, and general appearance of hair contain numerous chemicals. Although many of these products are safe with no long-term detrimental effects, certain processes can lead to permanent hair shaft damage.

Chemical Relaxants

Hair straightening using chemical relaxants is common especially in the African-American community, with a reported prevalence of up to 80% (3). Relaxants generally work by disrupting and reforming cortical disulfide bonds and can be either alkalotic or acidotic. During the relaxing process, numerous disulfide bonds in the hair are broken nonselectively, and when they are reformed, it is to a lesser degree, decreasing the overall tensile strength of the hair (4).

As a result of the very high or very low pH, skin irritation, hair loss, hair breakage, second-degree burns, and corneal burns have all been reported with chemical relaxants. Certain specific products have been associated with higher numbers of adverse events for unclear reasons. For instance, in the 1990s, a nationwide outbreak of alopecia, hair breakage, and scalp injuries occurred in men and women using a specific chemical relaxant (3). This product prompted 3422 people to call the FDA with complaints; a number that does not account for the countless others who were affected but did not take action. Upon close evaluation it was not clear whether the extreme acidity, the metallic salts (copper), or a combination of the two was responsible. The inability to clearly define what aspect of the relaxant caused such significant problems is worrisome, especially given the multitude of products still on the market and lack of close monitoring by any governmental organization.

Permanent Wave

Permanent wave solutions are used to add body and curl to straight hair, by reducing tensile strength and inducing the swelling of the hair shaft (4,5). These changes are caused by modifications of proteins within the hair cortex, specifically the microfibril, which accounts for 50–60% of the cortex, and the supporting matrix (5). As in hair straightening, the breaking and reforming of disulfide bonds play a key role. Permanent wave solutions remove covalently bound lipids from the surface of the hair shaft, reducing the overall sheen of hair and changing the surface of the hair from hydrophobic to hydrophilic. This process is responsible for treated hair's increased absorption of water and other styling products (6).

Bleaching

Bleaching lightens hair by oxidizing melanin granules within the cortex. Once melanin is oxidized, its photoprotective function is lost; bleaching therefore increases hair's susceptibility to UV-induced damage. Bleaching also causes disruption of disulfide bonds without reformation, and increases the porosity of cuticles leading to decreased tensile strength and a brittle appearance (6,7). Darker hair, with its increased melanin content, requires a longer bleaching time than lighter hair and will acquire more damage as a result.

Hair Dyes

Hair dyes are classified as gradual, temporary, semipermanent, or permanent, in accordance with how long their effects are expected to last. They come in both natural and synthetic forms; the synthetic forms are more popular given their more expansive color range and more predictable results. Permanent dyes account for approximately 70% of dye sales and exert their color changes by causing oxidation reactions within the hair shaft (7). To access the cortex of the hair shaft and effectively dye the hair, it is necessary to first disrupt the protective barrier of the cuticle with the application of an alkalotic solution, often ammonia (7). Although this disruption accounts for the lasting effects of the dye, it also causes irreversible damage to the cuticle making hair especially susceptible to future insult. Semipermanent dyes offer a less-damaging, but shorter-lasting option for hair coloring. They are made of small molecular weight molecules that can diffuse freely in and out of the cortex and do not require the initial cuticle disruption. Unfortunately, given their softer mechanism of action, they will only last through six to eight shampoos and are unable to change hair color more than three tones (7).

If additional hair treatments, such as relaxing or perming, are desired, it is recommended that these procedures are performed at least a few days prior to coloring. In this way, a stylist may take advantage of the damage already created in the hair shaft, enabling more color to penetrate the cortex and leading to longer lasting results.

MECHANICAL ALTERATIONS

After initial chemical treatments in a salon, clients use numerous mechanical styling aids to create their finished appearance. The most common mechanical alteration is cutting or trimming the hair. Trimming the ends of the hair does not affect the rate of hair growth, a common myth, but does lead to thicker, blunt hair ends which appear fuller and healthier (Fig. 3.3.1). Additionally, trimming the ends of hair can help reduce the appearance of split ends (Fig. 3.3.2). While cutting the hair on a regular basis can be advantageous for healthy hair, most other mechanical alterations lead to the damage of the hair shaft and cuticle.

Blow-Drying

The use of a blow-dryer to rapidly dry hair after washing is almost universal. Its widespread use, however, does nothing to lessen the detrimental effects that blow-drying can have. Studies using scanning electron microscopy have shown that blow-drying induces irreversible splitting throughout the inner and outer cuticle layers of the hair shaft, a loss of the protective cuticle, and a consequent fragmentation of the hair shaft (Figs. 3.3.3 and 3.3.4) (8). These effects are amplified when hair is dried more rapidly and leave the hair weaker with increased porosity and decreased shine. The use of leave-in conditioners or other moisturizing styling products prior to drying hair can help negate some of these consequences.

Hot Iron/Curling Iron

Although the use of a hot iron (for straightening hair) or a curling iron (for curling hair) will inevitably have detrimental

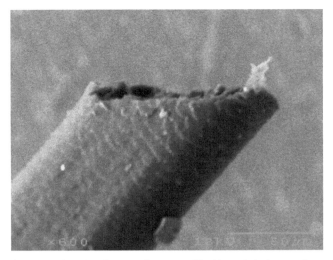

Figure 3.3.1 Scanning electron microscopy of freshly cut hair shows an intact cuticle and a healthy, unfrayed distal end. Source: Figure courtesy of John M. Olson, The Life Science Scanning Electron Microscopy Facility, University of California-Los Angeles.

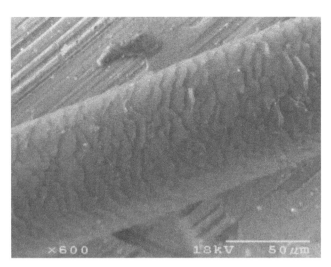

Figure 3.3.3 Scanning electron microscopy of untreated hair demonstrates a healthy, intact cuticle that provides protection to the underlying hair shaft. Source: Figure courtesy of John M. Olson.

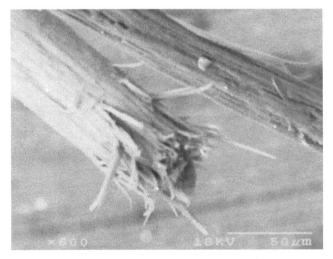

Figure 3.3.2 When hair is not subjected to regular cutting and undergoes environmental insults causing cuticle destruction, trichorrhexis nodosa, or split ends, develops as seen here. This makes hair appear lusterless and increases the difficulty of styling. Source: Figure courtesy of John M. Olson.

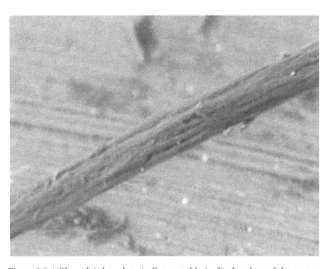

Figure 3.3.4 Blow-dried or chemically treated hair, displays loss of the protective cuticle and consequent fragmentation of the hair shaft. Source: Figure courtesy of John M. Olson.

effects on the hair shaft, there are scientifically proven safety measures that can be employed to minimize the damage. Research with scanning electron microscopy has shown that controlling the moisture content of hair is key to long-term protection (9). For instance, when a curling iron is applied to dry hair, cracking of the hair shaft becomes rapidly apparent. When the same process is performed in wet hair, not only is cracking seen, but bubbling and buckling of the cuticle also appear (9,10). This is likely caused by the formation of steam, and its attempt to escape from under the cuticle. Hence, it is important to ensure that hair is entirely dry prior to styling with an iron. In addition, the use of leave-in conditioners, especially low-molecular weight products that can penetrate the cortex, is recommended prior to styling.

Hair Extensions

Used for decades in the African-American community, hair extensions are now gaining popularity amongst all ethnic

groups in the United States. To date, research on the long-term effects of hair extensions has been conducted only in African-Americans because of the historically increased prevalence. Given the uniformity of the practice however, it is possible to extrapolate certain conclusions from the data that do exist and apply them to the community at large.

Extensions are synthetic hairpieces, mimicking real hair, that are attached to hair shafts in order to extend the length of hair and increase body. They are often heavy and are attached to a few hair shafts at a time. This process can increase traction on the hair shaft; ultimately, traction alopecia, similar to that seen in tight braids or dreadlocks, can develop. Although no randomized, clinically controlled trials exist, retrospective data from the United States and Nigeria have suggested that cicatricial alopecia, a common occurrence in African-American women, is much more prevalent in those with a history of using hair extensions (11–13). In addition, allergic contact dermatitis, secondary to the latex-based glues used to attach the hair, is common. More seriously, anaphylaxis during the application of hair extensions in people with latex allergies has also been reported (11).

Clearly, care should be taken prior to recommending hair extensions to any given client. Any history of latex allergy should be sought; and it may also be beneficial to give time to the hair to recover in between applications of repeated hair extensions.

INNATE INSULTS

Hormones

By the age of 50, nearly 50% of men and women will be affected by hair loss (14). A large percentage of these cases have classic clinical presentations, which are termed either male or female pattern hair loss; this hair loss is likely secondary to hormonal effects in genetically susceptible individuals. The influence of hormones in male pattern hair loss has been well studied and confirmed with clinical trials noting an increased hair growth with the use of finasteride, a 5α-reductase inhibitor. Pattern hair loss in women is a new area of research and key differences have been noted. In men, pattern hair loss peaks in the third and fourth decades of life and may continue over time; in women, there is a bimodal distribution of occurrence with one peak in the third decade and another in the fifth (15). In women with typical signs of hyperandrogenemia who also present with pattern hair loss, anti-androgen therapy can offer some improvement (15). However, most women with pattern hair loss do not have objectively increased levels of androgens and the pathophysiology in these women has not yet been clearly defined.

Substance Abuse

Substance abuse exerts a multitude of proven detrimental effects on the body. As with any process that affects one's overall health, it is reasonable to assume that these effects may be manifest outwardly in the form of cosmetic deterioration. One retrospective study examined the effects of various types of substance abuse on the graying process in human hair. It found that in patients who endorsed histories of substance abuse, hair graying occurred more rapidly at a younger age (16). It also found that the longer a study participant had used alcohol, amphetamines, or heroin, the more likely they were to have earlier graying.

Systemic Diseases

Systemic diseases and their treatments are well known to cause alterations in hair growth and texture. Table 3.3.1 offers a summary of diseases that may affect the hair and the resulting clinical manifestations. It is important to remember that virtually any process that places undue stress on the body can lead to telogen effluvium, causing transient diffuse hair loss.

This summary underscores the necessity of counseling to any patient who desires cosmetic enhancement of his or her hair, on the importance of general health maintenance.

CONCLUSIONS

UV radiation, chemical treatments, styling techniques, and systemic abnormalities can all affect the health of the hair.

Table 3.3.1 Hair Manifestations of Systemic Diseases

Systemic Disease	Possible Manifestations in Hair
Hypothyroidism	Thinning of lateral eyebrows, hair that is dry, coarse, and brittle, diffuse thinning of hair
Hyperthyroidism	Thinning of hair
Cushing's Syndrome	Hypertrichosis, increased lanugo on extremities, androgenetic alopecia in women
Sarcoidosis	Cicatricial alopecia
Amyloidosis	Alopecia
Lupus Erythematosus	Diffuse or patchy scarring or nonscarring alopecia
Zinc deficiency	Diffuse alopecia, graying of hair
Female androgen excess	Pattern hair loss, hirsutism
Anorexia nervosa	Hypertrichosis, lanugo
Syphilis	Diffuse hair loss, patchy alopecia of scalp and beard area, loss of eyelashes and lateral third of eyebrows
Various neoplasms	Paraneoplastic hypertrichosis, telogen effluvium, alopecia neoplastica

Protective strategies do exist and should be utilized abundantly by clinicians, stylists, and clients to minimize permanent hair damage.

REFERENCES

1. Nogueira AC, Dicelio LE, Joekes I. About photo-damage of human hair. Photochem Photobiol Sci 2006; 5: 165–9.
2. Draelos ZD. Sunscreens and hair photoprotection. Dermatol Clin 2006; 24: 81–4.
3. Swee W, Klontz KC, Lambert LA. A nationwide outbreak of alopecia associated with the use of a hair-relaxing formulation. Arch Dermatol 2000; 136: 1104–8.
4. Wolfram LJ. Human hair: a unique physicochemical composite. J Am Acad Dermatol 2003; 48(6 Suppl): S106–14.
5. Kuzuhara A. Analysis of structural changes in permanent waved human hair using Raman spectroscopy. Biopolymers 2007; 85: 274–83.
6. Sinclair RD. Healthy hair: what is it? J Investig Dermatol Symp Proc 2007; 12: 2–5.
7. Bolduc C, Shapiro J. Hair Care Products: waving, straightening, conditioning, and coloring. Clin Dermatol 2001; 19: 431–6.
8. Okamoto M, Yakawa R, Mamada A, et al. Influence of internal structures of hair fiber on hair appearance. III. Generation of light-scattering factors in hair cuticles and the influence on hair shine. J Cosmet Sci 2003; 54: 353–66.
9. Ruetsch SB, Kamath YK. Effects of thermal treatments with a curling iron on hair fiber. J Cosmet Sci 2004; 55: 13–27.
10. McMichael AJ. Hair breakage in normal and weathered hair: focus on the black patient. J Investig Dermatol Symp Proc 2007; 12: 6–9.
11. McMichael AJ. Ethnic hair update: past and present. J Am Acad Dermatol 2003; 48(6 Suppl): S127–33.
12. Nnoruka EN. Hair loss: is there a relationship with hair care practices in Nigeria? Int J Dermatol 2005; 44(Suppl 1): 13–17.
13. Khumalo NP, Jessop S, Gumedze F, Ehrlich R. Hairdressing and the prevalence of scalp disease in African adults. Br J Dermatol 2007; 157: 981–8.
14. Rogers NE, Avram MR. Medical treatments for male and female pattern hair loss. J Am Acad Dermatol 2008; 59: 547–66.
15. Olsen EA. Female pattern hair loss. J Am Acad Dermatol 2001; 45: S70–80.
16. Reece AS. Hair graying in substance addiction. Arch Dermatol 2007; 143: 116–18.

3.4 Aesthetic hair care
Corey Powell

KEY POINTS

- A basic hair care routine can result in healthy, beautiful hair
- Shampooing eliminates chemicals and grease from hair. But overshampooing removes healthy lipids leading to dry, brittle hair. Hair should ideally be shampooed no more than every other day
- Conditioners help replace the healthy lipids removed by shampoos. Instant conditioners can be used with each shampoo. Deep conditioners, which should be left in place for 20–30 minutes, should be used 1–2 times per week
- Household remedies such as apple cider vinegar, baking soda, avocados, and lemons/chamomiles can also be used as an alternative to expensive salon products

The positive correlation between the perception that people have about their physical appearance and the level of self-esteem and psychological mood is well documented (1). It has also been established that visits to a hair salon, and the beautification process that takes place there, can significantly contribute to feelings of joy and increased sociability while decreasing the feelings of anxiety, stress, and aggressiveness (1). Hairstyles frame the face and play a critical role in establishing an overall aesthetic effect (Fig. 3.4.1). For these reasons, hair care is an essential component of any cosmetic regimen (Fig. 3.4.2). A basic overview of daily treatments and styling modalities will be laid out in this chapter.

BASIC HAIR CARE GUIDELINES

The goal of any basic hair care regimen is to create healthy, attractive hair. Desirable hair is instantly recognizable by its sheen, smooth-texture, and clean-cut ends. No matter what treatments are utilized in a salon, daily hair care is necessary to maintain a healthy head of hair. By following a few basic hair care steps at home, hair will have increased longevity and remain vibrant between salon visits.

Shampooing

Hair should not be shampooed daily; innate lipids present in the cuticle of the hair shaft contribute to sheen and moisture. Excessive shampooing will remove the lipid layer leaving hair dull and dry. The goal of washing is to eliminate chemical and environmental buildup while retaining the natural structure of the hair shaft. Ideally, hair should be shampooed no more than every other day employing the following techniques:

Comb: Begin by combing hair from the ends to the scalp, removing any tangles or knots. Combing with a wide toothed comb has been proven to inflict less breakage of hair shafts than brushing.

Pre-shampoo treatment: Prior to wetting the hair, apply a pre-shampoo therapy. Natural oils are optimal for this step and different options exist for different hair types; for example, coconut, rice bran, hemp, pomegranate, and avocado oils all have beneficial effects. Begin applying the oil at the ends where the majority of damage occurs and work the oils into the hair using the hands, while moving toward the scalp.

Scalp brushing and massage: With the pre-shampoo therapy in place, first gently brush the scalp with a natural boar bristle brush. This will stimulate scalp circulation and remove dry, dead scalp, while loosening any dirt or buildup. After brushing, start massaging the scalp by using the index and middle fingers to perform gliding spiral movements from the hairline to the crown, slowly making your way around the entire circumference. Massage is restorative and revitalizing, further increasing blood flow to follicles and decreasing stress.

Shampoo: Place a quarter size portion of shampoo in the palm and add a small amount of water, rubbing the palms together to create suds. Begin at the scalp by applying the shampoo and gently exfoliating using your fingertips. Add water and more shampoo as needed to cleanse the entire length of hair, rinsing thoroughly when complete.

Protect: Squeeze out the excess water prior to applying the conditioner.

Conditioning

As a result of the excellent detergent action of shampoos, resident sebum is often removed from the hair shaft. To ensure that this action does not leave hair dry and brittle, a conditioner should be applied following every shampoo. For daily usage, instant conditioners are ideal. They should be left on for

(A)   (B)

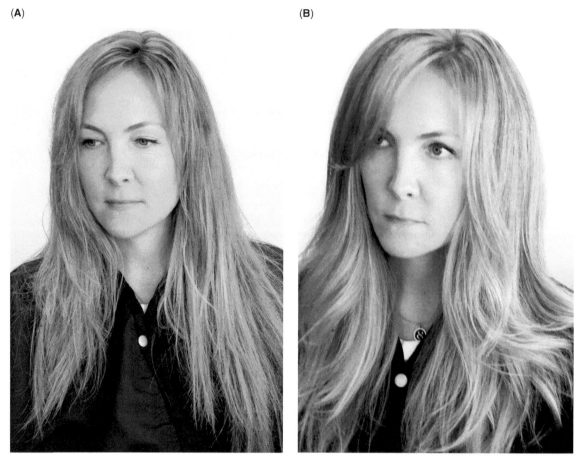

Figure 3.4.1 (**A** and **B**) Proper cleansing, conditioning, and styling of the hair can transform the overall appearance.

(A)   (B)

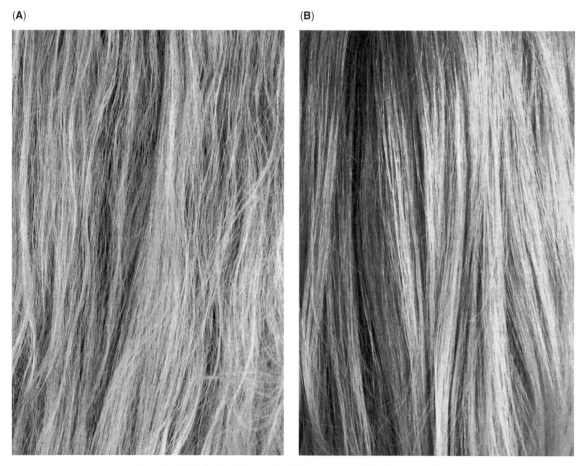

Figure 3.4.2 Hair before (**A**) and after (**B**) cleaning, conditioning, and styling.

one to three minutes and then thoroughly rinsed away. Most hair types also benefit from treatment with deep conditioning agents, applied one to two times per week. These agents must be left on for 20–30 minutes for maximum efficacy and are further augmented with heat. For hair that is naturally very oily, deep conditioning treatments should be spaced out over longer periods to avoid buildup of the product and weighed down hair.

General Grooming Tips

- Wet hair should never be brushed, as wet hair has a lower breaking point than dry hair (2). To initially style wet hair, a wide-toothed comb is preferred.
- Prior to blow drying, the hair should always be protected with either a leave-in conditioner or other styling aid to prevent permanent cuticle destruction and breakage.
- Look for leave-in products that contain ultraviolet (UV) protection to avoid the detrimental effects of photodamage.
- When overly dry hair shafts produce static electricity, this creates flyaway hairs. This unattractive look can be prevented with the addition of moisturizing products prior to drying (2).

PRODUCT DETAILS

Shampoos

Although the primary responsibility of any shampoo is to comprehensively cleanse the scalp and hair, consumers today have become accustomed to multifunctional product claims. The shampoo industry has evolved to provide shampoos that not only have optimal detergent properties, but that also condition, strengthen, and optimize appearance. Shampoo character can also have important effects on scalp health as well, contributing to the resolution of dandruff or eradication of microbes.

In 1933, when hair-specific shampoo was first introduced, it was primarily composed of alkyl sulfate surfactants (3). Surfactants, or detergents, are responsible for the cleansing ability of a shampoo. They work by reducing the surface tension between water and dirt, making dirt water-soluble and available for removal (3). The effectiveness of the early surfactants was noticeably diminished in hard water and often led to skin irritation. These ingredients have been replaced today primarily with anionic sodium alkyl ether sulfate surfactants.

Based upon the purported properties of a given shampoo, additional ingredients will also be included. A moisturizer or a humectant is added to leave hair silky and to replenish lipids stripped away by detergents. Numerous stabilizers are necessary to ensure that the shampoo remains active and free of contaminants; these include preservatives, UV absorbers, antioxidants, buffers, and dispersing agents (3). Fragrances, dyes, and liquid crystal all contribute to the cosmetic appeal of a product and help create distinguishing characteristics. When therapeutic effects are the goal, pharmaceutically active compounds are incorporated. Dandruff, seborrheic dermatitis, and psoriasis are examples of scalp conditions that commonly include medical shampoos in a treatment protocol.

Table 3.4.1 Classification of Shampoo Ingredients (3)

Surfactants	Alkyl sulfosuccinate, alkyl ether carboxylate, acyl peptides, olefin sulfonate, betaine, sulfonate betaine, fatty alcohol ethoxylate, sorbiton ether esters, alkyl polyglucosides
Moisturizers	Natural oils, fatty acid esters, alkanolamides
Humectants	Propylene glycol, polyethylene glycol, glycerin, sorbitol, lactate
Stabilizers	Organic acids, parahydroxybenzoic acid ester, salicylic acid, sorbic acid, methylparaben, DMDM hydantoin, benzophenone derivatives, ascorbic acid, alpha-tocopherol, butyl hydroxy-anisole, citrate, lactate, phosphate, polyvinyl-pyrolidone
Conditioners	Vegetable oils, wax, lecithin and lanolin derivatives, protein hydrolysates (collagen, silk, animal proteins), quaternary ammonium compounds, silicones, cationic polymers such as polyquaternium-10 and 16 or hydroxy-propyltrimonium chloride
Medications	Selenium disulfide, zinc pyrithione, piroctone olamine, ketoconazole, ciclopirox olamine

Abbreviation: DMDM, 3′-Demethoxy-3o-Demethylmatairesinol.

Recently, the use of conditioning agents have also become commonplace in shampoos. They maintain the softness and smoothness of hair by coating the shaft with a thin protective film. However, in naturally oily hair, it may be beneficial to avoid products with added conditioning agents, as they can intensify the greasy appearance. Table 3.4.1 classifies many ingredients that may be found in a shampoo according to their function.

Conditioners

Clinically, the use of conditioner is intended to prevent damage, improve texture, and ease styling of hair. Microscopically, conditioners leave behind a thin film that reduces friction between hair shafts by smoothing out cuticle scales, lessening the need for combing force, and decreasing damage incurred during grooming (4). Many different types of conditioners exist, all of which have specified purposes and should be chosen based upon hair care needs.

Instant conditioners are the most prevalent and are generally applied after every shampoo; they are rinsed off shortly after application. These agents' primary purpose is to improve the everyday manageability of hair. They are not restorative but will provide moderate protection against typical daily insults. Deep conditioners are more concentrated than instant conditioners and are designed to be left in place for 20–30 minutes for optimal effect. They may be used prior to chemical straightening or waving treatments to minimize damage and their effects are intensified with the addition of heat. Deep conditioners may actually help to enforce the structural integrity of the hair shaft through the delivery of amino acids and other low-molecular weight molecules that can penetrate into the cortex (5).

Blow drying lotions, or leave-in conditioners, have the same purpose as other conditioners but do not contain oil and may therefore remain in the hair with no need for rinsing. They should be applied after towel drying the hair and prior to styling (5).

Household Remedies

Surprisingly, numerous household goods may be just as beneficial for the hair as expensive salon products. Based upon the appearance and needs of one's hair, various treatments may be utilized:

Apple Cider Vinegar

Rich in alpha hydroxy acids (AHAs), apple cider vinegar is ideal for treating hair that is dull and lifeless secondary to excessive product buildup. It can also help to eradicate follicle-clogging bacteria to allow the release of sebum and promote restoration of a healthy shine.

Baking Soda

Similar to apple cider vinegar, baking soda can also be utilized to remove buildup from the hair shaft. Adding a teaspoon of baking soda to any shampoo before applying it to hair will improve the detergent activity of the shampoo.

Avocados

Avocados contain more than 25 essential nutrients, including the B-vitamins and the natural antioxidant, vitamin E. Avocado can be mashed and applied directly to the hair to work as a deep conditioner, promoting restoration of the hair shaft and increasing shine, manageability, and tensile strength.

Lemons/Chamomile

Lemons and chamomile, if applied prior to UV exposure, can hasten the bleaching of melanocyte granules, lightening blonde or brown hair. Unfortunately, this process also exposes the hair to harmful UV radiation and further insult from melanocyte degradation. If applied transiently in the shower, the acidity of lemon juice can help remove product buildup without any detrimental effects.

SAFETY CONCERNS

With the plethora of synthetic ingredients included in today's cosmetic formulations, there has been understandable concern regarding the long-term side effects of frequent usage. Considerable attention has been paid especially to the use of ammonium laureth sulfate, parabens, and phthalates. Although currently available data suggest that the degree of exposure to these chemicals during shampooing and conditioning is too miniscule to induce serious pathology, long-term studies are lacking.

The safety of ammonium laureth sulfate was most comprehensively reviewed in 1983 in *The Journal of the American College of Toxicology*. At that time it was concluded that although skin and eye irritations were common side effects, there was no reason to believe that the usage may lead to permanent toxicity.

CONCLUSIONS

The health and style of hair play an essential role in creating an aesthetically appealing appearance. Healthy, attractive hair requires both a skilled stylist and an individualized home care regimen. By adhering to a few basic guidelines, an ideal head of hair can be attainable by everyone.

REFERENCES

1. Picot-Lemasson A, Decocq G, Aghassian F, Leveque JL. Influence of hairdressing on the psychological mood of women. Int J Cosmet Sci 2001; 23: 161–4.
2. Sinclair RD. Healthy hair: what is it? J Investig Dermatol Symp Proc 2007; 12: 2–5.
3. Trüeb RM. Shampoos: ingredients, efficacy and adverse effects. J Dtsch Dermatol Ges 2007; 5: 356–65.
4. Trueb RM. Dermocosmetic aspects of hair and scalp. J Investig Dermatol Symp Proc 2005; 10: 289–92.
5. Bolduc C, Shapiro J. Hair care products: waving, straightening, conditioning, and coloring. Clin Dermatol 2001; 19: 431–6.

3.5 Excess hair
David Beynet

KEY POINTS

- Hair removal is one of the most common reasons for patients to present for a cosmetic consultation
- Over-the-counter options include topical depilatories, waxing, and trimming. While these are effective, they do not result in permanent hair reduction
- Medical therapies including eflornithine and systemic agents can also be effective for reducing hair
- Laser technologies revolutionized the field by allowing safe, permanent hair reduction. Laser hair removal (LHR) works best on dark terminal hairs in light skinned patients, though new technologies allow for the safe treatment of nearly all skin types
- Current limitations for LHR include the inability to effectively treat blond and vellus hairs

Both men and women commonly seek hair removal. Patients have their own reasons, be they purely cosmetic or for a medical condition. Common hair removal areas include chest and back (men), face and legs (women), and almost any other area where hair bothers a patient. Medical conditions such as pseudofolliculitis barbae and hirsutism can also be improved. Hair removal can greatly improve the self-image of patients. For example, the presence of terminal facial hair is a significant cause of psychological distress for women (1). Some men feel uncomfortable to take their shirt off at the beach because of excess amounts of body hair. A remedy for such conditions is safe, effective hair removal.

Regardless of the reason for the patient's desire for hair removal, there are many treatment options. There are topical depilatory creams, tweezing, and waxing to name a few of the over-the-counter (OTC) mechanisms for hair removal. These may work well for some patients and be all that is necessary. Other patients may desire a longer lasting solution or need to treat an underlying medical condition to get improvement. Some of the prescription or physician-based treatments include laser-based procedures, prescription anti-androgens, and topical eflornithine cream (Vaniqa™, SkinMedica Inc, Carlsbad, California).

HOME REMEDIES AND OTC HAIR REMOVAL TREATMENTS

Many patients with excess hair begin their treatment by shaving or trimming their hair. These options only remove the hair above the surface of the skin. Thus, these forms result in temporary improvement in the appearance of the hair. Shaving can also result in irritation of the skin when performed on a daily basis. Waxing or plucking of the hair results in complete epilation, indicating removal of the entire hair shaft including the portion below the skin. As a result, waxing and plucking

may postpone hair regrowth for a longer period than shaving or trimming. Similar to shaving, waxing and plucking may result in irritation of the skin, and are unfortunately, only temporary forms of hair removal.

Topical therapies can be of use in patients wishing to avoid repeated shaving or trimming of their unwanted hair. Numerous OTC topical depilatories are available. Depilatories remove only the hair above the surface of the skin, and thus result in only temporary improvement. The majority of these depilatories utilize the same or similar chemical groups to break down hair keratin. Topical depilatories typically contain potassium thioglycolate, or a similar thiol compound, and calcium hydroxide. The potassium thioglycolate and calcium hydroxide combine to form calcium thioglycolate. Calcium thioglycolate breaks down the disulfide bonds that link keratin fibers, thereby significantly weakening the hair fiber. The hair can then be easily separated from the skin surface by gently wiping the skin; chemical depilatories do not remove the part of the hair that lies beneath the skin. The advantages of topical depilatories is that they work for all hair types, including vellus and blonde hairs, they are inexpensive, and they can be performed safely at home by patients. Unfortunately, the calcium hydroxide and thiol compounds can be very irritating to the skin. Also, if these topical depilatories are left on the skin for too long of a period, they can cause irritant contact dermatitis.

Finally, electrolysis is an option for patients. In electrolysis or electrology, an ultra thin metal probe is inserted into the hair follicle to destroy the hair. If inserted properly, the electrolysis probe does not puncture the skin but rather slides down the hair shaft. Once the probe is placed properly, electric current is passed by one of the three modalities: galvanic, thermolysis, or blend. Regardless of the modality used, the electricity delivered damages the hair follicle, matrix, and stem cells, resulting in potentially permanent hair removal. Another advantage is that electrolysis can be performed on all hair types, including vellus and blonde hair types. Unfortunately, many treatment sessions are necessary in order to result in improvement, as each hair follicle is treated individually. Furthermore, the effectiveness of electrolysis may be dependent on the expertise of the practitioner.

MEDICAL TREATMENTS FOR UNWANTED HAIR

The prescription medication, eflornithine (Vaniqa™), is the first and only FDA approved product in its class that has been clinically proven to be safe and effective for hair growth reduction. In controlled clinical studies, eflornithine cream was shown to inhibit hair growth rate by 48%. This provided a clinically meaningful benefit to most of the patients and increased their self-confidence (2,3). At the biochemical level, eflornithine is a highly selective and irreversible inhibitor of ornithine decarboxylase, a key rate-limiting enzyme in the biosynthesis of polyamines, which are critical for anagen hair growth (4,5). Synergistic efficacy of eflornithine has also been reported in combination with laser hair removal (LHR) (4).

Systemic steroidal and non-steroidal anti-androgens, including spironolactone, flutamide, cyproterone acetate, finasteride, and cimetidine can be considered, particularly in the case of hirsute women (6). These medications may result in unintended systemic side effects when used to treat hirsutism. As a result, the use of these anti-androgens is now limited to only the severe cases where there is a documented, underlying androgen abnormality.

LASER HAIR REMOVAL (LHR)

LHR is a commonly performed cosmetic procedure for patients of all skin types. In 2006, nearly 1.5 million LHR treatments were performed in the United States alone (7). Initially, LHR was reserved for patients with light skin types (Fitzpatrick I–III) due to the increased incidence of adverse effects in patients with dark skin types. With the advent of lasers with longer wavelengths, longer pulse durations, and improved cooling mechanisms over the last decade, LHR can be safely performed in all skin types including dark skin (Fitzpatrick types IV–VI). LHR has the ability to significantly reduce the number of hairs and their rate of growth, while maintaining a low incidence of side effects (8–10).

LHR can be used on any area of the body for cosmetic reasons and can be used to treat medical conditions such as hirsutism, pseudofolliculitis barbae, and acne keloidalis nuchae. These conditions are often more prevalent in patients of color, and can safely be improved with laser therapy (11).

The mechanism of LHR is based on the theory of selective photothermolysis. In selective photothermolysis, a specific laser is utilized so that the wavelength produced by the laser is absorbed by the target chromophore. As the photons from the laser are absorbed by the target chromophore, heat is generated. This heat destroys the neighboring structures causing temporary or permanent damage (12). In LHR, the target chromophore is melanin, which is primarily found in the epidermis, hair bulb, and hair shaft. Melanin absorbs the photons emitted from the laser; this absorption leads to heat production in the hair follicle. This heat diffuses from the hair shaft

and hair bulb, causing permanent thermal destruction of the surrounding follicular structures and follicular stem cells. It is this destruction of the follicular stem cells that is thought to be the basis for permanent hair reduction.

Caution must be taken when treating patients with dark or tanned skin types. The epidermal melanin in high concentrations in these patients has two unwanted outcomes. The first is that a small number of photons ultimately reach their intended site, the follicular structures; this results in decreased efficacy. The second is that there is increased heating of the epidermis (13). This can lead to side effects such as hyperpigmentation, hypopigmentation, blistering, and scarring.

The melanin absorption spectrum ranges from approximately 300 to 1200 nm, with absorption decreasing as wavelength increases. Follicular structures are located at a depth of 2–4 mm within the dermis. The ideal laser should have a wavelength which can facilitate adequate photon absorption by melanin, as well as penetrate sufficiently into the dermis to heat the hair follicles. Laser wavelengths between 600 and 1100 nm are ideal for these functions (14).

In addition to wavelength, pulse duration is an important consideration in LHR. Relatively long pulse durations are necessary for effective hair removal due to the relatively large size of the hair follicle and its longer thermal relaxation time. Long laser pulse durations result in slow heating of the follicular unit and a greater diffusion of heat from the hair shaft and bulb. The greater diffusion of heat allows for destruction of the entire follicular unit, not just the pigmented components alone (15). This leads to a more effective LHR.

There has been a marked increase in the number of lasers for LHR since the first lasers were approved in 1996 (16). LHR is primarily done with the following light sources: the ruby laser (694 nm), the alexandrite laser (755 nm), the diode laser (810 nm), the neodymium:yttrium-aluminum-garnet (Nd:YAG, 1064 nm) laser, intense pulsed light , and intense pulsed light with radio frequency. The ruby laser is the most selective for melanin absorption but has a short penetration depth and a high incidence of side effects. The Nd:YAG laser has the deepest penetration but the least specificity for absorption by melanin (15). This may result in decreased efficacy; however, the Nd-YAG laser tends to lead to less adverse effects. The alexandrite and the diode lasers have benefits of both of these extremes.

In general, the safest lasers are those with long wavelengths, long pulse durations, and optimal cooling devices. The alexandrite, diode and Nd:YAG lasers are in general the preferred devices to perform LHR safely. The long wavelengths of these devices allow for decreased epidermal melanin absorption and increased penetration depth. The long pulse duration slows down the heating rate, and results in a low incidence of side effects such as depigmentation (10,17). Although the Nd:YAG has a safer side effect profile, the diode and alexandrite lasers may be more effective because of greater melanin absorption. A mean hair reduction hair ranging from 58% to 62% on facial sites and 66% to 69% on nonfacial sites has been reported after three treatments with the long-pulsed Nd:YAG compared with a 74–84% hair reduction with the diode laser (15). Patients with skin types I–III can be safely and effectively treated with either the long pulsed alexandrite (755 nm) or diode laser (810 nm) (Figs. 3.5.1, 3.5.2, 3.5.3, 3.5.4, 3.5.5). The Nd:YAG (1064 nm) is a safe method for a dark skin type and is

(A) (B)

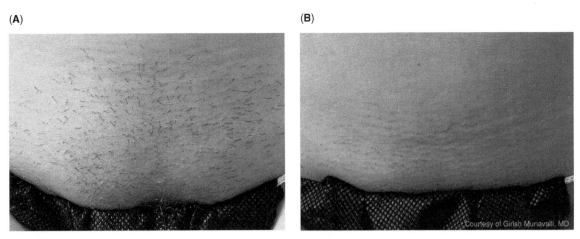

Figure 3.5.1 Improvement in the appearance of dark, terminal abdominal hairs before (**A**) and 6 months after 5 treatments with an 810-nm diode laser (Lightsheer® DUET, Lumenis, Santa Clara, California, U.S.A.) (**B**). *Source*: Photos courtesy of Girish Munavalli, MD.

(A) (B)

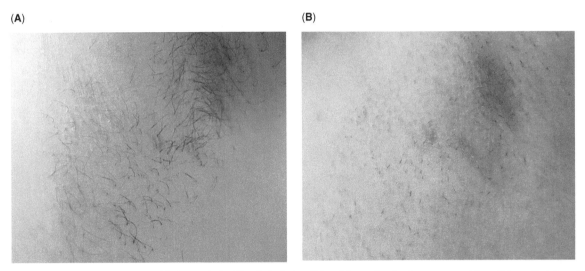

Figure 3.5.2 Improvement in the appearance of dark, terminal axillary hairs before (**A**) and 3 months after 5 treatments with an 810 nm diode laser (Lightsheer DUET) (**B**). *Source*: Photos courtesy of Shlomit Halamachi MD.

(A) (B)

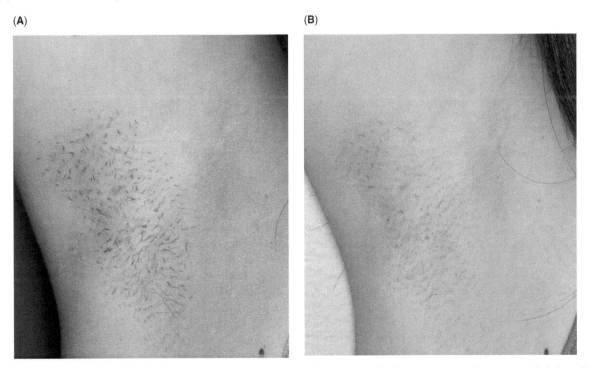

Figure 3.5.3 Improvement in the appearance of dark, terminal axillary hairs before (**A**) and 6 months after 3 treatments with an 810-nm diode laser (Lightsheer DUET) (**B**). *Source*: Photos courtesy of Suzanne Kilmer, MD.

(A)   **(B)**

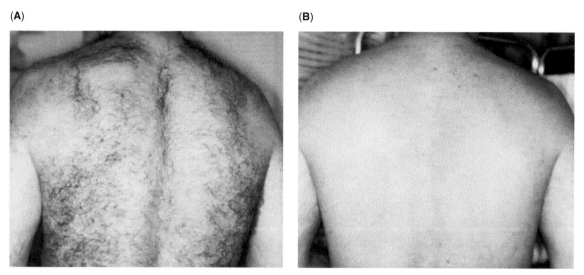

Figure 3.5.4 Improvement in the appearance of dark, terminal back hair before (**A**) and after 3 treatments with a 755-nm alexandrite laser (GentleLASE®, Candela, Wayland, Massachusetts, U.S.A.) (**B**).   *Source*: Photos courtesy of Marcelle Kutun, MD, CME, CLS.

(A)   **(B)**

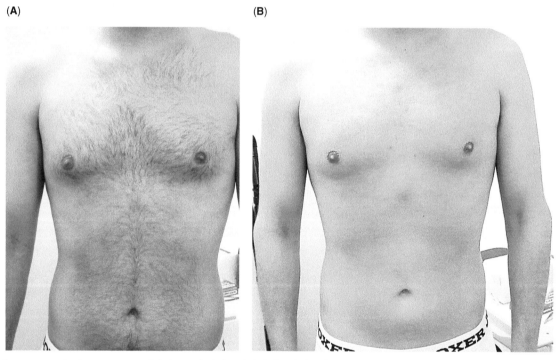

Figure 3.5.5 Improvement in the appearance of dark, terminal chest hair before (**A**) and after 3 treatments with a 755-nm alexandrite laser (GentleLASE) (**B**).   *Source*: Photos courtesy of Tony Ghidorzi, DO.

the laser of choice when performing LHR in these populations (Figs. 3.5.6, 3.5.7).

Efficient cooling devices reduce unwanted epidermal heating and thus help prevent laser-induced thermal damage. Epidermal thermal damage can result in pigmentary alterations, scarring, and blistering, especially in dark or tanned skin. Cooling devices also have the added benefit of decreasing the pain associated with the procedure. Current cooling devices use both evaporative and conductive mechanisms. These tend to provide more efficient epidermal cooling than

older techniques of using ice- or water-based gel. Dynamic cooling devices function by using a cryogen spray immediately prior to the laser pulse, which evaporates and instantaneously cools the epidermis (18). Conductive cooling devices include cooled sapphire laser windows, which cool the epidermis by conductive heat transfer. Conductive devices also lead to dermal compression, which has two benefits: compression brings follicular structures close to the area of maximal dermal laser penetration and compresses blood vessels, thereby decreasing the concentration of the competitive chromophore hemoglobin (13).

(A)   **(B)**

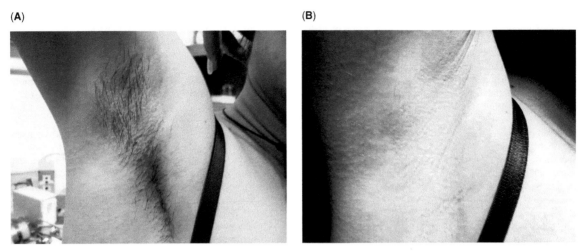

Figure 3.5.6 Improvement in the appearance of terminal axillary hairs in a type IV skin patient before (**A**) and after 3 treatments with a 1064 nm Nd:YAG laser (GentleYAG®, Candela) (**B**).   *Source*: Photos courtesy of Faye Jenkins, RN.

(A)   **(B)**

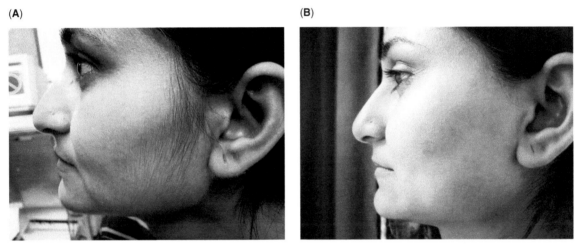

Figure 3.5.7 Improvement in the appearance of terminal facial hair in a type-IV skin patient before (**A**) and after 3 treatments with a 1064-nm Nd:YAG laser (GentleYAG) (**B**).   *Source*: Photos courtesy of Faye Jenkins RN.

In addition to the discussed side effects, there have been reported cases of paradoxical increased hair growth following LHR. The exact mechanism has not been established. It is important for physicians to monitor patients for possible increased hair growth following LHR, as this is typically a contraindication for further LHR.

LHR can be one of the most rewarding cosmetic procedures for patients. It is, however, important to set reasonable expectations for patients before beginning LHR treatments. First, patients must be aware that several treatment sessions are necessary to effectively perform LHR. These sessions should be scheduled sufficiently far apart that the hair has re-entered its anagen (growth) phase; if the sessions are too close together, the treatment will be ineffective. Typically, sessions are to be scheduled approximately every six weeks. Second, blonde and gray hairs probably will not respond to the treatment; vellus and fine hairs are similarly refractory to LHR. Finally, patients should not be tan at the time of their treatments. If a patient presents for their LHR session tan, then they should not be treated at that time. Unfortunately, despite our best efforts and treatments, there are some patients who do not respond well to hair removal treatments or who do not achieve permanent hair reduction.

CONCLUSIONS

Removal of excess hair is one of the most common reasons for patients to present to a cosmetic physician. Previously, patients were forced to undergo temporary, painful procedures such as waxing or plucking to remove excess body hair. In the last several years, new medical treatments have become available for removing hair. However, the introduction of safe, effective lasers for removing hair has revolutionized the field. Today, patients of all skin types can be effectively treated with lasers to remove dark, terminal hairs.

REFERENCES

1. Lipton MG, Sherr L, Elford J, Rustin MHA, Clayton WJ. Women living with facial hair: the psychological and behavioral burden. J Psychosom Res 2006; 61: 161–8.
2. Shander D, Ahluwalia GS, Morton JP. Management of unwanted facial hair by topical application of eflornithine. In: Elsner P, Maibach HI, eds. Cosmeceuticals and Active Cosmetics: Drugs vs. Cosmetics, 2nd edn. Boca Raton, Florida: Taylor & Francis Group 2005: 489–510.

3. Schrode KS, Huber F, Staszak H, et al. Randomized, double-blind, vehicle controlled safety and efficacy evaluation of eflornithine 15% cream in the treatment of women with excessive facial hair (Abstract). 57th Ann Meeting Am Acad Dermatol, San Francisco, CA, 1999.

4. Ahluwalia GS, Shander D. Synergy of eflornithine cream with laser and light-based systems for hair management. In: Ahluwalia GS, ed. Cosmetic Applications of Laser and Light-Based Systems. New York: William Andrew, Inc, 2009: 383–97.

5. Nancarrow MJ, Nesci A, Hynd PI, Powell BC. Dynamic expression of ornithine decarboxylase in hair growth. Mech Dev 1999; 84: 161–4.

6. Ahluwalia GS. Management of unwanted hair. In: Ahluwalia GS, ed. Cosmetic Applications of Laser and Light-Based Systems. New York: William Andrew, Inc, 2009: 239–52.

7. The American Society for Aesthetic and Plastic Surgery. [Available from: www.surgery.org]. (Accessed 23 January 2007).

8. Battle EF Jr, Hobbs LM. Laser-assisted hair removal for darker skin types. Dermatol Ther 2004; 17: 177–83.

9. Garcia C, Alamoudi H, Nakib M, Zimmo S. Alexandrite laser hair removal is safe for Fitzpatrick skin types IV–VI. Dermatol Surg 2000; 26: 130–4.

10. Greppi I. Diode laser hair removal of the black patient. Lasers Surg Med 2001; 28: 150–5.

11. Bridgeman-Shah S. The medical and surgical therapy of pseudofolliculitis barbae. Dermatol Ther 2004; 17: 158–63.

12. Anderson RR, Parrish JA. Selective photothermolysis: precise microsurgery by selective absorption of pulsed radiation. Science 1983; 220: 524–7.

13. Baugh WP, Trafeli JP, Barnette DJ Jr, Ross EV. Hair reduction using a scanning 800 nm diode laser. Dermatol Surg 2001; 27: 358–64.

14. Anderson RR, Parrish JA. The optics of human skin. J Invest Dermatol 1981; 77: 13–19.

15. Tanzi EL, Alster TS. Long-pulsed 1064-nm Nd:YAG laser-assisted hair removal in all skin types. Dermatol Surg 2004; 30: 13–17.

16. Galadari I. Comparative evaluation of different hair removal lasers in skin types IV, V, and VI. Int J Dermatol 2003; 42: 68–70.

17. Alster TS, Bryan H, Williams CM. Long-pulsed Nd:YAG laser-assisted hair removal in pigmented skin: a clinical and histological evaluation. Arch Dermatol 2001; 137: 885–9.

18. Nahm WK, Tsoukas MM, Falanga V, et al. Preliminary study of fine changes in the duration of dynamic cooling during 755-nm laser hair removal on pain and epidermal damage in patients with skin types III–V. Lasers Surg Med 2002; 31: 247–51.

3.6   Hair loss and hair transplantation
Paul J. McAndrews

KEY POINTS

- There are many causes for hair loss. In order to properly treat patients, physicians must attempt to determine the cause of their hair loss
- Androgenetic alopecia is the most common cause of hair loss
- Treatments include both medical and surgical approaches
- Topical minoxidil and oral finasteride have been shown to promote some regrowth of hair and slow the rate of hair loss for patients
- Effective hair transplants require (*i*) informed patients, (*ii*) artful precision to use the hair bank wisely and effectively, and (*iii*) performance of the procedure by a properly trained specialist

---

Not all types of hair loss are alike. Hair loss, like stomach pain, is a symptom not a diagnosis. There are many things that can cause stomach pain and the treatments are all different. Similarly there are multiple causes for hair loss and the treatments also differ. The most common form of hair loss is androgenetic alopecia (male or female pattern hair loss). However, in order to offer the best care to our patients we must evaluate for other potential causes. Once the cause of hair loss is established, we can then discuss the ideal medical and surgical approaches to hair loss with each patient individually.

APPROACH TO HAIR LOSS

In order to the understand hair loss, it is vitally important to understand what is normal hair growth. An average person has 100,000 to 150,000 terminal hair follicles on his or her scalp (1). Hair follicles produce approximately 1 cm of new hair growth in a month (2). All human hair grows in cycles. For scalp hair, the growing phase (anagen) accounts for 85–90% of the hair and lasts for approximately two to six years. The shedding phase (catagen) accounts for about 1% of the scalp and lasts for approximately three weeks. Finally, the resting phase (telogen) accounts for approximately 10% of the scalp and lasts approximately three months (3). It is typical for an average person to shed between 50 and 100 strands of hair per day (4). Shedding of the hair is normal since new strands of hair will begin growing in those follicles. This cycle continues to repeat itself throughout a person's life.

When a patient presents with the symptom of hair loss, it is important to first determine the correct cause of hair loss in order to properly treat it. Utilizing the following algorithm (Fig. 3.6.1), providers can simply and effectively assign a preliminary diagnosis to a patient's hair loss.

The first thing to determine is whether there is true hair loss or if the hair shaft is breaking. It is important to examine the hair that has fallen out and determine if there is a bulb. If there is no bulb at the end of the hair, the hair is breaking. This is usually caused by outside, environmental damage to the hair (e.g., blow-drying, straightening, perming, hair dye, bleaching, sun exposure, hair styling, etc.). Remember the hair is essentially a dead piece of protein string, and the more traumas it experiences the more likely it will break. The treatment for hair breakage is to avoid trauma, and the hair follicle will produce a new healthy hair with a passage of time.

If the hair is not breaking, the next step is to determine whether the hair loss is due to scarring. There are several dermatologic diseases that cause scarring of the scalp and may destroy the hair follicles. An examination by a dermatologist, and in some cases a scalp biopsy, may be needed to determine which type of hair loss is occurring. If it is a hair loss due to a scarring disorder, the disease needs to be treated promptly because once the hair follicle is destroyed the hair will never grow back. After the disease process is stopped, hair transplants can be used to fill in the bald spot created.

If the hair loss is not caused by a scarring disorder then the next step in the diagnostic process is to determine whether the patient is experiencing a significant increase in shedding. Excessive shedding, known as telogen effluvium, is usually caused by a preceding traumatic event, whether physical or psychological. A thorough medical history will often pinpoint the trigger. Laboratory testing may be necessary to rule out other physiological causes. In either case, the normal shedding cycle will return when the cause is identified and treated. In any case of shedding hair loss, hair transplantation is not an appropriate treatment option.

If examination reveals a non-breaking, non-scarring, and non-shedding hair loss disorder, then we need to determine whether the hair loss is diffuse or patterned through a careful physical examination. The two most common forms of patterned hair loss are alopecia areata and androgenetic alopecia. The treatments for these two diseases are very different and therefore the correct diagnosis is imperative.

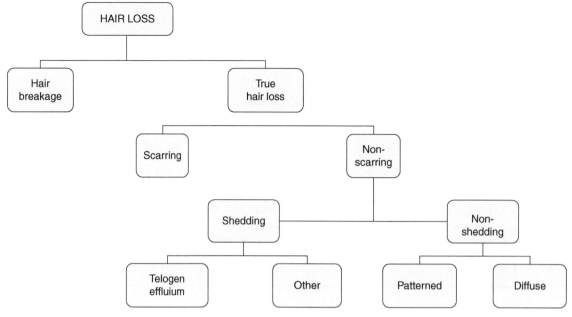

Figure 3.6.1 Hair loss diagnosis.

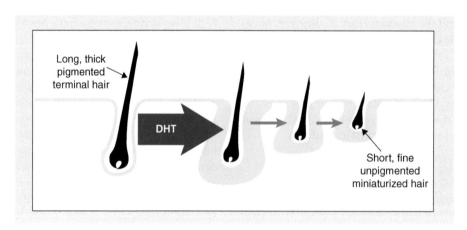

Figure 3.6.2 Hair miniaturization (DHT, dihydrotestosterone).

Androgenetic alopecia, the most prevalent type of hair loss for which patients seek professional treatment today, is a disease of aging that everyone experiences to some degree. A patient's genetics will determine the severity and extent of hair loss. Androgenetic alopecia can be inherited from either the mother's side or father's side of the family, or both. The hair around the sides and back of the scalp is usually "good" genetic hair that lasts a lifetime. Each person has a "genetic light switch" embedded in their DNA. We do not know when this proverbial switch will turn on for any individual. However, when it does, the patient begins to experience miniaturization of the susceptible hair follicles under the influence of the hormone dihydrotestosterone (DHT) (Fig. 3.6.2). During the miniaturization process, the hair shaft of the affected follicles becomes smaller and finer with each successive growth cycle until they are no longer noticeable to the naked eye. When you see a shiny bald man, he still has hair all over his scalp, but it is no longer visible to the human eye. Studies have shown that the human eye cannot tell a person is balding until the person has lost over 50% density (5). By the age of 25, 25%

of all men will be affected by male patterned hair loss. By age 40, this figure increases to approximately 50% (6). For women, one in four experiences a noticeable hair loss by the age of 50.

The extent of an individual's hair loss is normally classified using two scales. Male pattern hair loss is most commonly classified using the Norwood Scale and men may progress through these stages as they age (7). Female pattern hair loss is typically classified by the Ludwig Scale; however we do occasionally see women who present with male pattern hair loss.

SPECIAL CASES OF HAIR LOSS

While alopecia can pose a significant psychological burden on otherwise healthy individuals, physicians must be aware of the particularly difficult case of chemotherapy-induced alopecia. For such patients, the loss of hair is psychologically distinct from normal age-related alopecia. For the cancer patient, it is a very public stigma of their disease and thrusts them into the identity of a cancer patient. One study of women receiving chemotherapy found that for nearly half of the women, alopecia was the most traumatic side effect of their therapy, and over a quarter of the patients no longer felt like women (8). Some women have even described the loss of their hair as worse than the loss of a breast following breast cancer (9). The psychological changes involved are not always transitory either: even after remission of cancer and regrowth of their hair, nearly 25% of the women do not return to their baseline level of confidence. Because Western culture has traditionally placed a greater emphasis on women's hair, much of the literature on chemotherapy and body image has focused on women; however, recent research has revealed that men are also subject to the trauma of chemotherapy-induced alopecia (10). Even though hair loss may seem trivial compared with the threat of death, it is of the utmost importance that the physician understand and respect the damage that it can inflict upon body image and self-esteem.

Another situation which demands both vigilance and sensitivity on the part of the physician in a cosmetic practice is the case of a patient suffering from body dysmorphic disorder. While it is entirely natural for patients to want to improve their appearance, these individuals may obsess over their appearance, believing themselves to be ugly or deformed despite a normal appearance (11). Because it may be ultimately debilitating, suspicion of body dysmorphic disorder should be followed up on and, if warranted, the appropriate psychiatric referrals be made.

MEDICAL TREATMENTS FOR HAIR LOSS

Topical minoxidil solution (Rogaine™, McNeil-PPC Inc, Fort Washington, Pennsylvania), was the first product to show a proven efficacy in the treatment of androgenetic alopecia in both men and women; the U.S. Food and Drug Administration (FDA) approved topical minoxidil use for hair loss in men in 1986 and for women in 1991 as a prescription product. Interestingly, the hair growth effect of minoxidil was discovered serendipitously during its development as an oral treatment for refractory hypertension (12). The precise mechanism of action of hair growth for minoxidil is not known, though most research supports action via opening of potassium channels in dermal papilla cells (13). A significant increase in hair counts can be seen in patients following four months of twice-daily application; in clinical trials, data following 12 months of therapy shows a significant increase of terminal hairs compared with the placebo group (14,15). A 5-year follow-up of subjects who consistently used the 2% and 3% minoxidil solution showed that the effect peaked at one year with a slow decline in regrowth in subsequent years (16). Minoxidil was thus shown to provide benefit for both stimulation of new terminal hair growth, as well as for slowing the progressive miniaturization of the scalp hair that is seen in androgenetic alopecia. Unfortunately, discontinuation of topical minoxidil resulted in a loss of the hair gained during the treatment (17). Minoxidil 2% is now available over the counter (OTC) for both men and women. A higher 5% dose is also available OTC, but in the United States it is approved only for use in men (18).

Androgenic alopecia in men can also be treated by reducing the production of the active androgen, DHT, at the follicular level. Finasteride (Propecia™, Merck & Co, Inc., Whitehouse Station, New Jersey) is a competitive inhibitor of type 2, 5-α reductase, the enzyme responsible for the conversion of testosterone to DHT in hair follicles. It has been shown in clinical studies to help halt hair loss and to stimulate hair regrowth in androgenic alopecia (19,20). More specifically, finasteride treatment has been shown to increase the number of hairs in anagen phase and to increase the anagen to telogen ratio (21). In 1997, Propecia™ (finasteride 1 mg) was approved by the FDA for treatment of hair loss in men. Finasteride use is contraindicated in women because of the potential risk of undervirilization of a male fetus during pregnancy.

HAIR TRANSPLANTS

The medical and surgical treatments for androgenetic alopecia have vastly improved over the recent years; however, there is still no perfect treatment. In 1939, a Japanese doctor named Dr. Okuda published an article describing a micrograft hair transplant procedure into the eyebrow of his patients. Yet hair transplants were relatively unheard of until Dr. Orentreich published an article in 1959 on the punch grafting technique (22). Dr. Samuel Ayers and Dr. Mike Corbett were the first pioneers of hair transplants in the Western United States beginning in 1961. They developed the reputation as the "Hair Transplant Surgeon to the Stars" and patients would travel from around the world to have their hair transplants performed.

Today's hair transplant should look completely natural and undetectable, in the right hands. The "doll's hair" plugs of yesterday are gone. However, there are immense differences in "when and how" the hair transplant surgery is performed around the world. There is also a great deal of misinformation about hair loss and the treatments of hair loss in our society. Throughout the rest of this section, we will discuss the key attributes to a successful hair restoration procedure.

The three important attributes of a successful hair transplantation method are discussed in detail next.

(A) Informed decisions: It is imperative that patients become educated on hair loss and the limitations to the various treatments. This is critical for patients to have realistic goals and expectations.

(B) Artful precision: Techniques and technologies that maximize the survival of the limited amount of good genetic hair must be utilized to achieve a successful hair transplant. These techniques should be combined with the artistic design of the hairline that is unique for each individual patient.

(C) Unparalleled results: Excellent results are attained when an ethical doctor who has been properly trained directly applies these techniques himself—hands-on.

Informed Decisions

Informed decisions give patients the ability to make an educated choice. The most important concept for doctors performing hair transplants, and patients considering hair transplants, is to understand the limitations of hair transplants and the goals of a successful hair restoration procedure. There is a fixed and limited supply of good genetic donor hair that each patient has on the sides and the back of the scalp to transfer to the thinning area; this good genetic hair is known as the "hair bank."

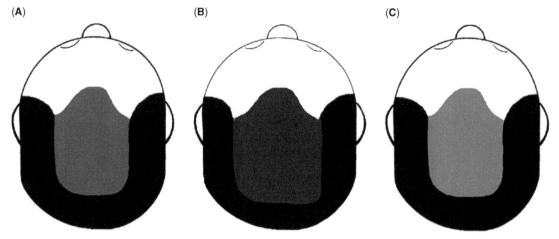

Figure 3.6.3 (**A**) Before a hair transplant, (**B**) after a hair transplant, and (**C**) 5 years after a hair transplant for a patient not using Propecia.

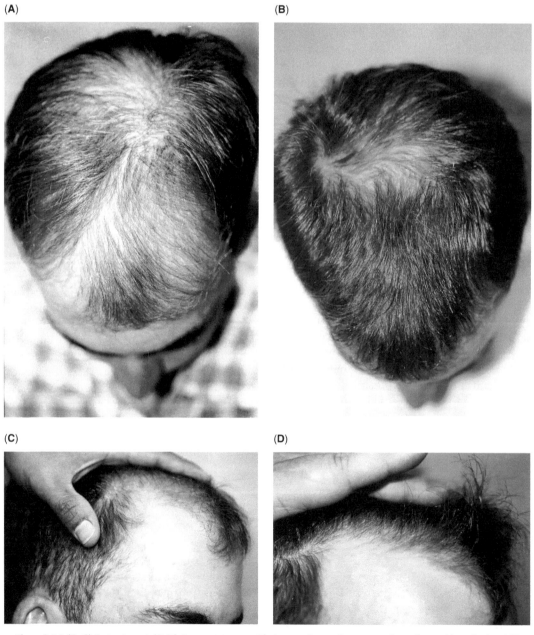

Figure 3.6.4 (**A, C**) Pretreatment, (**B, D**) 4 years status post 1 hair transplant and concurrently on finasteride and minoxidil.

Many people assume a good candidate for hair restoration is a patient with plenty of donor hair; this is not necessarily the case. What really makes a good candidate is a patient that has realistic goals about what can be accomplished. The number of grafts each patient will require ultimately depends on the patient's present extent of hair loss, the prediction of future hair loss, and the patient's individual hair restoration goals. One of the most vital components to setting realistic goals is an effective consultation. A patient needs to understand the progressive nature of androgenetic alopecia and the limitations to hair transplants in order to make an informed decision. This knowledge will help them understand the importance of not only creating a hairline that looks good today but also in the future as their hair loss progresses. If the patient has unrealistic expectations of what can be accomplished, he or she is not an appropriate candidate. While most patients can be educated and are able to adjust their expectations as necessary, others are not and should not undergo a

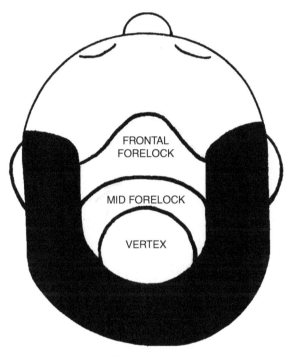

Figure 3.6.5 Areas of the scalp.

hair transplant procedure. It is therefore extremely important that the physician who will carry out the procedure perform this initial consultation, discuss the patient's expectations, and help the patient to make an informed decision.

Once the patients recognize their hair loss and decide to proceed with the hair transplantation procedure, it is important to maximize the potential benefits of medical therapies for alopecia. Medical forms of therapy can slow, stop, and/or somewhat reverse androgenetic alopecia and are an incredibly useful addition to hair transplantation procedures. The below scenario (Fig. 3.6.3A–C) exemplifies the need of assistance from medical therapies for hair loss. If a patient with 30% density (Fig. 3.6.3A) of hair came to a surgeon with the desire to create the look of a full head of hair, the surgeon would need to add approximately 20% density to achieve 50% total hair density. Patients with approximately 50% hair density (Fig. 3.6.3B) have the appearance of a full head of hair. The patient's initial goal was attainable; however with the progressive nature of androgenetic alopecia, this 50% hair density may not be able to be maintained. The average male experiencing androgenetic alopecia loses approximately 4% density per year (23). This means that in 5 years following the transplantation, the patient's hair density would again be 30% (his original 30% would have decreased to 10%, plus the 20% hair density transplanted) (Fig. 3.6.3C). This example illustrates the difficulty that the progressive nature of androgenetic alopecia poses, as well as the need for the early inclusion of medical treatment to retard the progression of hair loss. Finasteride is the most effective single treatment, but the combination of finasteride with topical minoxidil yields the best results.

By contrast, the next patient underwent a conservative hair transplant with the addition of oral finasteride and topical minoxidil (Fig. 3.6.4A–D). This patient presented at the age of 21, by which time he was devastated by his hair loss and its social effects. He strongly desired a hair transplant. The patient underwent a very conservative hair transplant in which approximately 900 follicular unit grafts were used from the existing frontal forelock only, but also began treating with minoxidil and finasteride. These pictures demonstrate his results four years after a single conservative hair transplant, with the addition of minoxidil and finasteride. The medical therapies have helped to prevent further hair loss and the need

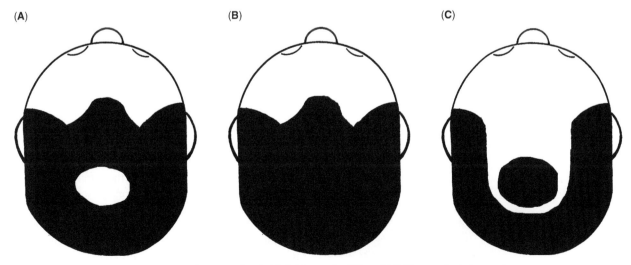

Figure 3.6.6 (**A**) Before hair transplant (HT), (**B**) I year after HT , and (**C**) 20 years after hair transplant.

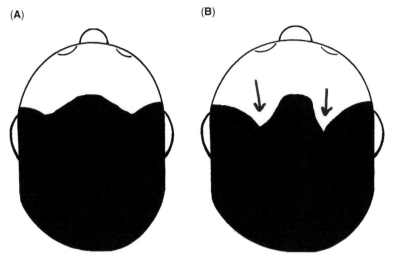

Figure 3.6.7 (**A**) Immature hairline and (**B**) mature hairline.

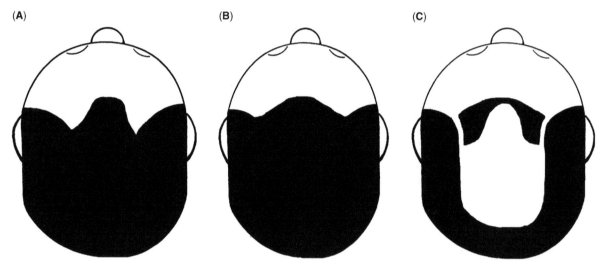

Figure 3.6.8 (**A**) Pre-hair transplant (HT), (**B**) 1 year post-HT, and (**C**) 20 years post HT.

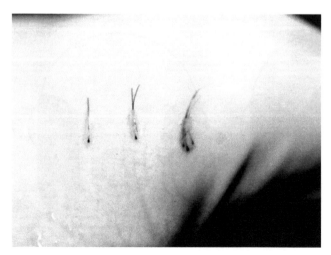

Figure 3.6.9 Grafts dissected into natural hair groupings (NHG).

for additional hair transplants, helping this patient to maintain a natural, full appearance.

Artful Precision

Artful precision dictates that it is imperative the physician use the limited donor supply as wisely and efficiently as possible. Hair transplantation surgery is as much art as it is science. The goal of a hair transplant is to artistically and naturally frame the face and to maintain a youthful appearance. Understanding how and why the hair grows, the different angles that the hair grows in different locations on the scalp, and how to use each and every follicular unit to its maximum potential are all a part of this artistic component. There is no such thing as one size fits all when designing the hairline. Every human being is unique and is framed slightly differently. The design of the hairline is determined by (*i*) each individual's age, (*ii*) extent of hair loss, and (*iii*) future prediction of further hair loss. We need to beware of creating a youthful appearance today, at the expense of looking unnatural tomorrow. The hair restoration surgeon must have the artistic ability to recreate what nature took away, designing a hair transplant that not only looks good today but that will also look good in the future.

Aesthetically, the most important area to have hair is in the frontal forelock because it frames the patient's face and maintains a youthful appearance (Fig. 3.6.5). Maintaining hair in the frontal forelock with a balding vertex is a naturally occurring balding pattern in men. In an extensively balding young man, the limited amount of good genetic hair should be reserved for the frontal forelock and the mid-forelock. However the hair in the frontal forelock is typically some of the last hair to miniaturize during the balding process. This can present a dilemma in young patients experiencing androgenetic alopecia because many times they desire to use their limited amount of good genetic hair to solve their acute problem (i.e., the vertex or the temporal recessions). Transplanting into the vertex will solve the acute problem for this balding male (Fig. 3.6.6A). For the next several years, this patient will be happy with his newly acquired hair in the vertex (Fig. 3.6.6B). When his existing hair in his frontal forelock and mid-forelock miniaturizes, he will be left with a very unaesthetic result that does not follow a natural balding pattern and he will become very unhappy (Fig. 3.6.6C). Unfortunately, by then, the physician may not have enough good genetic hair available to create a natural balding pattern in the more important frontal and mid-forelock areas. The doctor solved an acute problem for this patient, but long term has created a huge cosmetic detriment. Therefore, transplanting hair in the vertex of a young male is not a wise use of this very limited good genetic hair and it is prudent to refrain from transplanting hair in this area. Instead, these patients should be placed on the medical therapies, minoxidil and finasteride, as alternative options.

Before reaching puberty many men do not have frontotemporal triangles (Fig. 3.6.7A), but by the age of 25, the overwhelming majority of men develop temporal recessions (Fig. 3.6.7B). It is a very natural bald area in the aging face. However, it can be very disconcerting for the young man because it is usually the first sign of hair loss.

Hair transplant surgeons should also refrain from transplanting hair into this area because it will eventually create a very unaesthetic and unnatural balding pattern. An immature hairline will not naturally frame the face of an aging and balding man (Fig. 3.6.8A–C).

As the above cases demonstrate, every hair transplant procedure must be performed with the foresight of how it will look on that patient 10 or 20 years later. A good hair transplant procedure will stand the test of time and the patient will look natural today and in the future, even if they continue to experience additional hair loss. Using the precious and limited donor hair as wisely and efficiently as possible is the essential foundation of any treatment plan.

When it comes to the mechanics of the hair transplant, there are vastly different techniques and technologies used throughout the world. At present the best way to ensure the highest survival and best cosmetic results entails dissecting the hair into the natural hair groupings with the aid of a stereoscopic microscope. Hair typically grows in groups of one to four follicles surrounded by a

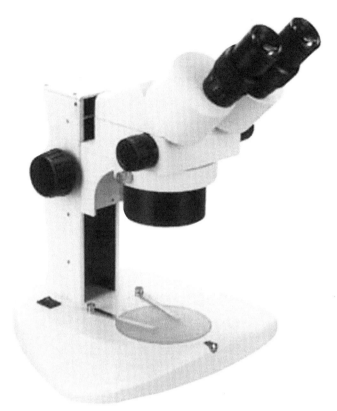

Figure 3.6.10 Stereoscopic microscope.

fibrous sheath, known as follicular units. Since hair naturally grows in these follicular units, it should be transplanted in the same way to give the most natural results (Fig. 3.6.9); this technique is known as a follicular unit transplant. A stereoscopic microscope aids to help preserve the follicular units intact during dissection to ensure increased survival and growth (Fig. 3.6.10). Separating every hair into single hair micrografts should not be performed, as this decreases the survival of the grafts.

Unparalleled Results

Unparalleled results are achieved when all of these important components are personally applied by a qualified, trained physician. There is an immense amount of detail and subtleties that are involved in the mechanics and artistry of a hair transplant, which makes it vitally important that the hair transplant surgeon has been properly and formally trained in the science and art of hair restorations in a residency or fellowship. A properly designed hairline should be age appropriate and should mimic nature considering the patient's overall extent of hair loss. It is necessary to create more conservative hairlines on younger patients or those patients with more extensive hair loss. The bad hair transplants seen in public everyday are a constant reminder that not every hair transplant surgeon has the training or artistic skill necessary to create a natural result.

CONCLUSIONS

In summary, it is important to understand that there is not a perfect treatment for hair loss, but the treatment options today are vastly improved. Ultimately, it is the combination of medical therapies and properly performed hair trans-

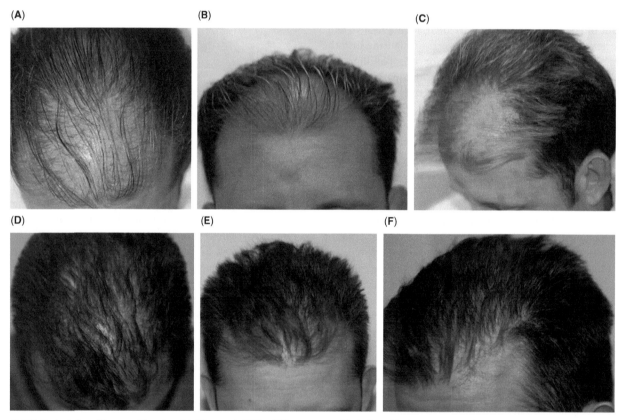

Figure 3.6.11 Patient 1, a 39–year-old male with Norwood II/IIIa diffuse patterned hair loss (**A–C**, pretreatment); status post 2400 grafts in 2 sessions (**D–F**, posttreatment).

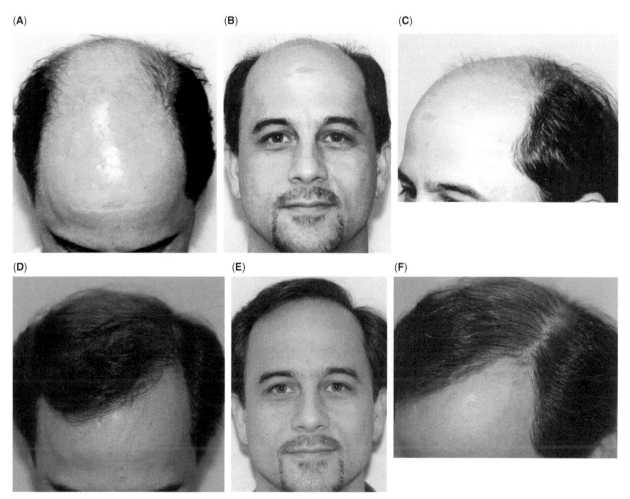

Figure 3.6.12 Patient 2, a 40–year-old male with Norwood VI hair loss (pretreatment, **A–C**); status post 3000 grafts in 2 sessions (**D–F**, posttreatment).

plants which can help our patients achieve their goals. Patients who are realistic about their goals are very satisfied and happy that they went forward with their hair transplant (Fig. 3.6.11 and 3.6.12).

REFERENCES

1. Headington JT. Transverse microscopic anatomy of the human scalp. A basis for a morphometric approach to disorders of the hair follicle. Arch Dermatol 1984; 120: 449–56.
2. Montagna W, Parakkal PF. The Structure and Function of Skin. New York: Academic Press, 1974.
3. Kligman AM. The human hair cycle. J Invest Dermatol 1959; 33: 307.
4. Olsen EA. Androgenetic Alopecia. In: Olsen EA, ed. Disorders of Hair Growth: Diagnosis and Treatment. New York: McGraw Hill, Inc., 1994: 257–83.
5. Hamilton JB. Patterned loss of hair in men: types and incidence. Ann NY Acad Sci 1951; 53: 708–28.
6. Rhodes T, Girman CJ, Savin RC, et al. Prevalence of male pattern hair loss in 18–49 year old men. Dermatol Surg 1998; 24: 1330–2.
7. Norwood OT. Male pattern baldness: classification and incidence. South Med J 1975; 68: 1359–65.
8. Munstedt K, Manthey N, Sachsse S, Vahrson H. Changes in self-concept and body image during alopecia induced cancer chemotherapy. Support Care Cancer 1997; 5: 139–43.
9. Freedman TG. Social and cultural dimensions of hair loss in women treated for breast cancer. Cancer Nurs 1994; 17: 334–41.
10. Hilton S, Hunt K, Emslie C, Salinas M, Ziebland S. Have men been overlooked? A comparison of young men and women's experiences of chemotherapy-induced alopecia. Psychooncology 2008; 17: 577–83.
11. Phillips KA. Body dysmorphic disorder: clinical aspects and treatment strategies. Bull Menninger Clin 1998; 62: A33–48.
12. Burton JL, Marshall A. Hypertrichosis due to minoxidil. Br J Dermatol 1979; 70: 593–5.
13. Buhl AE, Waldon DJ, Conrad SJ, et al. Potassium channel conductance: a mechanism affecting hair growth both in-vitro and in-vivo. J Invest Dermatol 1992; 98: 315–19
14. Olsen EA, Weiner MS, Delong ER, et al. Topical minoxidil in early male pattern baldness. J Am Acad Dermatol 1985; 13: 185–92
15. Olsen EA, Delong ER, Weiner MS. Dose-response study of topical minoxidil in male pattern baldness. J Am Acad Dermatol 1986; 15: 30–7
16. Olsen EA, Weiner MS, Amara IA, Delong ER. Five-year follow-up of men with androgenic alopecia treated with topical minoxidil. J Am Acad Dermatol 1990; 22: 643–6
17. Olsen EA, Weiner MS. Topical minoxidil in male pattern baldness: effects of discontinuation of treatment. J Am Acad Dermatol 1987; 17: 97–101
18. Olsen EA, Dunlap FE, Funicella T, et al. A randomized clinical trial of 5% topical minoxidil vs. 2% topical minoxidil and placebo in the treatment of androgenic alopecia in men. J Am Acad Dermatol 2002; 47: 377–85
19. Kaufman KD, Olsen EA, Whiting D, W, the Finasteride Male Pattern Hair Loss Study Group. Finasteride in the treatment of men with androgenetic alopecia. J Am Acad Dermatol 1998; 39: 578–89
20. Whiting DA, Olsen EA, Savin R, et al. Male Pattern Hair Loss Study Group. Efficacy and tolerability of finasteride 1 mg in men aged 41 to 60 years with male pattern hair loss. Eur J Dermatol 2003; 13: 150–60
21. Van Neste D, Fuh V, Sanchez-Pedreno P, et al. Finesteride increases anagen hair in men with androgenic alopecia. Br J Dermatol 2000; 143: 804–10
22. Orentreich N. Autographs in alopecias and other selected dermatological conditions. Ann NY Acad Sci 1959; 83: 463
23. Kaufman KD. Long-term 5 year multinational experience with finasteride 1mg in the treatment of men with androgenetic alopecia. Eur J Dermatol 2002; 12: 45–6.

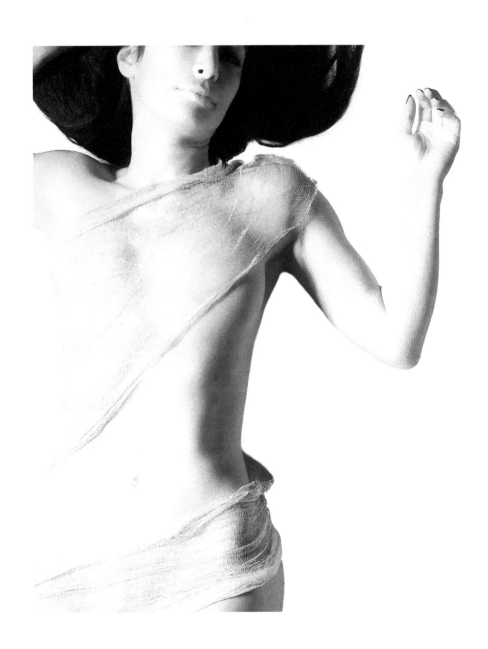

The search for the perfect body has long been an obsession for humans. Mainstream media feeds and reflects society's constant fixation on the ideal body. Unfortunately, over the last several decades, obesity has emerged as a troubling epidemic. As a result, weight loss and diet have emerged as national trends not only to improve people's cosmetic appearance but also to reduce the medical impact of obesity.

For many people, diet and exercise are simply not enough to achieve their desired appearance. Increasingly, patients are turning to medical interventions to treat their unwanted fat. In this section, we will discuss therapeutic options, both invasive and noninvasive, to help these patients achieve their ideal body.

4.2   The impact of obesity
Andrew L. DaLio

KEY POINTS

- Obesity is defined on the basis of a person's body mass index
- Obesity is an epidemic in America, with two-thirds of Americans being classified as overweight while one-third are obese
- Obesity is not only a cosmetic concern, but can have severe impact on our general health. Obesity has been correlated with heart disease, high blood pressure, stroke, diabetes, osteoarthritis, infertility, and several forms of cancer
- Body contouring procedures, in combination with lifestyle changes and a healthy diet, can help patients to reverse the impact of obesity and achieve their ideal body appearance

---

It should come as no surprise in a culture of super-sized, fast-food dollar menus, deep-fried Twinkies, and conspicuous consumption that obesity in America has reached epidemic proportions. The Center for Disease Control estimates that obesity and inactivity will soon supplant tobacco and tobacco-related-illnesses as the leading cause of death in America (1). It's a truism that almost borders upon cliché, but a visit to any suburban mall can leave no doubt: America has largely become a nation of fat people (2).

DEFINITIONS

"Overweight" and "obesity" are labels used to classify a range of weights that exceed what is generally considered to be a healthy norm. For adults, these classifications are based on the body mass index (BMI) (3). The BMI is a simple height and weight calculation that generally correlates the amount of body fat in an individual. However, the BMI formula can be misleading when applied to people with a higher percentage of muscle mass than a normal person, and should only be used as an indicator for further testing rather than the source for a definitive diagnosis.

An individual's BMI can be determined by dividing their weight in kilograms (kg) by the square of their height in meters (m²).

$$BMI = weight\ (kg)/\ height^2\ (m^2)$$

The same number can be calculated in feet (ft) and pounds (lbs) by dividing their weight in pounds (lbs) by the square of their height (ft²) and multiplying the result by 4.88.

$$BMI = [weight\ (lbs)/\ height^2\ (ft^2)] * 4.88$$

The standard weight categories associated with BMI ranges (for adults) are as follows:

BMI	Weight Status
<14.9	Starvation
15.0–18.4	Underweight
18.5–22.9	Normal
23–27.9	Overweight
30 and above	Obese

OBESITY IN AMERICA

Surveys conducted by the National Center for Health Statistics estimate that two-thirds of adults in the United States are overweight, one-third are obese, and that the average adult's waistline keeps growing each year (4). The obesity rates among African-Americans and Latinos are even higher, and the overall obesity rate varies according to income, disproportionately affecting the poor and lower-income Americans (4). In a recent *Time/ABC News* poll, 58% of Americans indicated they would like to lose weight, but only half of those surveyed were actually trying to slim down (5). By some estimates, Americans spend more than $30 billion a year on weight loss products and services, but the real economic costs of obesity, in terms of healthcare costs, lost productivity, etc. easily exceed $100 billion annually (6,7). Most of the overweight people recognize the problem, yet they are not taking the necessary steps to actually lose weight and keep it off.

There are a number of well-documented causes for weight gain and obesity, but in the simplest terms, an increase in BMI results from an imbalance of caloric consumption and energy expenditure—in other words, eating too much and not getting enough exercise. While genetics, overall health, and a host of other factors play a significant role in governing the body's ability to burn calories, an increase (or a decrease) in BMI must always be the result of an imbalance of energy.

In order to maintain a certain weight, the energy "in" must equal the energy "out."

Every calorie counts and there are no quick fixes. A trendy 30-day diet cannot undo a lifetime of poor nutritional choices. Eating habits are—by their very nature—habitual. The body develops a physiological and psychological dependence on consuming certain volumes and types of food, and regardless of whether or not these habits are healthy, they are incredibly difficult to change. It takes an enormous amount of will power and self-discipline to lose weight.

Genetics may play a role in governing the body's ability to efficiently burn calories, and more importantly, it may affect the distribution of fat throughout the body, but genetics alone cannot explain the rapid increase in the overall obesity rate in America. Obesity may have strong genetic determinants, but the genetic composition of the human population does not change rapidly. And the rapid change in obesity rates must reflect major changes in nongenetic factors. The rise in obesity reflects a social and cultural phenomenon, but obesity itself—an individual's weight—must always be the result of his or her lifestyle choices. Personal choice—in the form of diet and exercise (or the lack thereof)—is all that ultimately governs an individual's weight (8).

Apart from aesthetic concerns and rising healthcare costs, obesity has other implications. The BMI serves as an important marker for a number of obesity-related illnesses. In the simplest terms, the human body operates like a machine. It is designed to work within certain tolerances and only under certain conditions. An increase in weight beyond the normative BMI range increases the strain on the body's systems. And much like any machine, the body is more likely to fail if more strain is exerted on any of its systems.

OBESITY, THE METABOLIC SYNDROME, AND OUR GENERAL HEALTH

Excess weight correlates with a number of generalized health problems such as heart disease, high blood pressure, stroke, type 2 diabetes, incontinence (bladder control problems), osteoarthritis, infertility, and several forms of cancer. And to make matters worse, the overall complication rate for many of the surgeries necessary to correct these problems increases along with the BMI (9).[1]

In other words, the more overweight the persons are, the more likely they are to develop a serious—and potentially life threatening—medical condition, and the less likely it becomes that surgery will be able to correct the problem (10,11).

While surgical procedures such as gastric bypass can be used to address the underlying cause of obesity, physicians and their patients are increasingly turning to less invasive cosmetic procedures to minimize the impact of obesity. Body contouring procedures such as liposuction and abdominoplasty, carried out in conjunction with a sensible weight loss regimen, can refine the shape and contours of the body once a normal BMI has been achieved.

DIFFERENCES BETWEEN CELLULITE AND EXCESS FAT

The difference between excess fat and cellulite is a source of confusion, amongst both physicians and patients alike. Excess fat simply addresses the concern of being overweight while cellulite addresses the appearance of skin due to underlying adipose tissue anatomy. Cellulite is the dimpling of skin seen most commonly on the buttock and thighs of postpubescent women (12). Most likely, the appearance of cellulite is due to the fibrous septae structure of postpubescent female adipose tissue; these weak fibrous septae facilitate fat herniation into the dermis, creating the dimpled appearance of cellulite. It is important to note that unlike excess volume of subcutaneous fat, the presence of cellulite has no negative implications on one's overall health. Cellulite is estimated to be present in 85–95% of postpubertal women and is more common in Caucasian than in Asian women (13,14). The preponderance of cellulite suggests its role as a normal, structural phenotype rather than an abnormal pathologic condition.

Western media directs a large amount of attention to the treatment of cellulite, thus spawning tremendous commercial interest in the development of cellulite therapies. Ads can be found for topical creams, massage, exercise programs, and a variety of technologies. As excess fat and cellulite are different entities, it is important to note that a technology or procedure that effectively treats excess fat may have no effect on the formation of cellulite, and vice versa. Unfortunately, much of the public marketing confuses cellulite formation with being overweight, creating great ambiguity as to which treatments may or may not be effective.

GOALS OF BODY CONTOURING PROCEDURES

Just as the goal of an overweight person on a diet is to achieve a normal BMI, the goal of the plastic surgeon is to restore a patient's normal appearance. "Normal" in this context may be a somewhat relative term. Our perception of physical attractiveness varies according to age, culture, and geography, but there are some standards which appear to be nearly universal.

In men, an attractive healthy physique is a tall, symmetrical stature; a V-shaped torso with a slim waist; a waist-to-shoulder ratio of 0.75 or lower; a smooth, clean complexion; thick hair; and clear eyes.

In women, an attractive figure constitutes a waist-to-hip ratio of 0.70 with symmetrical facial features; full lips; relatively full breasts; a clear complexion; thick hair; and clear eyes.

What makes these qualities attractive may be debatable, but a tour through any major art gallery will confirm that they are both universal and timeless. Consider Michelangelo's *David*, sculpted in 1504; or the *Venus de Milo*, created sometime between 130 and 100 BC. Both exhibit qualities that we find attractive even today and the movie stars of yesteryear could easily grace the covers of today's fashion magazines.

Of course, cosmetic surgery cannot turn anyone into a fashion model, any more than a gym membership can turn an armchair quarterback into a professional football player. But it can increase a person's overall attractiveness and beauty. In the case of a formerly overweight or obese patient

---

[1]Recent studies conducted at the Memorial Sloan–Kettering Cancer Center and elsewhere have noted exceptions to this rule; however, further study will be needed to determine whether the decrease in complication rates associated with >25 BMI is a result of earlier diagnosis and treatment, changes in perioperative technique, or postoperative care. Regardless, there can be no doubt that a patient with a normal BMI has a greater chance of a positive surgical outcome with a lower risk of complications than an overweight or obese patient.

who has gone through the rigors necessary to reduce his or her BMI, such a change can directly impact his or her overall quality of life and make it easier for them to maintain a healthy weight.

In general, breast and body contouring procedures should only be performed on patients within 20% of their ideal weight or with a BMI less than 25. A BMI higher than 25 increases the likelihood of surgical complications and would decrease the long-term benefits of an elective cosmetic procedure.

CONCLUSIONS

Obesity is an epidemic in America that unfortunately shows no signs of dissipating anytime soon. Unfortunately, obesity is much more serious than just a cosmetic concern, as it can have severe impacts on patient's general health and greatly reduce their life expectancy. While many patients present to cosmetic surgeons to "cure" their obesity, it is important to remember that the only real cure is for the patient to lose weight. Body contouring procedures should be viewed as an additional treatment, with exercise and a healthy diet, to help patients achieve their cosmetic goals.

REFERENCES

1. Mokdad AH, Marks JS, Stroup DF, Gerberding JL. Actual causes of death in the United States, 2000. JAMA 2004; 291: 1238–45.
2. Ogden CL, Carroll MD, McDowell MA, Flegal KM. "Obesity among adults in the United States – no change since 2003–2004." NCHS data brief no 1. Hyattsville, MD: National Center for Health Statistics, 2007.
3. Gadzik J. 'How much should i weigh?' - Quetelet's equation, upper weight limits and BMI prime. Conn Med 2006; 70: 81–8.
4. Centers for Disease Control and Prevention. National Center for Health Statistics. "National Health and Nutrition Examination Survey." 2002.
5. ABC NEWS/AOL Poll. Overweight in America – 12/13/05: conducted December 13–15, 2005. Data collection and tabulation by ICR-International Communications Research of Media, Pa.
6. Finkelstein EA, Fiebelkorn IC, Wang G. National medical spending attributable to overweight and obesity: how much, and who's paying? Health Aff 2003; W3: 219–26.
7. Larkin M. "Ways to win at weight loss." FDA Consumer. Publication No. (FDA) 98–1287
8. Hill JO, Trowbridge FL. Childhood obesity: future directions and research priorities. Pediatrics 1998; 101: 570–4.
9. Barrera R, Arslan V, Gebrayel N, Melendez J. Body mass index as a predictor of complications and length of hospital stay after thoracic surgery. Nutr Clin Pract 2000; 15: 181–4.
10. O'Brien JM Jr, Phillips GS, Ali NA, et al. Body mass index is independently associated with hospital mortality in mechanically ventilated adults with acute lung injury. Crit Care Med 2006; 34: 738–44.
11. Pasulka PS, Bistrian BR, Benotti PN, Blackburn GL. The risks of surgery in obese patients. Ann Intern Med 1986; 104: 540–6.
12. Avram MM. Cellulite: a review of its physiology and treatment. J Cosmet Laser Ther 2004; 6:181–5.
13. Nürnberger F, Müller G. So-called cellulite: an invented disease. J Dermatol Surg Oncol 1978; 4: 221–9.
14. Draelos ZD. In search of answers regarding cellulite. Cosmet Dermatol 2001; 14: 55–8.

4.3   Approach to cellulite and fat

4.3.1   Lasers and noninvasive body contouring treatments
Daniel I. Wasserman, Mathew Avram, and Andrew Nelson

KEY POINTS

- While invasive technologies remain the gold standard for fat removal, emerging non-invasive technologies may represent effective treatment options for the proper patient
- Physical technologies attempt to modulate fat through massage, mobilizing the fat into lymphatics for drainage
- Nonspecific technologies such as radiofrequency, ultrasound, and nonspecific lasers heat the dermis and fat, resulting in fat modulation
- Fat-specific lasers are being developed, but are not commercially available at present
- Cryolipolysis, that is, controlled cold exposure, can be used to cause apoptosis of fat and slow removal of excess adipose tissue
- All of these noninvasive treatments for fat and cellulite should be considered as new, emerging technologies. It is important to closely evaluate these technologies from an evidence-based perspective before incorporating them into your practice

---

For decades, fat has been considered a "neglected subject" within medicine (1). However, with advances in research and clinical applications, the field of fat has undergone significant change. It is now clear that excess fat not only has significant cosmetic implications, but is also a cause of serious medical illnesses. Weight loss and diet have emerged as national obsessions, not just in the United States but around the world. As a result, there have been many industrious attempts to treat unwanted fat both invasively and noninvasively.

Liposuction remains the gold standard for reducing unwanted fat. Unfortunately, while liposuction is extremely effective, it remains an invasive procedure associated with patient discomfort, the need for general or tumescent anesthesia, risk of bruising, and prolonged healing time. In the last decade, there has been a significant shift in cosmetic procedures toward noninvasive, minimal downtime techniques as patients become more reluctant to undergo invasive surgeries. Less invasive physical modalities to treat fat have been developed and many more are in the process of being released to market. These devices employ several approaches for the treatment of fat, including a reduction in the overall volume of fat, improvement in the appearance of cellulite, and skin tightening without the reduction of fat.

This chapter will focus on those therapies that employ light or light-related technologies for the treatment of undesired fat and the appearance of cellulite. Because noninvasive treatments of fat and cellulite are still in their infancy, it is important to critically appraise these technologies. These new technologies are making a slow, steady progress toward an effective, safe, noninvasive treatment for fat and cellulite.

PHYSICAL TREATMENTS FOR CELLULITE

Endermologie (LPG systems, Cedex, France) is an FDA-cleared device for the treatment of cellulite. Endermologie is a hand-held device which utilizes both negative and positive pressure to knead and roll the skin. The combination of these two pressures results in physical manipulation and deep massage of the tissue, necessitating the use of a special LPG suit to protect the skin (2). Typically, treatments are performed twice weekly, with a treatment session lasting approximately 45 minutes. It is purported that Endermologie modulates and improves cellulite by breaking down subcutaneous fat, while also improving blood and lymphatic flow (3,4). Many of the more recent technologies for the treatment of fat and cellulite utilize a similar massage mechanism as Endermologie, in combination with other therapeutic modalities.

A recent clinic study of 33 women treated with Endermologie for 15 sessions demonstrated a statistically significant improvement in the appearance of cellulite, as assessed by a visual scale (2); however, only five of the 33 patients had actually demonstrated clinical improvement. Furthermore, there was no untreated control area for comparison in this study. Statistically significant improvements were also noted in the circumference of the treated areas, but these improvements were modest. The treatments were well tolerated, with common mild adverse events such as pain (33% of treated patients) and ecchymosis (9%) developing when higher negative pressure settings were utilized. Overall, this study shows modest potential for Endermologie as a treatment of cellulite.

RADIOFREQUENCY

At the turn of the 20th century, Nikola Tesla first recognized the heating of biological tissues with radiofrequency (RF) current. Subsequent collaboration between the physicist William T. Bovie and surgeon Harvey Cushing produced the first widely accepted RF generator (5). These contributions laid the foundation for the application and implementation of RF devices in medicine.

RF is the electromagnetic wave frequency between audio and infrared that ranges from approximately 1.0×10^5 nm to about 3.0×10^{13} nm. RF treatments can be defined as the destruction or modulation of biological tissues using electricity from an unmodulated, sinusoidal wave, alternating current at wavelengths that fall into the range for RF signaling. The ionic influences near the device applicator attempt to drive the ions to follow the changes in direction of the alternating current. This ionic flow causes molecular frictional heating low enough to confine energy transmission to a controllable tissue mass without generating excessive radiation, and without stimulating neuromuscular reaction and electrolysis (6). This heat energy is generated so that the tissue, rather than the device itself, is the source of heat (7). Aside from their role in a variety of medical subspecialties, RF devices represent a growing segment of the cosmetic industry specifically geared toward the treatment of subcutaneous fat and/or cellulite.

RF devices nonspecifically heat the dermis in order to produce a remodeling effect, possibly altering native collagen or stimulating the production of neocollagen (6). Adipose tissue may be heated more readily than the dermis due to its inherent high electrical resistance. The heat transfer coefficient of fat is much lower than that of the dermis so the heat produced in the dermis spreads better than that accumulated by adipocytes (8). When heated by a nearby RF source, adipose tissue can rise in temperature approximately seven fold in comparison with that of the dermis (9). Thus heat can be confined to fat effectively. The application of RF for the improvement of cellulite is based on the modulation of the adipose layer's fibrous septae scaffolding in order to create a better appearance of the natural outpouchings of the underlying fat chambers.

The most frequently studied RF devices for the treatment of fat are the VelaSmooth™ (Syneron Medical Ltd, Yokneam, Israel) and VelaShape™ (Syneron Medical Ltd, Yokneam, Israel) which combine massage, vacuum suction, bipolar RF, and infrared light (700–2000 nm). (Figs. 4.3.1.1,4.3.1.2,4.3.1.3)

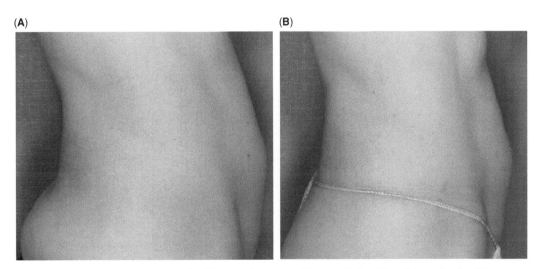

(A)   (B)

Figure 4.3.1.1 Clinical improvement in the appearance of the abdomen of a 60-year-old woman before (**A**) and 3 months after (**B**) treatment with VelaShape. Baseline circumference 87 cm; 3 month follow-up circumference 84 cm.   *Source*: Photos courtesy of Dr Lori Brightman.

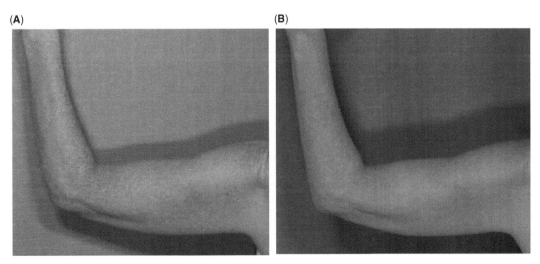

(A)   (B)

Figure 4.3.1.2 Clinical improvement in the appearance of the arms of a 55-year-old woman before (**A**) and 6 months after (**B**) 5 treatments with VelaShape. 5 treatments, radiofrequency level 3, infrared level 2, Vacuum level 1, and treatment duration 7 minutes 45 seconds. Baseline circumference: 27.75 cm; mean 6 month follow-up circumference: 26.9 cm.   *Source*: Photos courtesy of Dr Lori Brightman.

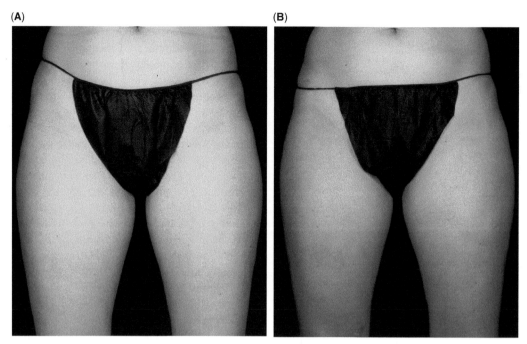

Figure 4.3.1.3 Clinical improvement in the appearance of the thighs of a 41-year-old woman before (**A**) and 6 months after (**B**) treatments with VelaShape. 5 treatments, radiofrequency level 3, infrared level 2. Vacuum level 1, treatment duration 3 minutes 53 seconds and 10 minutes 10 seconds. Mean baseline measurement: 58.5; mean 6 month follow-up measurement: 56.8 cm.   *Source*: Photos courtesy of Dr Lori Brightman.

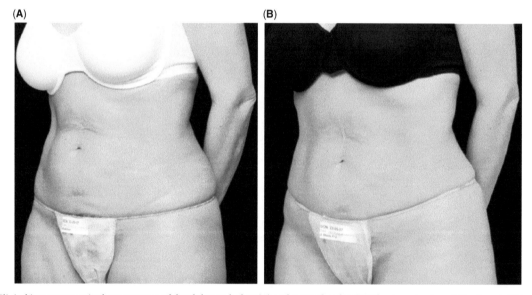

Figure 4.3.1.4 Clinical improvement in the appearance of the abdomen before (**A**) and 4 months after (**B**) Thermage treatment. Treatment: 300 pulses, Treatment level range 2.0–5.0. Baseline measurement: 79.2 cm; 4 month follow-up measurement: 78.5 cm.   *Source*: Photos courtesy of Dr Lori Brightman.

Sadick and Mulholland first evaluated two patient groups (a total of 35 patients) with a twice-weekly treatment for four weeks or eight weeks, with no control group (10). Nearly two-thirds of the total patients treated had improvement of up to 50%; however, histological analyses failed to demonstrate any difference between treated and untreated skin. Several studies have since demonstrated this very modest but often temporary improvement (11–14). Nootheti et al. performed a head-to-head study of VelaSmooth™ (Syneron Medical Ltd, Yokneam, Israel) versus TriActive™ (Cynosure Inc, Westford, Massachusetts, USA) for the treatment of lower extremity (thigh) cellulite in 20 patients twice a week for 6 weeks (15). TriActive combines mechanical massage with 808-nm diode laser light to stimulate fibroblasts and collagen production. Both devices demonstrated a modest improvement in upper and lower thigh circumferences, but there was no statistically significant difference between the outcomes of the two devices. Cellulite appearance, based on average improvement in smoothness, was mildly improved overall for both devices, but again lacked statistically significant difference between the two devices. The perceived grade change of cellulite was calculated by comparing the values from before and after treatment; this was again modest and failed to reveal any statistical difference between the two devices. Bruising incidence and intensity were 30% higher in the VelaSmooth (seven subjects) than in the TriActive system (one patient).

Unipolar RF devices have also been developed for the treatment of cellulite and fat. Thermage™ (Solta Medical Inc, Hayward, California, USA) utilizes monopolar capacitively coupled RF energy to tighten and contour skin; in clinical practice, Thermage may show modest improvements in skin tightening and contouring (Fig. 4.3.1.4 A&B). Goldberg et al., using a new unipolar volumetric RF device, treated 30 patients for six sessions, every other week. Each session consisted of a total of 150–170 W for 30 seconds (16). A mean decrease in leg circumference of 2.45 cm was reported, but the authors failed to reveal individual or group data and did not use any negative controls. Histologic comparisons between pretreatment and post-treatment biopsies revealed an increase in dermal fibrosis; however, MRIs failed to demonstrate any change in the panniculus, and post-treatment histological photographs were not provided.

The heat generated by RF devices can result in adverse events related to overheating most often related to pulse stacking, grid overlap, or aggressive settings. The latter is often a result of users' attempts to decrease the number of passes required by increasing the delivered amount of energy per pass. Damaged fibrous septae adjacent to adipose tissue appeared to be particularly susceptible to RF heat damage, which may in turn provide some of the therapeutic benefit seen in the treatment of cellulite (17). In a retrospective review of 757 treatment sessions across 259 patients treated for facial wrinkles and facial rejuvenation, the adverse events that were observed in greater than 1% of the total number of sessions were erythema 24 hours post treatment (1.22%), second-degree burn (2.70%), and severe pain (11.49%) (18).

While RF is an exciting technology for the treatment of fat, its unpredictable results, guarded patient tolerance, combined with its treatment cost prevents it from being more widely accepted. Refinements to this technology, however, may produce more clinical benefit in the future.

ULTRASOUND

The application of ultrasound technology, for uses other than the more traditional role of imaging, has been a rapidly expanding area of medical technologies. Well-known examples include noninvasive focused ultrasound for the ablation of tumors and shock wave therapy for renal calculi. Nonfocused ultrasound has traditionally been used for physiotherapy. As ultrasound technology continues to develop, aesthetic applications for this approach have been growing.

Recently, focused, noninvasive ultrasound technologies have begun to emerge as nonsurgical alternatives to the removal of fat. Currently, there are no FDA-approved ultrasound devices for the removal of subcutaneous fat commercially available in the United States. The Ultrashape™ Contour I (Ultrashape, Tel Aviv, Israel) is being used in Europe and the United Kingdom. The system focuses ultrasound waves to deliver concentrated acoustic energy into a focal volume at a precise depth in the subcutaneous tissue without damaging neighboring structures due to their differential susceptibility to mechanical stresses (19).

In a phase II, prospective, nonrandomized, controlled trial of 164 patients, 137 underwent one treatment to the abdomen, thighs, or flanks; they demonstrated mean circumference reductions of 2.3 cm, 1.8 cm, and 1.6 cm respectively, at 12 weeks. There was no statistical difference between the treatment sites, but there was a statistical difference from baseline at all time points except day 1. Approximately 77% of the observed circumference reduction took place within 14 days of treatment. Internal controls of untreated thighs revealed significant differences between the untreated and treated thighs. Interestingly, there was no statistically significant weight reduction in either the treated or untreated groups (20).

In a prospective, noncontrolled trial using Ultrashape Contour I, patients found similar improvements in the circumference of all treated areas in all patients after three treatments. The outer thighs and abdomen demonstrated the greatest degree of improvement with cumulative mean reductions and standard deviations of 4.60 ± 2.12 cm and 4.15 ± 2.30 cm respectively (17). Additional studies are needed in order to reproduce and substantiate the results seen to date. There is no peer-reviewed literature on other ultrasound technologies currently being developed for the treatment of fat.

Ultrasound in Combination with Liposuction

Surgical adjuncts using ultrasound were developed for both invasive and noninvasive assistance of traditional liposuction (ultrasound-assisted liposuction). Both of these external and internal approaches have been commercialized for use. Despite having direct effects on subcutaneous fat, their role is to assist the mechanical debridement of fat in liposuction. A full discussion of these technologies is beyond the scope of this chapter.

LASERS AND LIGHT SOURCES

The selective destruction of fat using light sources is a very active area of research. At this time, the only commercial laser devices using laser to specifically remove fat are in the setting of laser-assisted liposuction. There are several wavelengths currently being marketed, all with the promise to facilitate the removal of fat, allow for faster procedure time, decrease the physical demands on the surgeon, and improve postoperative patient morbidity (21).

Many lasers have been studied and marketed as fat modulating lasers. However, these lasers do not specifically target adipose tissue, but rather target the dermis. In reality, the clinical effects of these technologies are likely due to nonspecific heating of the dermis and subcutis, which may cause remodeling of the collagen. This remodeling is thought to improve the appearance of excess fat and cellulite. As these devices do not specifically target the fatty tissue, their clinical effects are limited.

Intense-pulsed light (IPL) therapy and lasers in the visible and near infrared portion of the electromagnetic spectrum have been shown to induce new collagen formation and improve facial rhytides (22–24). In a split-sided, nonrandomized, unblinded study, Fink et al. used a combination treatment of retinyl cream and IPL for the treatment of cellulite. A majority of patients reported improvement, however, there was no objective observer and all patient results were judged by patient self-improvement ratings (25). The use of IPL has been employed for fat-related treatments, not to selectively remove fat, but to induce dermal changes with the production of new collagen. The new dermal collagen, and possibly thicker

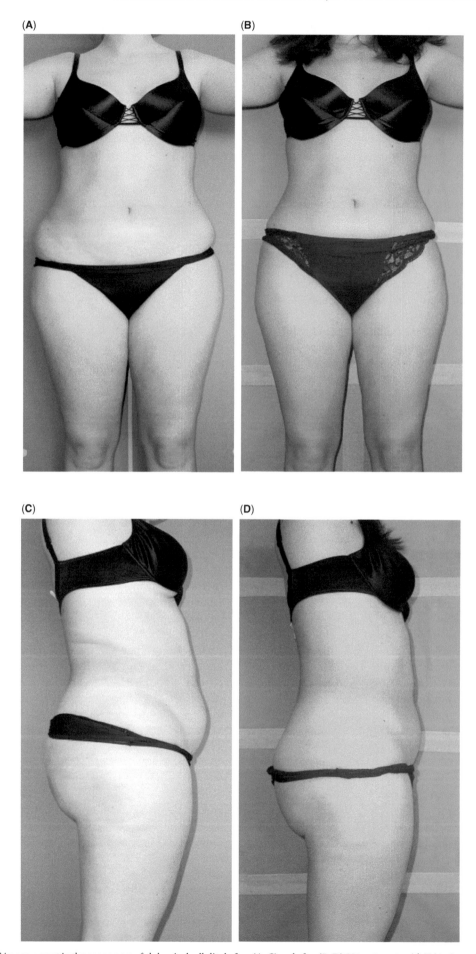

Figure 4.3.1.5 Clinical improvement in the appearance of abdominal cellulite before (**A, C**) and after (**B, D**) 20 treatments with TriActive.   *Source*: Photos courtesy of Andrea Pelosi, Milan.

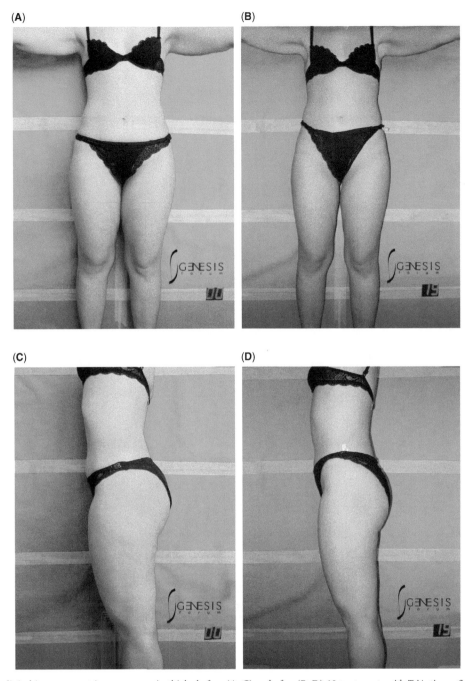

Figure 4.3.1.6 Marked clinical improvement in appearance in thighs before (**A**, **C**) and after (**B**, **D**) 19 treatments with TriActive.   *Source*: Photos courtesy of Andrea Pelosi, Milan.

dermis, assists to blunt the visual appearance of fat. Unless IPL devices are able to induce true fat destruction, their role in fat-related disorders should be viewed, at best, as limited.

The TriActive device (Cynosure, Westford, Massachusetts, USA) is FDA cleared for the treatment of cellulite. This device combines the suction massage mechanism of Endermologie with low-intensity diode laser (808 nm) pulsation and superficial contact cooling. It is thought that this combination improves the appearance of cellulite by increasing lymphatic drainage, improving blood flow, and simultaneously tightening skin in the treated areas. Patients are typically treated with the device twice weekly. In any given treatment, approximately 15–30 passes with the device are performed (Figs. 4.3.1.5 and 4.3.1.6). In clinical studies, the TriActive device has been shown to have a modest effect in improving the appearance of

cellulite (26). A second clinical study demonstrated that 25% of patients treated with the TriActive device showed clinical improvement in the appearance of cellulite following 12 treatments; furthermore, improvements in the thigh circumference were noted. The device was well tolerated, although approximately 20% of patients reported mild bruising following the treatment (27).

The SmoothShape device (Eleme Medical, Merrimack, New Hampshire, USA) also combines a suction and mechanical massage mechanism similar to Endermologie with laser treatments. The SmoothShape device utilizes a dual wavelength laser system to treat subcutaneous fat. The 915 nm laser output is thought to be relatively preferentially absorbed by lipids, thereby resulting in fat liquefaction. The second wavelength, 650 nm, is thought to modify the permeability of the fat cell

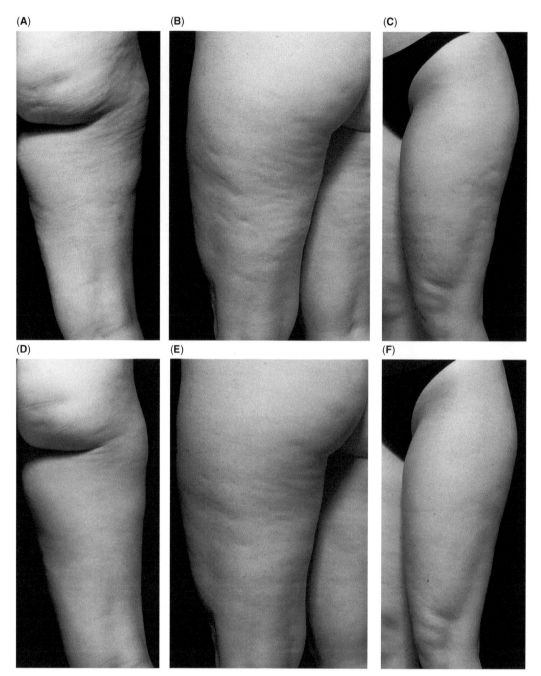

Figure 4.3.1.7 Clinical improvement in thigh circumference and texture before (**A,B,C**) and after (**D,E,F**) 8 treatments with SmoothShape.   *Source*: Photos courtesy of Khalil A. Khatri, MD.

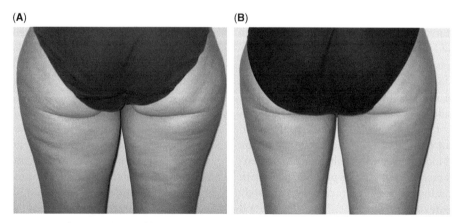

Figure 4.3.1.8 Clinical improvement in the upper thigh and buttocks before (**A**) and after (**B**) 9 treatments with SmoothShape, resulting in a smoother skin and reduction in thigh circumference.   *Source*: From Ref. (28).

membrane, thereby facilitating the liquefied fat to be mobilized into the interstitium. Patients are typically treated two to three times weekly with the SmoothShape device, with multiple passes of the device being performed in any given treatment (Figs. 4.3.1.7 and 4.3.1.8). In a recent clinical study, the SmoothShape device was shown to result in a significant improvement in the thickness of the subcutaneous fat pad dimensions, as assessed by MRI (28). In the clinical study, one leg was treated with the laser while the other served as a control, which was treated with massage alone. The authors observed a 1.19-cm² improvement from baseline in the leg treated with the SmoothShape device compared to a 3.82 cm² increase in the untreated control leg; 82% of the patients in the study responded to treatment. The device was well tolerated, with the only reported adverse event being an occasional increase in urinary frequency.

FAT-SPECIFIC LASERS

At present, no commercial laser device targeting fat specifically with selective photothermolysis has been FDA approved. The absorption spectrum of lipid rests within the infrared portion of the electromagnetic spectrum as a result of their large amounts of CH and CH₂ bonds. For most of lipid's absorption spectrum, water acts as the dominant target. Using a tunable free electron laser, Anderson et al. detailed the absorption spectrum of lipid-rich subcutaneous fat. They demonstrated lipid's selective absorbance at 1210 nm and 1720 nm (29). In addition, the subcutaneous fat was selectively destroyed at 1210 nm, while nonselective thermal injury was seen throughout the entire dermis as near as 1250 nm.

The 1210-nm band provides for a particularly attractive wavelength to treat fat. The near- and mid-infrared spectral region of about 900–2800 nm encompasses the most tissue-penetrating optical wavelengths (30). The greatest penetration is seen around 1200 nm, paralleling one of lipid's absorption peaks. Anderson et al., in the above study, observed a selective fat destruction up to at least 0.5 cm in depth. Development of a laser at this wavelength is currently underway. Whether focused energy at this wavelength can selectively ablate subcutaneous fat deposits or thermally damage subcutaneous fat pockets and their associated fibrous structures poses important questions when considering the prospect of body contouring versus cellulite treatment with the use of a 1210-nm laser.

COMBINATION DEVICES

Many new devices have been developed which combine several therapeutic technologies in an attempt to achieve greater clinical efficacy. Typically, these devices utilize a physical manipulation and suction mechanism to massage the tissue; in addition, they also incorporate RF energy as well as a laser or light source. VelaSmooth, combining bipolar RF energy with an infrared light source, represents one such example. In the future, we expect that more devices will continue to use this multitechnology-based approach in order to maximize the potential efficacy of these devices. Perhaps by combining the effects of multiple modalities, a synergistic improvement will be possible. This continues to be an active area of research in noninvasive body contouring technologies.

CRYOLIPOLYSIS

Cryolipolysis™ (Zeltiq Aesthetics, Pleasanton, California, USA) is a new technology based on the clinical observation that cold exposure, under the proper circumstances, can result in localized panniculitis with the reduction and clearance of fat. This phenomenon known as "popsicle panniculitis" was initially observed in children(31,32).

Cryolipolysis utilizes controlled fat cooling, "energy extraction," to cause apoptosis of the adipocytes. Approximately two days following the treatment, this adipocyte apoptosis causes localized inflammation of the fat layer. As this inflammation clears over the next several weeks, macrophages engulf the adipocytes and the excess fat is slowly eliminated from the body. The entire process takes approximately three to four months to observe the full clinical effect of cryolipolysis. The Zeltiq CoolSculpting system is commercially available and is presently FDA cleared for the noninvasive reduction of fat, skin cooling, and other various indications.

Initial clinical trials have demonstrated promising results for cryolipolysis. A multicenter, prospective, nonrandomized clinical study evaluating the use of cryolipolysis for fat layer reduction of the flanks (i.e., love handles) and back (i.e., back fat pads) was conducted at 12 sites (33). Each patient was treated

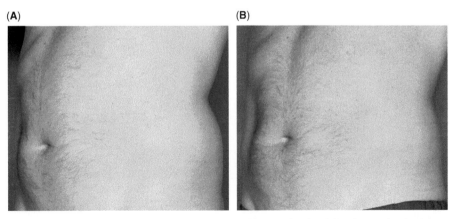

Figure 4.3.1.9 Clinical improvement in the appearance of the abdomen of a 56–year-old man at baseline (**A**) and 2 months after (**B**) a single treatment with Zeltiq. Breeze device, Vacuum, Massage 60 minutes each. Baseline: 88 cm; FU 2-month circumference: 86 cm. *Source*: Photos courtesy of Dr Lori Brightman.

on one side, while the contralateral side served as a control. The majority of patients had a clinical change following their treatment, as assessed by physician observation and digital photography four months post treatment. A subset of the patients underwent ultrasound imaging to further determine the effect of cryolipolysis; an average reduction of 22.4% was noted in the thickness of the fat layer following cryolipolysis. Cryolipolysis has also been shown to significantly reduce abdominal fat, particularly in the periumbilical area (Fig. 4.3.1.9) (34). The best cosmetic results with cryolipolysis are achieved in those patients with a modest, discrete fat bulge. Cryolipolysis therefore appears to be a promising new technology for noninvasive fat treatment in the proper patient.

Cryolipolysis is well tolerated by patients in clinical practice. Following treatment, the skin is cool and firm. Bruising may develop, as the device utilizes a vacuum system to increase its efficacy. Cryolipolysis has also been shown to cause temporary numbness and altered sensation in the treated area, which can last up to a few weeks. Finally, no clinically significant alterations in lipid profiles or liver function tests have been observed following cryolipolysis.

CONCLUSIONS

Many of the emerging technologies for the treatment of unwanted fat and cellulite offer limited gains for the patient. The technologies employed are exciting new ways for noninvasive cosmetic enhancements, but still fall short of their advertised rewards. As new devices continue to be released to the public, it is important to understand the mechanisms of these devices in order to properly anticipate the clinical and histological gains that patients seek. Noninvasive fat and cellulite treatments, at present, should be considered as new, emerging technologies and should be regarded with a healthy dose of skepticism before they enter mainstream medical practice.

REFERENCES

1. Wells HG. Adipose tissue, a neglected subject. JAMA 1940; 114: 2177–83.
2. Tülin Güleç A. Treatment of cellulite with LPG endermologie. Int J Dermatol 2009; 48: 265–70.
3. Ersek RA, Mann GE 2nd, Salisbury S, et al. Noninvasive mechanical body contouring: a preliminary clinical outcome study. Aesthetic Plast Surg 1997; 21: 61–7.
4. Chang P, Wiseman J, Jacoby T, et al. Noninvasive mechanical body contouring: (Endermologie) a one-year clinical outcome study update. Aesthetic Plast Surg 1998; 22: 145–53.
5. Ni Y, Mulier S, Miao Y, Michel L, Marchal G. A review of the general aspects of radiofrequency ablation. Abdom Imaging 2005; 30: 381–400.
6. Zelickson BD, Kist D, Bernstein E, et al. Histological and ultrastructural evaluation of the effects of a radiofrequency-based nonablative dermal remodelling device. Arch Dermatol 2004; 140: 204–9.
7. Organ LW. Electrophysiologic principles of radiofrequency lesion making. Appl Neurophysiol 1976–1977; 39: 69–76.
8. de Felipe I, Redondo P. Animal model to explain fat atrophy using nonablative radiofrequency. Dermatol Surg 2007; 33: 141–5.
9. Chou CK. Radiofrequency hyperthermia in cancer therapy. In: Bronzino JD, ed. The biomedical engineering handbook. Boca Raton (FL): CRC Press, 1995: 1424–30.
10. Sadick NS, Mulholland RS. A prospective clinical study to evaluate the efficacy and safety of cellulite treatment using the combination of optical and RF energies for subcutaneous tissue heating. J Cosmet Laser Ther 2004; 6:187–90.
11. Alster TS, Tanzi EL. Cellulite treatment using a novel combination radiofrequency, infrared light, and mechanical tissue manipulation device. J Cosmet Laser Ther 2005; 7: 81–5.
12. Wanitphakdeedecha R, Manuskiatti W. Treatment of cellulite with a bipolar radiofrequency, infrared heat, and pulsatile suction device: a pilot study. J Cosmet Dermatol 2006; 5: 284–8.
13. Sadick N, Magro C. A study evaluating the safety and efficacy of the Vela Smooth system in the treatment of cellulite. J Cosmet Laser Ther 2007; 9: 15–20.
14. Kulick M. Evaluation of the combination of radio frequency, infrared energy and mechanical rollers with suction to improve skin surface irregularities (cellulite) in a limited treatment area. J Cosmet Laser Ther 2006; 8: 185–90.
15. Nootheti PK, Magpantay A, Yosowitz G, Calderon S, Goldman MP. A single center, randomized, comparative, prospective clinical study to determine the efficacy of the VelaSmooth system versus the Triactive system for the treatment of cellulite. Lasers Surg Med 2006; 38: 908–12.
16. Goldberg DJ, Fazeli A, Berlin AL. Clinical, laboratory, and MRI analysis of cellulite treatment with a unipolar radiofrequency device. Dermatol Surg 2008; 34: 204–9.
17. Narins RS, Tope WD, Pope K, Ross EV. Overtreatment effects associated with a radiofrequency tissue-tightening device: rare, preventable, and correctable with subcision and autologous fat transfer. Dermatol Surg 2006; 32: 115–24.
18. de Felipe I, Del Cueto SR, Pérez E, Redondo P. Adverse reactions after nonablative radiofrequency: follow-up of 290 patients. J Cosmet Dermatol 2007; 6: 163–6.
19. IMoreno-Moraga J, Valero-Alte´s T, Martinez Riquelme Asarria-Marcosy MI, Royo de la Torre J. Body contouring by non-invasive transdermal focused ultrasound. Lasers Surg Med 2007; 39: 315–23.
20. Teitelbaum SA, Burns JL, Kubota J, et al. Noninvasive body contouring by focused ultrasound: safety and efficacy of the Contour I device in a multicenter, controlled, clinical study. Plast Reconstr Surg 2007; 120: 779–89.
21. Mann MW, Palm MD, Sengelmann RD. New advances in liposuction technology. Semin Cutan Med Surg 2008; 27: 72–82.
22. Goldberg DJ. New collagen formation after dermal remodeling with an intense pulsed light source. J Cutan Laser Ther 2000; 2: 59–61.
23. Bjerring P, Clement M, Heickendorff L, Egevist H, Kiernan M. Selective non-ablative wrinkle reduction by laser. J Cutan Laser Ther 2000; 2: 9–15.
24. Prieto VG, Diwan AH, Shea CR, Zhang P, Sadick NS. Effects of intense pulsed light and the 1,064 nm Nd:YAG laser on sun-damaged human skin: histologic and immunohistochemical analysis. Dermatol Surg 2005; 31: 522–5.
25. Fink JS, Mermelstein H, Thomas A, Trow R. Use of intense pulsed light and a retinyl-based cream as a potential treatment for cellulite: a pilot study. J Cosmet Dermatol 2006; 5: 254–62.
26. Boyce S, Pabby A, Chuchaltkaren P, Brazzini B, Goldman MP. Clinical evaluation of a device for the treatment of cellulite: TriActive. Am J Cosmet Surg 2005; 22: 233–7.
27. Nootheti PK, Magpantay A, Yosowitz G, Calderon S, Goldman MP. A single center, randomized, comparative, prospective clinical study to determine the efficacy of the VelaSmooth system versus the TriActive system for the treatment of cellulite. Lasers Surg Med 2006; 38: 908–12.
28. Lach E. Reduction of subcutaneous fat and improvement in cellulite appearance by dual-wavelength, low-level laser energy combined with vacuum and massage. J Cosmet Laser Ther 2008; 10: 202–9.
29. Anderson RR, Parrish JA. Selective photothermolysis: precise microsurgery by selective absorption of pulsed radiation. Science 1983; 220: 524–7.
30. Du Y, Hu XH, Cariveau M, et al. Optical properties of porcine skin dermis between 900 nm and 1500 nm. Phys Med Biol 2001; 46: 167–81.
31. Rotman H. Cold panniculitis in children. Arch Dermatol 1966; 94: 720–1.
32. Duncan WC, Freeman RG, Heaton CL. Cold panniculitis. Arch Dermatol 1966; 94: 722–4.
33. Dover J, Burns J, Coleman S, et al. A Prospective Clinical Study of Noninvasive Cryolypolysis for Subcutaneous Fat Layer Reduction – Interim Report of Available Subject Data. American Society for Laser Medicine & Surgery, Annual Meeting, 2009.
34. Rosales-Berber IA, Diliz-Perez E. Controlled cooling of subcutaneous fat for body reshaping. To be presented, 15th World Congress of the International Confederation for Plastic, Reconstructive and Aesthetic Surgery. New Delhi, 2009.

4.3.2 Liposuction
Andrew L. DaLio

KEY POINTS

- Liposuction is an effective treatment to remove localized excess fatty tissue
- Technique can be performed in different body areas, including abdomen, buttocks, arms, legs, and neck
- Multiple techniques have been developed such as dry, wet, super-wet, and tumescent methods. Most of the liposuction cases are performed using super-wet or tumescent techniques
- Common complications associated with liposuction include bruising and hematoma formation, superficial contour irregularities, seromas, and altered sensation
- Potentially dangerous complications can be deep venous thrombosis formation, abdominal penetration, fat embolism, and significant fluid volume shifts following the procedure

---

Liposuction is consistently among the most common cosmetic surgical procedures performed in the United States (1). Simply put, it is a procedure whereby a cosmetic surgeon, using various techniques, removes excess fat from a patient's body. The fat comes out in the form of blood-tinged, yellow slurry with the consistency of cake batter. It's enough to make anyone want to skip dessert.

Fat distribution varies remarkably between men and women. Men tend to accumulate fat relatively evenly around their entire trunk, whereas women tend to build fatty deposits in focal areas such as the lower abdomen, flanks, hips, buttocks, and thighs (Fig. 4.3.2.1). Differences in the distribution of fat predetermine the natural zones optimal for elective liposuction.

However, not all fatty deposits are created equally: the location and composition of the fatty deposit determine whether it is amenable to liposuction. Typically, there is a deep layer composed of loose fatty tissue with few fibrous septae, and a superficial layer composed of much more dense fat within dense, firm fibrous septae. The deep layer can easily be removed through liposuction; however, the superficial layer must be approached with caution to avoid developing superficial contour irregularities postoperatively.

DIFFERENCES BETWEEN TREATING CELLULITE AND FAT

The septae holding fat and subcutaneous tissue together often causes a surface rippling or dimpling of the skin commonly referred to as "cellulite." Cellulite develops more frequently in women than men. The most accepted explanation for this is that, as women gain weight and their adipocytes hypertrophy,

their septae become inflexible and the fatty deposits between these fibrous bands begin to bulge.

Cellulite is not the cause for a person being overweight. Postadolescent women with an ideal body weight almost invariably exhibit some regional component of cellulite (2). In men, the septae are more tightly woven, which prevents the bulging appearance. Additionally, skin of men's thighs tends to be thicker than that of women, thus masking the rippling or dimpling associated with the increased buildup of fatty cells in the thigh region.

Liposuction is not a treatment for cellulite, and it can sometimes exacerbate the appearance of cellulite by "deflating" the underlying deep fatty layers and causing the skin to appear more rippled (3). Some surgeons advocate the use of aggressive pre- and postoperative massage to ameliorate the appearance of cellulite, and cosmetic companies recommend the use of topical or systemic therapy, but there is no scientific evidence to support the effectiveness of either of these approaches (4).

LIPOSUCTION TECHNIQUE

The basic goal of liposuction is to remove the right amount of fat to achieve a smooth, contoured appearance without disturbing the neighboring tissue, blood vessels, and connective tissue. In general, the surgery is performed using a cannula (a hollow tube) and an aspirator (suction device). Cannulas range tremendously in size and shape, which affect the volume and rate of fat removal, but the smaller cannulas typically have lower complication rates (5). The most common complication is an overresection of fat in one focal area, which results in superficial contour abnormalities. This can be avoided by using multiple access ports (small incisions

(A)   **(B)**

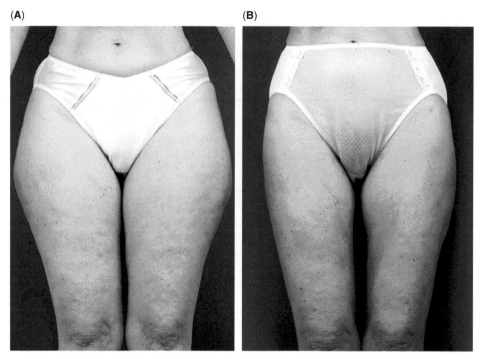

Figure 4.3.2.1 (**A**) A 62-year-old woman with inherent maldistribution of subcutaneous tissue. Note the classic "pear shape" of her body, with a fairly lean waist and upper torso, but significant subcutaneous tissue in the gluteal and hip area. (**B**) Postoperative result 1 year after she underwent 4-L liposuction of the hip, buttocks, and inner thighs.

used to insert the cannula into the fatty deposit) with cross-tunneling or overlapping cannula movement. The edges of the zone area are typically feathered with very small cannulas and minimal suctioning. This result of this technique will be a more even and smooth contour.

Liposuction can be performed under local anesthesia using lidocaine or bupivicaine as nerve blockers to numb the affected area, or under general anesthesia, in which case local nerve blockers are not necessary.

Subcutaneous tissue infiltration using saline or Ringer's lactate solution, coupled with epinephrine as a vasoconstrictor, promotes the ease of fat aspiration, minimizes blood loss, helps achieve a more even contour, and allows for a much larger volume of lipoaspirate (fat removal) than cases done without infiltration.

There are four basic liposuction infiltration volume techniques.

Dry (no infiltrate)
Wet (200–300 cc per treated area)
Super wet (1 cc infiltrate per 1 cc estimated lipoaspirate)
Tumescent (2–3 cc infiltrate per 1 cc estimated lipoaspirate)

Most commonly, liposuction is performed using the super-wet or tumescent technique. This approach requires approximately 20 minutes for maximal vasoconstriction prior to beginning the actual aspiration and offers an ideal balance between hemostasis and fluid retention while minimizing the impact of lidocaine toxicity. The traditional maximum dose of lidocaine with epinephrine is 7 mg/kg. In wet, super-wet, and tumescent liposuction methods, the lidocaine and epinephrine are injected into subcutaneous tissue, which delays absorption,

and much of the lidocaine is removed as part of the lipoaspirate. This raises the accepted maximum safe dosage to approximately 35 mg/kg. Under these conditions, absorption by the body may take anywhere from 12 to 36 hours.

Depending on the extent of the procedure, patients should be able to resume normal activities 2–14 days after surgery. A compression garment should be worn for two to four weeks to maintain the body's contours and minimize swelling and bruising. Over-the-counter pain medication should be sufficient to manage any postoperative discomfort.

POTENTIAL COMPLICATIONS ASSOCIATED WITH LIPOSUCTION

The overall complication rate in standard liposuction cases is quite low. Nevertheless, while liposuction may be a straightforward cosmetic procedure, there is the potential for significant morbidity. Some of the most potentially devastating complications are mentioned below:

Penetration of the underlying abdominal fascia with a perforation of the abdominal structure: Fascia is the soft connective tissue that permeates the human body. If the cannula is inserted too deeply, it can puncture the fascia beneath the targeted fatty deposit and potentially damage the underlying internal organs (such as the intestines). Any organ damage will require hospitalization and additional surgery to repair, and in rare instances, can potentially be fatal.

Deep venous thrombosis and subsequent pulmonary embolism: A deep venous thrombosis is a blood clot that forms in one of the body's deep veins, typically in the legs or pelvic region. If a clot forms in one of

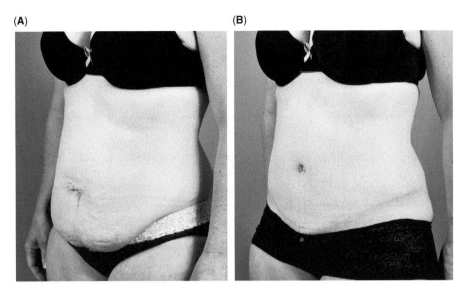

Figure 4.3.2.2 (**A**) A 48-year-old G2P2 woman with a moderate abdominal pannus. (**B**) Postoperative results 1 year after a full abdominoplasty with liposuction of the lateral abdominal and flank areas.

the major arteries or dislodges and becomes stuck in one of the arterial branch points, it can block the flow of blood through the circulatory system, resulting in chest pain, difficulty breathing, circulatory collapse, and sudden death.

Fat embolism: A fat embolism, much like a deep vein thrombosis, results from a blockage of fat entering the circulatory system and disrupting the flow of blood throughout the body. The mortality rate for an untreated fat embolism is approximately 1 in 10.

Fluid imbalance with either over- or underhydration: Fat stores much of the body's fluids. If too much fat is removed without an appropriate volume of fluid (saline) being replaced, potentially fatal dehydration could set in. If too much fluid is added to the body, it could cause organ damage to the heart, lungs, or kidneys.

However, the overall complication rate for liposuction is less than 0.7 % and as per the Food and Drug Administration reports the death rate is less than three per 100,000 procedures. Compared with car accidents, which result in 16 deaths per 100,000, liposuction is statistically safer than driving in rush hour traffic (6).

The more common complications resulting from liposuction are nowhere near as life-threatening. Some of these are listed below:

Hypoesthesia (a partial loss of sensation): Can be either temporary or permanent.

Seromas: A seroma is a pocket of clear fluid (much like a bruise) that builds up after surgery and will require drainage to heal properly.

Ecchymoses and hematomas: These are two different types of bruising. Ecchymoses are the result of damage to the capillaries which deliver the blood supply, and hematomas are bruises that develop as a result of internal bleeding. Hematomas may require additional surgery to correct.

Superficial contour irregularities.

CONCLUSIONS

Liposuction remains one of the most common and sought after surgical cosmetic procedures. In the right hands, liposuction can result in dramatic improvements in a patient's appearance and can help remove particularly troubling areas of excess fatty tissue (Fig. 4.3.2.2). Unfortunately, in the wrong hands, liposuction can result in many complications, both relatively minor cosmetic complications and potentially life-threatening outcomes. With this in mind, it is important that only proper patients are selected for liposuction and the procedure is performed by an experience cosmetic physician who specializes in the procedure.

REFERENCES

1. American Society of Plastic Surgeons website 2007. [Available from: http://www.plasticsurgery.org/media/statistics]
2. Ortonne JP, Zartarian M, Verschoore M, Queille-Roussel C, Duteil L. Cellulite and skin ageing: is there any interaction? J Eur Acad Dermatol Venereol 2008; 22: 827–34.
3. Iverson RE, Pao VS. Liposuction. Plast Reconstr Surg 2008; 121(Suppl 4): 1–11.
4. van Vliet M, Ortiz A, Avram MM, Yamauchi PS. An assessment of traditional and novel therapies for cellulite. J Cosmet Laser Ther 2005; 7: 7–10.
5. Coleman WP, Hendry SL. Principles of liposuction. Semin Cutan Med Surg 2006; 25: 138–44.
6. Liposuction information. US Food and Drug Administration: Center for Devices and Radiological Health, 2002.

The epidemic of obesity is now driving the field for patients seeking to lose their extra weight and regain their health. There are hit shows on television documenting the struggles of these patients as they lose weight. Unfortunately, many patients cannot achieve their ideal body through diet and exercise alone. Even if they do lose weight, patients may be left with extra, sagging skin. While some people may benefit from noninvasive laser therapies, or limited liposuction, there are still a large number of patients who will require more invasive, surgical correction.

ABDOMINOPLASTY

Most cultures consider a relatively narrow waist physically attractive, and scientists studying the perception of physical attractiveness have found that both sexes use the waist to hip ratio (WHR) when judging the attractiveness of women. In addition to being a mark of female beauty, it is viewed as an indicator of generalized good health and fertility (1). In Western cultures, a WHR of 0.7 is considered ideal. The classic measurement of 36-24-36 will yield a WHR of 0.67.

However, very few people are blessed with the genetics for a naturally ideal WHR. Poor dietary habits, childbirth, and BMI fluctuations resulting from negative changes in diet and exercise can all result in an increased abdominal girth and a less than desirable appearance. Ideally, diet, exercise, and lifestyle changes should be enough to restore the body's contours; when they are not, surgery can be used to rejuvenate the waistline.

Some changes in abdominal appearance are a natural part of the aging process. Potential patients will have to undergo a physical examination to determine whether an abdominoplasty will produce the desired results. The examination will focus on the quality of skin, the thickness of the subcutaneous layer (the fat and muscle beneath the skin), how it varies from one area to another, the integrity of the underlying musculofascial layer (the muscles and connective tissue that give the abdomen its form), and how the intra-abdominal fat affects the overall appearance of the abdomen. In men, the volume of intra-abdominal fat can often exceed the amount of fat present in the subcutaneous layer and may inhibit the ability of an abdominoplasty to yield the desired results.

Surgical Techniques for Abdominoplasties

Abdominoplasty can be of multiple types. They vary depending on the extent of the surgery and the desired outcome. However, as surgical procedures, they can be divided into three subcategories, which are discussed next.

The Full Abdominoplasty

The full abdominoplasty begins with an extended transverse crescent-shaped incision over the lower abdomen, with an extensive undermining and elevation of the abdominoplasty flap up to the level of the xiphiod and bilateral costal margins. The umbilicus is circumscribed and freed from the surrounding skin. The underlying musculofascial layer is imbricated and tightened as needed. Excess skin is excised, the wound is closed in layers, and the umbilicus is exteriorized in its appropriate anatomic position (Fig. 4.4.1).

In other words, a wide incision is made from hip to hip; the skin and fat are detached from the muscles of the abdomen; and the navel is detached from the muscle, fat, and connective tissue holding it in place. The surgeon then tightens the abdominal wall by repositioning the muscle and tissue into overlapping layers; skin from the upper abdomen is pulled down to tightly cover the belly; the excess skin and fat are cut away; the belly button is repositioned; and everything is sewn back together.

Liposuction can sometimes be used to aspirate (remove) fat from the lateral abdominal areas, but doing so increases the risk of ischemic postoperative complications. Ischemic complications are generally the result of trauma to the tissue which damages the blood vessels. An ischemic complication in an abdominoplasty could inhibit the body's ability to naturally restore blood flow to the skin and connective tissue pulled down over the abdomen and could require additional surgeries.

The Mini Abdominoplasty

As its name implies, the mini abdominoplasty is similar to the full abdominoplasty in terms of its surgical technique but has a much smaller scope. Rather than recontouring the entire abdomen, the surgeon targets the specific area around the patient's navel. By tightening the skin and muscle tissue under the belly button, the surgeon can redefine the shape of a patient's abdomen and achieve a more contoured appearance.

Ideal candidates for this procedure have mild skin and fascial laxity in the infraumbilical region of the abdomen. The procedure begins with a limited transverse abdominal incision. The abdominoplasty flap is elevated up to the umbilicus, and the fascial layer is imbricated as needed. A small segment of excess skin is removed and the wound is closed over drains in a layered fashion.

The Circumferential Lower Body Lift

This procedure essentially combines the full abdominoplasty with an anterior abdominoplasty and a flank-thigh-buttock lift. It is indicated for patients with marked laxity of the entire lower trunk, lateral thigh, and buttock areas. Surgically, it is much like a full abdominoplasty, except the excision involves a donut-shaped resection of skin from the anterior abdomen, across the lateral thigh and buttock areas, and tapering to the posterior midline. The procedure typically requires patient repositioning in order to circumferentially resect skin from the lower torso.

Imagine the skin as a poorly tailored suit of clothing: the circumferential body lift would be the equivalent of taking in the waist, tucking in the shirt, and tightening the belt.

Potential Complications Associated with Abdominoplasties

Abdominoplasties have a relatively high complication rate. Roughly one in three patients will experience some form of postoperative complication, although the majority of complications are relatively minor and related primarily to wound healing (2). Two in five patients will require some form of surgical revision in order to achieve the desired aesthetic outcome (2), and men are nearly three times more likely than women to experience postoperative complications (3).

The most common complications associated with abdominoplasty surgery are follows (4):

- Contour deformities such as an asymmetrical appearance or localized bulging. Patients may require additional surgery to correct these.
- Ischemic complications of the skin flaps and umbilical stalk: As described earlier, this is due to a loss of blood flow to the abdominal flap which may necessitate additional surgery in order for correction.

(A)   **(B)**

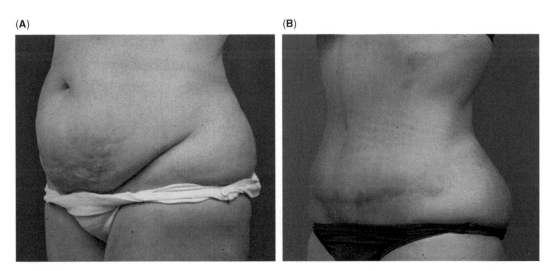

Figure 4.4.1 A 55-year-old G3P3 woman presented with a severe abdominal pannus. (**A**) Preoperative presentation. (**B**) One-year postoperative results following full abdominoplasty.

- Wound dehiscence: This is the opening of a wound around the sutures that typically results from poor wound care. Additional risk factors include age, BMI, and a history of tobacco use.
- Scarring: Abdominoplasty leaves an abdominal scar, particularly a more prominent or visible scar than would be aesthetically desirable.
- Sensory nerve entrapment syndromes: Damage to abdominal nerves during surgery may result in a continuous sensation of pain or loss of sensation in the affected area.
- Bleeding: The wound may continue to bleed postoperatively and may require drainage or additional surgery to correct.
- Localized infection: As with any surgery, there is a risk for infection that may inhibit the body's natural ability to heal and may result in increased scarring.
- Persistent seromas: A seroma is a pocket of clear serous fluid that sometimes develops in the body after surgery. When small blood vessels are ruptured, blood plasma can seep out. The body naturally absorbs the fluid over time (often taking days or weeks); however, a knot of calcified tissue sometimes remains.

Systemic complications such as deep venous thrombosis, pulmonary embolism, fat embolism, and complications arising from general anesthesia are rare but they have the potential to be life threatening. However, despite its inherent risks, abdominoplasty procedures have been shown to have a substantially positive impact on the self-perception and overall quality of life of post–weight loss patients (5).

BRACHIOPLASTY

The brachioplasty, or upper-arm lift, is a surgical procedure to remove the excess skin and fat from the upper arm. As the body ages, the skin in this area tends to become loose and flabby. Approximately 75% of patients who undergo this procedure have typically experienced a massive weight loss and as a result have excess, redundant skin (6). The primary issue with this procedure is the length of the scar that inevitably results from the excision. It typically extends from the medial antecubital fold (elbow) to the posteromedial axillary fold (armpit). Partly because of this scarring, the popularity of surgical brachioplasty remains low, accounting for less than 1% of all cosmetic surgical procedures performed in the United States (6).

Surgical Technique for Brachioplasty

Surgically, the underlying principles of the brachioplasty are similar to the abdominoplasty. The procedure begins with a crescent incision down the length of the upper arm. The excess skin and fat are cut away. The fascial layer is imbricated (or layered) to tighten the appearance of the arm, and the skin flap is closed tightly over the now much more compact upper arm.

Liposuction can be used to remove excess fat from the upper arm region; however, depending on the elasticity of the skin, liposuction alone (without a brachioplasty) can increase the degree of skin ptosis or droopiness in the area. Liposuction in this area should therefore only be performed in a conservative fashion using small cannulas to target specific fatty deposits.

Potential Complications of Brachioplasty

While brachioplasties are typically a much smaller and therefore less risky procedure compared with abdominoplasties, there are some inherent risks.

- Bleeding, bruising, and hematoma formation: If the bleeding is severe, this may require additional surgery or the placement of a drain to correct
- Localized infection: If limited, these may be controlled with antibiotics. However, if the infection is more severe or does not respond to antibiotics alone, this may require an additional surgery to wash out the affected area
- Scarring
- Contour deformity
- Altered sensation and potential nerve damage

MEDIAL THIGH LIFT

Like the brachioplasty, the medial thigh lift is a procedure ideal for patients who have had a massive weight loss, and as a result, have excess skin. Youthful skin is elastic and stretches as the body grows. And it will stretch to contain excess body fat as fat is added to the body. However, when a person loses weight, their skin still retains its stretched-out shape. The medial thigh lift serves as a way of removing the excess skin that hangs loose over the thigh.

Surgical Technique for Medial Thigh Lift

The medial thigh lift can be performed with a variety of incisions tailored to the shape and contour of the leg. The classic design removes a crescent shaped segment of skin with the resulting scar confined to the groin and perineal-thigh crease (the inner area of the thigh where the thigh meets the pelvis). Other incision designs include a vertical excision extending from the knee to the groin, and a T-shaped incision, combining the two.

The procedure follows the same surgical principles as the brachioplasty and the abdominoplasty: the excess skin and fat are removed, the underlying connective tissue is layered to tighten the overall contour of the leg, and the flap is closed tightly over the thigh.

Potential Complications of Medial Thigh Lifts

The procedure is not without its perils. The primary complications of the medial thigh lift include the following:

- Significant wound breakdown: This results from the wound around the incision and operative cavity failing to heal properly and may require additional reconstructive surgery to correct.
- Scarring.
- Fluid accumulations in the form of ecchymoses and hematomas: Ecchymoses are a result of damage to the capillaries which supply blood, and hematomas are bruises that develop as a result of internal bleeding. Both cause superficial discoloration of the skin and may require additional surgery for correction.

- Localized infection: As with any surgery, there is a risk for infection that may inhibit the body's natural ability to heal and may result in increased scarring.
- Changes in skin sensation: Damage to the nerves may result in persistent sensations of pain or a loss of sensation in the affected region.

CONCLUSIONS

Body contouring surgeries can be a wonderful technique to help patients improve their appearance. With the rising incidence of obesity, there is a growing population who has undergone significant weight gain and loss, who will likely require a body contouring surgery. These procedures can be performed following significant weight loss that leads to excessive loose skin, or can be performed to help tighten specific regions of the body. While these procedures can be extremely successful, they do carry the risks of any surgical procedure. Thus, these procedures should be performed by a cosmetic surgeon who specializes in this area in order to achieve the best possible results.

REFERENCES

1. Singh D. Adaptive significance of female physical attractiveness: role of waist-to-hip ratio. J Pers Soc Psychol 1993; 65: 293–307.
2. Hensel JM, Lehman JA, Tantri MP, et al. An outcomes analysis and satisfaction survey of 199 consecutive abdominoplasties. Ann Plast Surg 2001; 46: 357–63.
3. van Uchelen JH, Werker PM, Kon M. Complications of abdominoplasty in 86 patients. Plast Reconstr Surg 2001; 107: 1869–73.
4. Stewart K, Stewart D, Coghlan B, et al. Complications of 278 consecutive abdominoplasties. J Plast Reconstr Aesthet Surg 2006; 59: 1152–5.
5. Stuerz K, Piza H, Niermann K, Kinzl JF. Psychosocial impact of abdominoplasty. Obes J 2008; 18: 34–8.
6. American Society of Plastic Surgeons website 2007. [Available from: http://www.plasticsurgery.org/media/statistics]

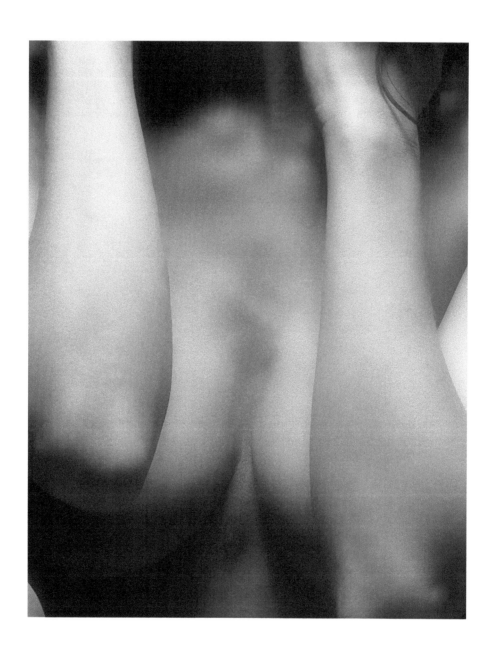

KEY POINTS
- Surgical procedures to reshape the breast are one of the most common reasons that women visit cosmetic surgeons
- Breast augmentation involves the insertion of either silicone or saline implants
  - These implants can be inserted above or below the pectoralis muscle through a variety of surgical approaches (inframammary, periareolar, transaxillary, and periumbilical)
  - Many patients will require surgical revision to improve the cosmetic outcome, due to capsular contracture, malposition, or improper selection of implant size
- Reduction mammoplasty is used to surgically improve macromastia and reshape the breast
  - If the patients are obese, they should attempt to achieve their ideal BMI prior to reduction mammoplasty for best results
  - Multiple surgical techniques can be utilized including the Wise pattern reduction, vertical line incision, central breast mound reduction technique, and in extreme cases breast amputation with free nipple grafting
- Mastopexy, breast lifts, can be performed to tighten the breast skin
  - This can be performed with or without an associated breast augmentation
  - Surgical approach very similar to mastopexy, but depends on the severity of the breast ptosis
- All breast contouring surgeries carry inherent risks. The most common risks include bruising, hematoma formation, scarring, infection, altered nipple sensation, contour deformities, and asymmetry of the breasts

Artists, sculptors, painters and poets have all debated the ideal proportions of the female breasts. Researchers and cosmetic surgeons have almost determined its exact geometric proportions. Unfortunately, few women are blessed with these "ideal" proportions. Many patients are self-conscious about the size of their breasts, while others may have medical conditions which alter their breasts. As a result, breast contouring surgery is one of the most common reasons to visit a cosmetic surgeon. When performed properly, breast contouring surgery can help patients improve their self-image, self-confidence, and happiness.

THE IDEAL BREAST

While the nuances of the ideal breast change over time, there are general guidelines that should be followed in order to determine the final shape of the breast:

The nipple position should be at, or slightly above, the inframammary crease.

In an ideal breast, an isosceles triangle should be able to describe the area between the two nipples and the suprasternal notch. The actual size of the triangle is arbitrary, but a hypotenuse of 18–21 cm will yield an ideal result.

The areolar diameter should be between 35 mm and 40 mm.

The distance from the areolar border to the inframammary crease should range between 4 cm to 8 cm, with a larger breast having larger distances.

In order to understand how breast surgeries are performed, it is useful first to know how the nerves and blood supply are structured within the breast.

Sensory innervation to the nipple is supplied by the lateral cutaneous branch of the fourth intercostal (T4) nerve. In other words, this is the nerve that communicates sensation and stimulation from the nipple to the brain. In breast reduction surgery, there is a 15% risk that the surgery will either damage the nerve or otherwise impair its ability to communicate with the brain, resulting in a change in nipple sensation (1).

There are three primary sources of blood supply feeding the breast. The internal mammary artery supplies blood to the medial portion of the breast, the lateral thoracic artery to the lateral portion, and perforators from the thoracoacromial artery and the lateral third, fourth, and fifth intercostal arteries supply a much less significant portion. While there is significant collateralization between these arteries, it is estimated that the internal mammary artery supplies 60% of the blood to the breast, while the lateral thoracic artery supplies 30% of the breast's blood, and the thoraco-acromial and intercostal arteries supply the remaining 10%.

The venous and lymphatic drainages of the breast lay closely parallel to each other. The majority of the drainage (approximately 80%) flows to the axilla, while the remaining 20% flows to the internal mammary region.

BREAST AUGMENTATION

Breast augmentation is now the most common cosmetic surgical procedure performed in the United States (2). More than two million women (1% of the total female population in the United States) have breast implants. However, augmentation mammoplasty remains mired in social and political controversies, and the Food and Drug Administration (FDA) closely scrutinizes the use of silicone gel implants while researchers continue to study their safety and longevity.

(A) **(B)**

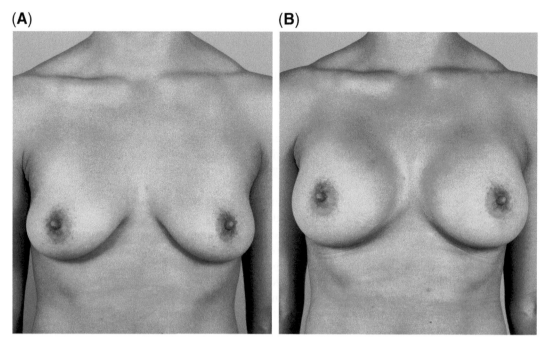

Figure 4.5.1 (**A**) A 27–year-old woman of 5' 7" (1.7 m) in height and 165 lbs (75 kg) in weight requested elective breast augmentation. (**B**) One year postoperative result following placement of bilateral subpectoral saline implants, placed via 4-cm inframammary incisions. The implants were Mentor Moderate Profile 375-cc implants, overfilled to 400-cc volume.

The majority of patients who consult for breast augmentation are young women who simply (for aesthetic and social reasons) want larger breasts (Fig. 4.5.1). However, women also consult for breast augmentation after they have given birth; post-partum breast augmentation can restore volume to the breast or correct any ptosis that has occurred as the result of the pregnancy or lactation. And patients with moderate or severe forms of developmental breast anomalies (such as asymmetry, ptosis, or agenesis of the breast) often request implant augmentation in conjunction with other reconstructive procedures.

Women who are contemplating breast augmentation should be made fully aware of the immediate and long-term risks associated with both saline and silicone implants. Unlike most other cosmetic procedures, which typically only carry a short-term postoperative risk for complication, breast augmentation is unique in that the risk for complications extends over the life of the implant (3). One in five women will require some form of reoperation within the first three years of augmentation. The most common reason for reoperation is to improve the aesthetic result: the implant may be poorly positioned, giving the breast a less-than-desirable contour, or the implant selected may have been the wrong size—either too large or too small— for the desired postoperative shape of the breast.

Types of Implants

The two current implant options for breast augmentation are saline- and silicone-filled implants. Both types of implants have a silicone elastomer shell, a type of plastic designed to stretch rather than rupture that will not break down in the naturally occurring heat of the human body. As their names imply, silicone implants are filled with a liquid silicone gel, while saline implants are filled with saline (salt water). Both implant types come in a variety of sizes, shapes, and surface textures; silicone gel implants also come with varying degrees of gel cohesiveness.

In 1992, the FDA restricted the use of silicone gel implants due to concerns over a possible link between gel implants and autoimmune diseases affecting connective tissue. It was thought that implant rupture or silicone leakage could have a toxic effect on the body and cause a litany of diseases (4). Subsequent large-scale clinical trials failed to substantiate any such link. In 1999, the National Academy Institute of Medicine issued a report with the following conclusion: "In an overall consideration of the epidemiological evidence, the committee noted that because there are more than 1.5 million adult women of all ages in the United States with silicone breast implants, some of these women would be expected to develop connective tissue diseases, cancer, neurological disease or other systemic complaints or conditions. Evidence suggests that such diseases or conditions are no more common in women with breast implants than women without implants" (5).

In other words, women with silicone gel implants were no more likely than women without implants (of any variety) to develop any substantial health problems, and any problems they did acquire were naturally occurring rather than the result of implant rupture or silicone migration. In light of the Institute of Medicine's findings and the massive amounts of research data collected during the intervening years, the FDA reapproved the use of silicone gel implants in 2006. And they are now available for breast reconstruction in women of all ages and for breast augmentation in women 22 years and older (6).

In 2007, plastic surgeons in the United States performed 347,524 breast augmentations, using silicone gel implants in 35% of the procedures. By comparison, in 1994, the first full statistical year after the FDA curtailed the use of silicone implants, only 6% of breast augmentations were performed with silicone gel implants (2).

What all of this means is, statistically, silicone gel implants have been proven to be used in breast augmentation as safely as saline implants. While they are equally safe to use, the different fillers have different textures and will give the breast a different postoperative feel. Women considering breast augmentation should carefully consider both types of implants in order to make an informed decision.

Surgical Techniques for Breast Augmentation

Just as there is a variety of implant styles, there are a number of ways the surgery can be performed. The placement of the implant, the depth of the surgical pocket created to hold the implant, and the type of incision used will all have an effect on the final aesthetic appearance of the augmented breast.

Placement of Implants

Breast implants may be placed either subpectorally (under the pectoralis muscles at the base of the breast) or subglandularly (under the breast gland only, and on top of the pectoralis major muscle).

The principal advantage of subpectoral placement is that it statistically lowers the risk of capsular contracture. Capsular contracture is part of the body's natural immune response to foreign objects. The actual mechanism that causes this is largely unknown, but essentially, the implant pocket begins to contract around the implant and squeeze it to the point where the implant may shift position within the breast. The subpectoral placement also has the advantage of allowing better overall soft tissue coverage and a more natural transition in the upper poles of the breast. And if a mastopexy (breast lift) becomes necessary in the future, the subpectoral placement increases the vascular viability of the nipple and areola region and decreases the likelihood of postmastopexy complications.

Subglandular placement of the implants can achieve better and more natural aesthetic results in cases of breast ptosis. Subglandular implantation is also much less painful and patients enjoy a faster overall recovery period.

Incisions for Implants

The most common incision used is an inframammary approach, which places the incision transversely at the level of the inframammary fold (IMF), along the base of the breast. The incision offers a well-concealed scar underneath the fold of the breast, with no visible scarring on the breast itself.

The periareolar approach places the incision at the junction of the areola and normal nonpigmented breast skin. The advantage of this approach is that it conceals the scar along the border of the areola, and there is no visible scarring on the breast itself. The disadvantage to this approach is that it results in a higher incidence of diminished nipple sensitivity, and there is also the potential that a periareolar incision will damage the ductal structures of the breast, inhibiting the person's ability to breastfeed in the future. Another disadvantage of this approach is that it limits the ability to revise the surgery to improve the aesthetic results, and attempted revisions can result in a tethering or inversion of the resulting scar when the periareolar incision is repeatedly reopened.

The transaxillary approach allows placement of the implant through the axilla (armpit), with no scars whatsoever on the breast itself. Surgical visualization, however, is poor and this approach increases the likely need for surgical revision to correct implant malposition. Surgical revisions via transaxillary incision are extremely difficult to perform and often require a secondary incision resulting in surgical scarring of the breast.

The transumbilical approach is the least frequently used surgical approach. The scar is limited to the periumbilical region (navel). The disadvantage to this approach is that it only allows for the use of saline implants. Revisions cannot be performed using this approach, and a secondary incision, with resulting surgical scarring, would be necessary to correct any malposition of the breast implant. Nevertheless, for certain patients and experienced surgeons, it is a viable option.

Potential Complications Associated with Breast Augmentation

Like all surgical procedures, breast augmentation carries its inherent risk for operative and postoperative complications. The potential complications are discussed in detail.

Hematoma

Postoperative bleeding resulting in a hematoma typically occurs within the first 24 hours after surgery; however, delayed bleeding (while unusual) can occur for as long as two weeks after surgery. The risk of hematoma development is 1–2%. Additional surgery may be necessary in order to evacuate the accumulated blood and prevent any further bleeding. If left untreated, large hematomas may cause pressure necrosis of the overlying tissue and compromise the viability of the skin.

Infection

Most postoperative infections occur within the first five days after surgery and typically result from an invasion of *Staphylococcus aureus* bacteria. When the infection involves only a superficial cellulitis, antibiotics will often eradicate the infection. However, when there is an associated peri-implant fluid collection, the chances of salvaging the implant with antibiotics diminish and it often becomes necessary to remove the implant in order to eradicate the infection and allow the breast to heal. Postoperative infections also increase the likelihood of capsular contractures.

Changes in Nipple Sensation

Surgical transection of small sensory nerves during the dissection of the implant pocket may result in changes in nipple sensation. Nerve damage can occur regardless of the surgical approach used. The change in sensation may be temporary, but in as many as one in seven cases, the loss of sensation can be permanent.

Capsular Contracture

All patients who undergo breast augmentation will develop a fibrous capsule (or shell) around the breast implant. This is the body's normal response to any foreign body. The fibrous capsule may hypertrophy, thereby contracting around the implant. The extent of the capsular formation varies tremendously and often occurs asymmetrically. The shell around one implant may be thicker than the shell around the other implant, creating a noticeable visual deformity. Capsular formation is unpredictable and may occur years after the implant is placed. A new or prolonged peri-implant inflammatory reaction, regardless of the etiology, has been suggested to have a role in the process of capsular formation. This inflammation can be due to low-grade infections, trauma, bleeding, fluid accumulation, silicone gel bleed, and a number of other possible factors. Symptoms of capsular contracture include the following:

Hardening of the breast
Pain or discomfort ranging from mild to severe
Extreme sensitivity to touch or pressure
Distortion or malposition of the breast implant
Distortion of the breast itself

Capsular formation is clinically graded using the Baker classification, shown in Table 4.5.1.

Factors which increase the risk of capsular contracture include the following:

Periareolar incisions. Statistically, this placement technique has the highest incident rate of triggering capsular contracture.
Smooth textured implants have a higher incidence rate for capsular contracture than textured implants.
Subglandular placement of implants has a higher incidence rate for contracture than subpectoral implantation.

Implant Rupture

Breast implants are designed to withstand the physical and chemical rigors that result from placement within the human body. And they have the potential to remain intact and in place for decades; however, rupture of either saline or silicone implants remains a significant local complication.

When a saline implant ruptures, the saline is quickly absorbed by the surrounding tissue and the implant can easily be removed or exchanged. Rupture rates for saline implants are 3–5% during the first three years after implantation, and 7–10% through the first five years after augmentation (7).

Silicone implant ruptures are more difficult to detect and more problematic when they occur. Overall rupture rates vary widely depending on the year of the implant's manufacture and how long it has been placed in the body. In general, ruptures occur at a rate of 0.3–1.0% per year of implantation. In other words, after 10 years, 3.0–10% of silicone gel implants will have ruptured (7).

Ruptures may be intra capsular, where the silicone gel leakage is confined to capsular tissue surrounding the implant, or the rupture may extend beyond the fibrous capsule and thus be classified as "extracapsular." Extracapsular rupture may lead to silicone migration and cause local complications within the breast tissue (such as silicone granulomas, foreign body reactions, and distortions of the breast).

When either intracapsular or extracapsular ruptures are detected, the consensus agreement is to recommend a removal of the implant with or without replacement.

Implant Malposition (Immediately Postoperative)

Implant asymmetry and malposition in the immediate postoperative period generally results from errors in surgical dissection and implant placement. When surgical errors are suspected, surgical revision may be necessary to correct the problem. Preexisting asymmetry should be carefully documented and photographed during the preoperative examination.

Impaired Mammographic Visualization

Implants do not increase the risk of breast cancer development, nor do they delay the detection of breast cancer. However, the presence of breast implants can impair the visualization of breast tissue, making it more difficult to visualize the size, location, and extent of a suspect mass during mammography.

In a recent article published in 2004, in the Journal of the American Medical Association, researchers found that among asymptomatic women (i.e., women with breast cancer who exhibit no symptoms), breast augmentation decreased the sensitivity of screening mammography from 66.8% to 45% and radiologists were one-third less able to visualize the suspected breast mass. However, breast implants have been shown to have no impact on the development of tumor size, estrogen-receptor status, or nodal status (8).

REDUCTION MAMMOPLASTY

Reduction mammoplasty, or breast reduction, is a surgical procedure which reduces the overall volume of the breast and reshapes its contours into a more aesthetically pleasing form (Fig. 4.5.2). Overly large, heavy, or pendulous breasts can cause neck pain, back pain, shoulder grooving from the supportive brassiere straps, and maceration of the skin along the IMF.

Macromastia (or overly large, heavy breasts) can result from disproportionate glandular development, which causes the breasts to grow to a disproportionate size relative to the rest of a woman's body, and it can occur as a result of generalized obesity. The breast itself is primarily composed of fatty tissue and muscle. As a person's BMI increases, the breast becomes a natural locus for fat buildup, and the fat cells within the breast tend to hypertrophy. Treating macromastia in an obese woman with proportionate macromastia (where the volume of fat in the breast is proportionate with her overall BMI) may not be treating the underlying cause of the disorder. Subsequent weight loss could then undermine the aesthetics of the newly reduced breast and require additional surgery to correct.

Weight loss alone will not always correct macromastia resulting from generalized obesity. Many women with overly

Table 4.5.1 The Baker Classification System for Capsular Contracture

Grade I	No palpable or visible anomaly is found.
Grade II	Breast appears normal, but is palpably firm.
Grade III	Breast appears abnormal and is visibly firm.
Grade IV	Patient complains of associated breast pain.

(A)   **(B)**

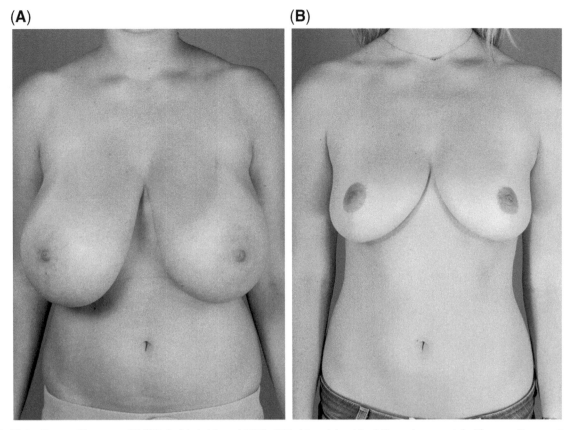

Figure 4.5.2 (**A**) An 18-year-old woman of 5' 3" (1.6 m) in height and 118 lbs (54 kg) in weight with a 34F cup size presented with severe disproportionate macromastia. (**B**) One-year postoperative result following bilateral reduction mammoplasty, utilizing the central parenchymal reduction technique and Wise pattern skin reduction pattern. The patient underwent resection of 833 g of tissue from the right breast and 814 g of tissue from the left breast.

large breasts who successfully lower their BMI still require reduction mammoplasty in order to reduce the volume of their breasts. However, it is important to achieve a reasonable BMI prior to surgery in order to optimize the final results.

Surgical Technique for Reduction Mammoplasty

Among the various breast reduction techniques, the most commonly used technique in the United States is the inferior parenchymal pedicle technique. This is also known as the keyhole or Wise pattern reduction, and involves an inverted T-shaped incision which encircles the areola. The excision extends downward, following the natural curvature of the breast. Excess fat, tissue and skin are removed, and the nipple is repositioned. With this technique, the blood supply to the nipple areolar complex is maintained through an inferiorly based breast parenchymal flap.

The vertical scar technique has been gaining widespread popularity due to the absence of the horizontal portion of the inverted T incision. The breast is reduced by removal of the lateral and inferior breast tissue, leaving the upper poles of the breast largely untouched.

The central breast mound reduction technique, initially described by Hester in 1985, has the advantage of maintaining the breast's underlying vascular supply, as well as its lactiferous ducts and nerves, with the option of utilizing various skin reduction techniques to address the macromastia and breast ptosis (9).

In very severe cases of macromastia, breast amputation with free nipple grafting may be necessary. However, this technique results in complete nipple denervation (loss of nerve sensation) and the inability to breast feed postoperatively.

Potential Complications of Reduction Mammoplasty

The severity and frequency of complications resulting from breast reduction surgery depends on the surgical technique used, the degree of macromastia, and the comorbid medical conditions of the individual patient. Complications arising from mammoplasty include the following:

Inability to breast feed: Breast reduction surgery may damage or close off the lactiferous ducts which supply breast milk to the nipple.

Breast asymmetry: The surgery may result in an unevenness of size or shape of the breasts. Additional surgeries may be necessary to correct this.

Ischemic complications of the skin flaps and nipple areolar complex: This is a loss of blood flow that may necessitate additional surgery for correction.

Delayed wound healing.

Bleeding: Postoperative bleeding resulting in a hematoma typically results within the first 24 hours after surgery; however, delayed bleeding (while unusual) can occur for as long as two weeks after surgery. The risk of hematoma development is 1–2%. Additional surgery may be necessary in order to evacuate the accumulated blood and prevent any further bleeding.

Infection: Most postoperative infections occur within the first 5 days after surgery and typically result from an invasion of *S. aureus* bacteria, which can be wiped out with antibiotics. More severe infections within the wound may require additional surgery to clear up.

Fluid accumulation in the form of ecchymoses, hematomas, and seromas: Ecchymoses are the result of damage to the capillaries which deliver the blood supply, and hematomas are bruises that develop as a result of internal bleeding. A seroma is a pocket of clear serous fluid that sometimes develops in the body after surgery. When small blood vessels are ruptured, blood plasma can seep out.

Despite the associated risks and scars, studies have demonstrated that breast reduction procedures result in a high level of patient satisfaction and patients report an improvement in both their overall health and their psychological functioning (10).

MASTOPEXY

The mastopexy, or breast lift, is a surgical procedure in which the cosmetic surgeon tightens the overall shape of the breast and reduces any excess skin (Fig. 4.5.3). A mastopexy can be performed alone or in conjunction with an augmentation procedure to add volume to the breast.

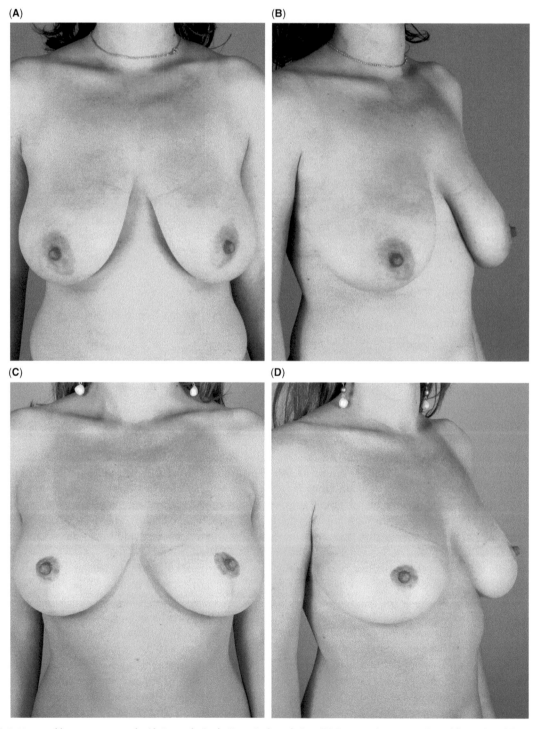

Figure 4.5.3 (**A**) A 48-year-old woman presented with Regnault Grade II ptosis; frontal view. (**B**) Preoperative presentation; oblique view. (**C**) Postoperative result following bilateral mastopexies via standard Wise pattern skin excision and internal parenchymal suture suspension; frontal view. (**D**) Postoperative result; oblique view.

As a woman ages, the weight of her breasts begins to pull downward on the skin enveloping the breast. As a result, the skin naturally develops a certain amount of laxity, it begins to stretch, and the breast begins to sag. The larger the breast, the more pronounced this ptosis becomes. Changes in BMI, pregnancy, and lactation can exacerbate the breasts' tendency to sag.

Ptosis in the breast refers to the descent of the nipple areolar complex and its position relative to the IMF. The common classifications were developed by Regnault in 1976, and are shown in Table 4.5.2 (11).

Mastopexy Surgical Technique

The severity of the ptosis determines the complexity of the mastopexy. Surgically, the procedure is very similar to the mammoplasty: both procedures utilize the same skin reduction and tightening components in order to establish a more aesthetically pleasing breast contour.

Table 4.5.2 The Regnault Classification of Breast Ptosis

Pseudoptosis	A pronounced drooping of the breast, but the nipple remains above the level of the IMF
Grade I Ptosis	The nipple lies at the level of the IMF
Grade II Ptosis	The nipple lies below the level of the IMF, but above the lowest contour of the breast
Grade III Ptosis	The nipple lies at the lowest contour of the breast

Patients, who desire to have both their skin envelope tightened and breast volume increased, can undergo a combination mastopexy-augmentation technique (Fig. 4.5.4). However, this combined procedure increases the risk of ischemic complications resulting from the disruption of the blood supply to the central breast mound, skin flaps, and nipple areolar complex (12). A conservative approach that stages the two procedures will often yield a better result: the ptosis can first be corrected with a mastopexy, and the augmentation can then be performed once the breasts have had a chance to properly heal.

For patients with mild ptosis, a limited skin reduction technique (via a circumareolar or limited vertical skin incision) may be adequate. However, the potential contour improvements should be weighed against the severity of the scars.

For patients with moderate, Grade III ptosis, a more aggressive skin tightening procedure involving an incision similar to the Wise pattern used in reduction mammoplasty may be necessary.

Potential Complications of Mastopexy

Complications from mastopexy procedures are similar to those of reduction mammoplasty and typically include the potential for the following:

Diminished or absent nipple sensation: Transection (severing) of small sensory nerves during surgery may result in changes in nipple sensation. Nerve damage can occur regardless of the incision used. The change in sensation may be temporary, but in as many as one in seven cases, the loss of sensation can be permanent.

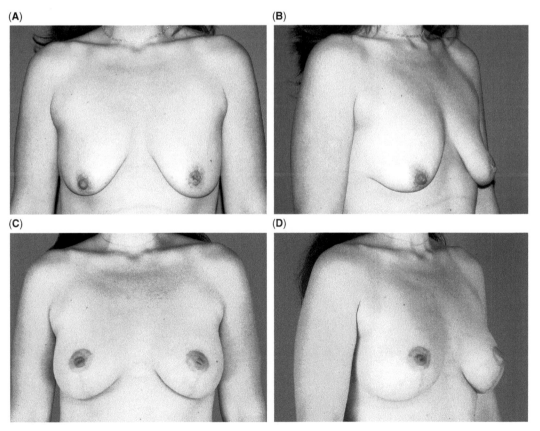

Figure 4.5.4 (**A**) A 43-year-old woman requested a combined 1-stage breast augmentation and mammoplasty procedure to restore shape and volume to her breasts; frontal view. (**B**) Preoperative presentation; oblique view. (**C**) One year postoperative result following the placement of bilateral subpectoral saline implants, model Inamed Style 10 270 cc implants, in combination with vertical mastopexies. (**D**) Postoperative result; oblique view.

Ischemic complications of the skin flaps and nipple areolar complex: This is a loss of blood flow that may necessitate additional surgery for correction.

Bleeding: Postoperative bleeding resulting in a hematoma typically results within the first 24 hours after surgery; however, delayed bleeding (while unusual) can occur for as long as two weeks after surgery. The risk of hematoma development is 1–2%. Additional surgery may be necessary in order to evacuate the accumulated blood and prevent any further bleeding.

Infection: Most post-operative infections occur within the first 5 days after surgery and typically result from an invasion of *S. aureus* bacteria, which can be wiped out with antibiotics. More severe infections within the wound may require additional surgery to clear up.

Unsatisfactory scarring: In this context, there will be a more prominent or visible scar than is aesthetically desirable.

CONCLUSIONS

Breast contouring surgeries can be extremely rewarding procedures, both for patients and cosmetic surgeons. Surgeries including breast augmentation, reduction mammoplasty, and mastopexy can all be utilized to help patients achieve their "ideal" breasts. These procedures can dramatically improve a patient's self-image and self-confidence. Furthermore, these procedures can reverse or limit medical conditions associated with macromastia. Unfortunately, these procedures are not without perils and revision procedures are often necessary to help patients achieve their ultimate goals. That said, in the hands of an experienced cosmetic surgeon, breast contouring surgeries often result in the happiest patients.

REFERENCES

1. Schlenz I, Kuzbari R, Gruber H, et al. The sensitivity of the nipple-areolar complex: an anatomic study. Plast Reconstr Surg 2000; 105: 905–9.
2. American Society of Plastic Surgeons website 2007. [Available from: http://www.plasticsurgery.org/media/statistics]
3. Handel N, Cordray T, Gutierrez J, Jensen JA. A long-term study of outcomes, complications, and patient satisfaction with breast implants. Plast Reconstr Surg 2006; 117: 757–67.
4. Kessler DA. Commissioner of FDA Statement on Silicone Gel Breast Implants. 1992.
5. Bondurant S, Ernster V, Herdman R. eds. Committee on the safety of Silicone Breast Implants, Institute of Medicine. Safety of Silicone Breast Implants. Washington DC: National Academy Press, 1999: 215–32.
6. FDA Approves Silicone Gel-Filled Breast Implants After In-Depth Evaluation. United States Food and Drug Administration, US Dept of Health and Human Services. FDA NEWS. P06-189 November 17,2006
7. Diseases. FDA Breast Implant Consumer Handbook – 2004 (2004-06-08). From Inamed and Mentor labeling at FDA's. [Available from: http://www.fda.gov/cdrh/breastimplants/]
8. Miglioretti DL, Rutter CM, Geller BM, et al. Effect of breast augmentation on the accuracy of mammography and cancer characteristics. JAMA 2004; 291: 442–50.
9. Hester TR, Bostwick J, Miller L, Cunningham SJ. Breast reduction utilizing the maximally vascularized central breast pedicle. Plast Reconstr Surg 1985; 76: 890–8.
10. Faria FS, Guthrie E, Bradbury E, Brain AN. Psychological outcome and patient satisfaction following breast reduction surgery. Br J Plast Surg 1999; 52: 448–52.
11. Regnault P. Breast Ptosis. Definition and Treatment. Clin Plast Surg 1976; 3: 193–203.
12. Handel N. Secondary mastopexy in the augmented patient: a recipe for disaster. Plast Reconstr Surg 2006; 118(7 Suppl): 152S–63S.

KEY POINTS

- Ethnic patients have differing facial features from Caucasians, and as a result, may have different ultimate goals for their cosmetic procedures
- The increasing melanin concentration of ethnic skin may guard the skin against the effects of ultraviolet light and photodamage
- Many ethnic patients develop solar lentigines, flat and pigmented seborrheic keratoses, as well as mottled hyperpigmentation as they age
- Facial aging in ethnic groups also occurs as a result of loss of hard and soft tissues, which include bone remodeling, gravitational redistribution of soft tissue, and fat atrophy

The concept of beauty has persisted throughout history. Historically, attractive facial features were once an evolutionary gauge measuring the fitness and suitability of a mate. Facial symmetry and aesthetics were seen as signs of sexual maturity, fertility, and emotional expressiveness (1). There is a wide range of characteristics defining a beautiful face, which differ for ethnic groups. For example, skin color, hair texture, and structural differences in the eyes, nose, and lips are a few of the global defining features of ethnic beauty (2). Many key differences exist in the facial structures of racial ethnic groups, and these differences must be taken into account when treating patients.

BEAUTY IN ETHNIC GROUPS

The African-American face often reflects a multiracial heritage, with ancestors of African, Native American, and Northern European descent. Furthermore, skin tone is a reflection of racial mixing and can range in color from olive to shades of brown and black (3). The African-American face is often characterized by a broader nasal base, decreased nasal projection, bimaxillary protrusion, orbital proptosis, and enhanced facial convexity. There is often a prominence of soft tissue in the midface, lips, and chin (4).

The Asian population is exceedingly diverse. It includes Indians, Chinese, Japanese, Koreans, Vietnamese, Thai, Cambodians, Malays, Indonesians, Filipinos, and Polynesians. Characteristic features of the Asian face are a wider intercanthal distance relative to a shorter palpebral fissure, lack of upper eyelid crease, broad nasal base, and small mouth. Asians typically have prominent mandibular angles with hypertrophic masseteric muscles, giving rise to a wider appearing lower face (5).

Many Hispanics living in North, Central, and South America reflect racial mixtures of European, Native American, and African descent. As a result, characteristic Latin features span a broad range. Hispanic skin color ranges from white to olive to brown. Common features of the Hispanic face are an increased bizygomatic distance with a greater convexity angle, bimaxillary protrusion, and a broader nose. These features can give the face a broad, somewhat rounded profile (6).

In European ancestry, an oval face is generally considered most aesthetically desirable. However, in African-American and Asian decent, a fuller, rounded face is frequently considered more attractive. In Caucasians, an upturned, pointed nose is seen as appealing as opposed to the wider and longer nose of darker racial ethnic groups (7). In nearly half of the Asian population, there is an absence of an upper eyelid crease, which is the most frequent request for cosmetic alteration in this group (8). Observations such as these have enhanced the understanding and impact of diverse facial morphologies in the perception of beauty (4).

THE AGING PROCESS

The aging face is a consequence of many elements of time, including photodamage, volumetric loss, and gravitational soft tissue and bone movement, resulting in fine wrinkles, skin laxity, pigmentary alterations, textural changes, and loose skin. Signs of aging are unique to each individual and are influenced by genetic and environmental factors. Aging in fair-skinned patients most commonly result from photodamage, manifest as wrinkles, skin laxity, dyschromia, and textural changes (9). In contrast, darker ethnic populations may be relatively protected from ultraviolet photodamage, but experience soft tissue and gravitational changes which are the predominant signs of cutaneous aging in these patients (10). These differences in the aging process ultimately have a significant impact on the goals and approach to helping ethnic patients achieve their ideals of beauty.

Extrinsic Aging (Photodamage) in Ethnic Skin

Photodamage results from long-term effects of sun exposure. Clinically, photodamage is displayed as wrinkling, textural roughness, mottled dyspigmentation, and telangiectasias. There is an increased incidence of premalignant and malignant skin lesions on photodamaged skin, including actinic keratoses, basal cell carcinomas, squamous cell carcinomas, and melanoma. Histopathological features of sun damage are characterized by alterations in the epidermis and dermis. There may be a hypertrophy or atrophy of the epidermis. Keratinocyte atypia with loss of polarity is often noted. In the dermis, there may be solar elastosis and degeneration of collagen. The pathogenesis of dermal changes includes enhanced matrix metalloproteinase enzyme activity leading to the degradation of collagen (11).

Photoaging affects all skin types. However, signs of photodamage may differ in lighter and darker toned ethnic skin. The sun exposed skin of Caucasians is far more susceptible to the deleterious effects of ultraviolet light than skin of more darkly pigmented racial ethnic groups. This was elucidated in a study by Montagna and Carlisle (12); the study compared the morphology of facial skin of 19 black and 19 white women between the ages of 22 and 50. Four-mm punch biopsies were obtained from the malar eminence of each subject and evaluated histologically. The researchers observed that the dark skin rarely displayed epidermal atrophy, and there was minimal evidence of solar elastosis. Overall, compared with white skin, dark skin showed minimal evidence of photodamage.

In dark skinned populations, photoaging is more often noticed in African-Americans than in Africans or African-Caribbeans, likely because of the heterogeneous mixture of African-American descent. In African-Americans, photoaging appears primarily in lighter-complexioned individuals and may not be apparent until the fifth or sixth decade (13). Clinically, photoaging in this population includes fine wrinkling, mottled pigmentation, and aggregation of dermatosis papulosa nigra (7).

The classic features of photoaging in East and Southeast Asians are discrete pigmentary changes, including solar lentigines, flat and/or pigmented seborrheic keratoses, and mottled hyperpigmentation. Toyoda and Morohashi assessed epidermal melanocyte morphology and alterations in the sun-exposed skin of 15 Japanese women in the age range 58–81 years (14). The investigators compared skin from the sun-exposed crow's feet area with the sun-protected skin from the post-auricular region of the same patient. Compared with the sun-protected skin, the sun-exposed skin showed a statistically significant increase in melanocyte number, nuclear heterogeneity, and signs of cell activation. In addition, melanocytes in sun-exposed skin contained larger intracytoplasmic vacuolar structures, and were closely opposed to neighboring keratinocytes.

Photoaging in the Hispanic population is displayed by a broad constellation of findings with signs relative to ancestral lineage. In fair-skinned Hispanics, photodamage probably occurs in the same frequency and degree as in Caucasians with wrinkling predominating over pigmentary alteration. Darker skinned Hispanics have clinical manifestations of photoaging similar to South Asians and African-Americans, including fine wrinkling and mottled pigmentation (15).

Intrinsic Aging in Ethnic Skin

Besides photodamage, facial aging occurs as a result of loss of hard and soft tissues, which include bone remodeling, gravitational redistribution of soft tissue, and fat atrophy. While darker skin is less prone to developing the fine lines associated with photoaging in lighter skin types, ethnic skin ages predominantly through intrinsic changes. In darker skin, aging occurs in the deeper muscular layers of the face, seen as sagging of the malar fat pads toward the nasolabial folds (7). Additionally, ethnic skin types have a higher probability of pigmentary changes with aging.

The first signs of aging occur in the upper third of the face. Ptosis of the upper eyelid appears during the fourth decade in darker racial ethnic groups, whereas fair-skinned patients display ptosis slightly earlier, beginning in the third decade (16). Brows of Hispanics tend to be implanted at a lower level with respect to the supraorbital rim, and nasolabial folds may be prominent.

Many dark skinned patients have excess skin in the upper eyelids and dark circles infraorbitally. As aging progresses, wrinkles in dark skinned ethnic patients appear as a result of expression and muscle contraction, mainly on the upper third of the face (17).

In the middle and lower face, aging appears as tear trough deformity, infraorbital hollowing, and malar fat pad ptosis resulting in a prominence of the nasolabial fold. All darker racial ethnic groups may display bimaxillary protrusion combined with infraorbital hyperplasia, contributing to more pronounced midface aging (7).

Darker racial ethnic groups experience jowl formation and pronounced melomental lines in the lower face. In the mentum area, darker skinned patients may display significant signs of aging. Fat can accumulate in the submandibular region as a result of a lower projection of the chin. This phenomenon often leads to rounding of the jaw line commonly noted in African-American patients. Generally, signs of aging in the lower face occur later in dark skinned patients and are less pronounced than in white skin races, with the exception of the accumulation of fat in the mentum region (4).

In lighter skin populations, the lips characteristically become thinner and flattened with a diminution of the philtrum, accentuating perioral wrinkles. These changes are less commonly seen in African-Americans, due to their characteristic voluminous lips. Therefore, a loss of lip volume is an uncommon complaint amongst African-Americans, and there is little demand for lip augmentation in this population (17).

CONCLUSIONS

The ideals of beauty can vary greatly between different patients and ethnicities. As a result, there is no one single approach to treatment for these patients. While dark skin patients may have less likelihood of developing photodamage, intrinsic changes and loss of facial volume contribute to the aging process. It is important to have an understanding of the variations between differing ethnicities, and their aging process, in order to provide ideal cosmetic treatments.

REFERENCES

1. Perrett DI, May KA, Yoshikawa S. Facial shape and judgements of female attractiveness. Nature 1994; 368: 239–42.
2. Porter JP, Lee JI. Facial analysis: maintaining ethnic balance. Facial Plast Surg Clin North Am 2002; 10: 343–9.
3. Grimes P. Beauty: an historical and societal perspective. In: Grimes P, ed. Aesthetics and Cosmetic Surgery for Darker Skin Types. Philadelphia: Lippincott Williams & Wilkins, 2008: 8–9.
4. Sutter RE, Turley PK. Soft tissue evaluation of contemporary Caucasian and African American female facial profiles. Angle Orthod 1998; 68: 487–96.
5. Yu CC, Chen PK, Chen YR. Botulinum toxin a for lower facial contouring: a prospective study. Aesthetic Plast Surg 2007; 31: 445–51.
6. Ramirez O. Facial surgery in the Hispano-American Patient. In: Matory W, ed. Ethnic Considerations in Facial Aesthetic Surgery. Philadelphia: Lippincott-Raven Publishers, 1998: 307–20.
7. Matory W. Definintions of beauty in the ethnic patient. In: Matory W, ed. Ethnic Considerations in Facial Aesthetic Surgery. Philadelphia: Lippincott-Raven Publishers, 1998: 61–3.
8. Rosenthal E. Ethnic ideals: rethinking plastic surgery, in New York Times. 1991.
9. Grimes P, Hexsel D, Rutowitsch M. The aging face in darker racial ethnic Groups. In: Grimes P, ed. Aesthetics and Cosmetic Surgery for Darker Skin Types. Philadelphia: Lippincott Williams & Wilkins, 2008: 27.
10. ??? (Listed as Carruthers Botox article, but doesn't seem correct).

11. Gilchrest BA. A review of skin ageing and its medical therapy. Br J Dermatol 1996; 135: 867–75.
12. Montagna W, Carlisle K. The architecture of black and white facial skin. J Am Acad Dermatol 1991; 24(6 Pt 1): 929–37.
13. Taylor SC. Skin of color: biology, structure, function, and implications for dermatologic disease. J Am Acad Dermatol 2002; 46(2 Suppl Understanding): S41–62.
14. Toyoda M, Morohashi M. Morphological alterations of epidermal melanocytes in photoageing: an ultrastructural and cytomorphometric study. Br J Dermatol 1998; 139: 444–52.
15. Munavalli GS, Weiss RA, Halder RM. Photoaging and nonablative photorejuvenation in ethnic skin. Dermatol Surg 2005; 31(9 Pt 2): 1250–60.
16. Harris MO. The aging face in patients of color: minimally invasive surgical facial rejuvenation-a targeted approach. Dermatol Ther 2004; 17: 206–11.
17. Grimes P, Hexsel D, Rutowitsch M. The aging face in darker racial ethnic groups. In: Grimes P, ed. Aesthetics and Cosmetic Surgery for Darker Skin Types. Philadelphia: Lippincott Williams & Wilkins, 2008: 34.

5.2 Hyperpigmentation and skin-lightening agents

Quyn S. Rahman and Stefani Takahashi

> **KEY POINTS**
>
> - Hyperpigmentation is one of the most common and challenging conditions to treat in ethnic skin
> - Hyperpigmentation can result from ultraviolet light, medications, topical agents, and inflammatory skin conditions
> - Skin-lightening agents work by inhibiting enzymes in the melanin synthetic pathway
> - Topical hydroquinone is one of the most commonly utilized lightening agents
> - Combination agents including topical hydroquinone, steroids, and retinoids can also be used for hyperpigmentation. These combination agents may be more effective, but typically are more expensive as well
> - Many natural ingredients, such as vitamin C, melatonin, licorice, soy, and others can also be used as skin-lightening agents

Pigmentary disorders in dark skin types can be recalcitrant and a challenge to improve. The abnormal dark pigmentation of the skin contributes to the aged appearance and is one of the most common concerns in our ethnic patients. Hyperpigmentation often results from chronic exposure to ultraviolet light, which can be a factor in melasma, solar lentigines, and ephelides. Hyperpigmentation also occurs secondary to medications, photosensitizing cosmetics, and inflammatory skin disorders. Hyperpigmentation appears to be more severe in darker skin types, likely due to the release of inflammatory mediators triggering melanocyte proliferation and melanogenesis (1). Postinflammatory hyperpigmentation (PIH) is common in individuals with Fitzpatrick skin types IV through VI and is unfortunately a frequent sequel to many inflammatory diseases of the skin. While PIH typically ultimately fades naturally, it may persist for months; as a result, it is a common presenting complaint of patients of color (2). Many agents are available for our patients, both to reduce the likelihood of developing hyperpigmentation as well as to reduce its appearance.

Knowledge of the melanin production pathway is necessary in understanding the mechanism of action of skin-lightening agents. The pathway begins with the conversion of the amino acid tyrosine to dihydroxyphenylalanine and, then, to dopaquinone by the copper-dependent enzyme tyrosinase. Dopaquinone becomes dopachrome, then dihydroxyindole, and, finally, eumelanin. Skin-lightening agents work by inhibiting or altering the key steps in the melanin synthesis pathway.

HYDROQUINONE

The most commonly used skin-lightening agent is hydroquinone (HQ). It is available over the counter in strengths up to 2%, by prescription in strengths of 3% and 4%, and in concentrations of up to 10% through compounding pharmacies. HQ is the most potent inhibitor of melanogenesis in vitro and in vivo. It inhibits the enzyme tyrosinase, probably by interfering with copper binding, thereby reducing the conversion of dihydroxyphenylalanine to melanin. Other possible mechanisms include selective cytotoxicity of melanocytes and inhibition of DNA and RNA synthesis (3).

HQ is applied typically by the patient to the hyperpigmented areas once or twice daily. Most patients display improvement in hyperpigmentation after one to three months of use. However, it is important to emphasize to patients that it will take several months for them to note the improvement, and that the improvement may be subtle. Newer HQ formulations are available, which are combinations of hydroquinone, glycolic acid, retinoids, fluorinated steroids, and/or vitamin C. Studies have shown that combination formulations, such as HQ with fluocinolone and tretinoin, may have superior efficacy when compared with HQ alone (4). These combination HQ formulations may be more costly than HQ alone.

Although HQ is considered safe, there are potential side effects of which patients should be aware. Acute complications of HQ are frequently encountered and are transient. They include contact dermatitis and paradoxical hyperpigmentation and hypopigmentation. Rarely, chronic adverse events such as exogenous ochronosis can develop. Ochronosis is characterized by sooty hyperpigmentation, erythema, papules, papulonodules, and colloid milia in sun-exposed skin. Exogenous ochronosis is related to long-term HQ use (5). Alternating the use of HQ with another depigmenting agent in four-month cycles may decrease the risk of exogenous ochronosis and skin irritation.

NATURAL INGREDIENTS TO TREAT HYPERPIGMENTATION

Recently, the use of natural ingredients for skin-lightening and whitening has been gaining popularity. There has been a cultural shift in favor of 'natural' products, which are often perceived as a safer alternative by many patients. These agents induce hypopigmentation by inhibiting the transfer of melanosomes to keratinocytes or inhibiting tyrosinase, which is an essential enzyme in the melanin synthesis pathway. Ingredients such as arbutin, azelaic acid, glycolic acid, kojic acid, licorice extract (glabridin), mequinol, paper mulberry, soy, vitamin C, niacinamide, and melatonin are natural agents used to induce hypopigmentation.

Arbutin is a glycosylated hydroquinone, derived from cranberry, blueberry, and bearberry leaves. Arbutin acts by competitively inhibiting tyrosinase and inhibiting melanosome maturation. It is less cytotoxic to melanocytes compared with HQ (6). The concentration of arbutin necessary for skin lightening has not been determined yet.

Azelaic acid is a naturally occurring dicarboxylic acid derived from *Pityrosporum ovale*. It inhibits mitochondrial oxidoreductase activation and DNA synthesis, as well as tyrosinase. Azelaic acid has minimal effect on normal pigment and the maximum effect on heavily pigmented melanocytes. It is well studied and has been used successfully in the treatment of rosacea, solar keratosis, and PIH (7).

Glycolic acid is an alpha-hydroxy acid derived from sugarcane. In low concentrations, glycolic acid produces desquamation of pigmented keratinocytes, and in higher concentrations, its application results in epidermolysis. Glycolic acid 30–70% can enhance the penetration of other topical skin lighteners such as hydroquinone, enhancing its efficacy (8). On darker skinned patients, glycolic acid should be started at low concentrations to avoid skin irritation or PIH.

Kojic acid is a tyrosinase inhibitor found in the *Aspergillus oryzae* fungus. It is used as a skin-lightening agent in concentrations of 1–4%. Lim et al. found 2% kojic acid compounded with 10% glycolic acid and 2% HQ to be more effective than 10% glycolic acid and 2% HQ without kojic acid in treating epidermal melasma (9). Irritant contact dermatitis is a common side effect of kojic acid and can be reduced by combining this agent with a topical corticosteroid.

Glabridin, the principal active compound of licorice root extract, is used in concentrations of 10–40% in skin-lightening products. The depigmenting effect of glabridin has been shown to be 16 times greater than HQ and faster acting (10).

Mequinol (4-hydroxyanisol) is approved for the treatment of solar lentigines. The combination of 2% mequinol and 0.01% tretinoin is available for the treatment of solar lentigines and has been proven effective. The combination of mequinol and tretinoin enhances depigmentation activity as compared with each component separately (11). Its mechanism of action is thought to be a tyrosinase substrate leading to competitive inhibition of melanogenesis.

Paper mulberry extract is a popular skin-lightening agent in Europe and South America. It is isolated from the root of the *Broussonetia papyrifera* tree. Paper mulberry has been compared favorably with HQ and kojic acid (12). It produces little to no skin irritation and, therefore, may be used favorably in dark skin types.

Unpasteurized soymilk contains two serine protease inhibitors, Bowman–Birk inhibitor and soybean tryptase inhibitor, which cause depigmentation through the reduction in melanin transfer. With twice-daily dosing for 12 weeks, soy has proven to be effective in improving mottled hyperpigmentation and solar lentigines (13).

Vitamin C reduces dopaquinone by interacting with copper ions at the tyrosinase activity site. The stable derivative of vitamin C, magnesium L-ascorbic acid-2-phosphate (MAP) has been shown to lighten pigmentation (14). Topical vitamin C may protect against phototoxicity and improve melasma and PIH (15).

Niacinamide, the amide form of vitamin B3, inhibits the transfer of melanosomes to epidermal keratinocytes. Niacinamide has been used to treat photodamage and hyperpigmentation.

Melatonin is a hormone secreted by the pineal gland in response to sunlight. It has been shown to inhibit melanogenesis in a dose-dependent manner. It is sold as an antioxidant in a cream formula. The concentration needed for depigmentation in human skin has not been established.

TOPICAL RETINOIDS

Retinoids, which include vitamin A and its derivatives, have been used topically for decades in the treatment of acne, photoaging, and hyperpigmentation. All-trans retinoic acid, adapalene, and tazarotene are topical retinoids commonly employed for these purposes, and all can be effectively used to treat hyperpigmentation in ethnic skin.

Topical Retinoids for Hyperpigmentation

Topical retinoids can be used alone, or combined with topical steroids, and/or hydroxyphenols in the treatment of PIH. When used in combination therapy, a greater and more rapid effect may be noted. A triple drug combination of fluocinolone acetonide 0.01%, HQ 4%, and tretinoin 0.05% applied once daily has been shown to be efficacious in the treatment of PIH. The topical corticosteroid suppresses melanocyte secretion of melanin. HQ inhibits tyrosinase, blocking melanin biosynthesis, and enhances the degradation of melanosomes. Tretinoin enhances epidermal turnover, which causes a dispersion of keratinocyte pigment granules. Together, these topical medications work synergistically to improve hyperpigmentation.

In a study by Grimes and Callendar, 74 patients from darker racial ethnic groups with acne-induced PIH were treated with tazarotene 0.1% cream (16); once daily application of tazarotene was effective in treating PIH when compared with the vehicle. Statistically significant reductions in overall disease severity, intensity, and area of hyperpigmentation within 18 weeks were noted. Side effects were minimal and included erythema, peeling, dryness, and burning.

Melasma is an acquired facial hyperpigmentation that is more prevalent in African-Americans, Hispanics, and Asians. It presents as light to dark brown patches with irregular borders symmetrically placed on the face. Melasma is associated with factors such as UV radiation, hormones, and the lability of melanocytes (17). Tretinoin as well as triple combination therapy with a tretinoin, corticosteroid, and HQ has been shown to lighten melasma in African-American patients with few side effects.

Topical Retinoids for Treating Photoaging

Photodamage presents in darker racial ethnic groups as rhytides, telangiectasias, solar comedones, dyspigmentation, and actinic keratoses (18). The melanin content and melanosomal dispersion pattern in darker skin may provide some inherent photo protection when compared with lighter complexions. However, darkly pigmented skin can still experience photodamage, albeit, at a later stage. In black skin, photodamage presents as hypo- or hyperpigmentation. In Asian skin, photoaging includes depigmentation in addition to epidermal atrophy, cellular atypia, and disorderly epidermal differentiation (17).

Topical retinoids have been shown to improve fine wrinkling, increase dermal collagen, and repair elastin fiber formation. These properties make retinoids a suitable option for the treatment of photodamage in darker skin types. Early epidermal changes with retinoid use include increased epidermal mucin and compaction of the stratum corneum. These alterations may be seen as improvement in texture and fine wrinkles. Long-term topical tretinoin therapy can cause epidermal hyperplasia in atrophic skin, dispersion of melanin granules, destruction of dysplastic keratinocytes, production of new dermal collagen, angiogenesis, decreased elastolysis, and comedolysis (19). Clinically, the skin is smoother, with fewer fine lines and wrinkles and a more even tone. Topical alphahydroxy acid formulations can be combined with topical retinoid therapy to enhance the penetration in photodamaged skin; however, an increased irritation may ensue (20).

Tretinoin 0.1% cream has also been shown to lighten lentigines caused by photoaging in Chinese and Japanese populations. Griffiths et al. evaluated 23 Chinese and 22 Japanese patients in a vehicle-controlled study of 40 weeks' duration (21). Compared with the 33% of the vehicle-treated patients, 90% of the tretinoin-treated patients had significantly lighter lentigines. This clinical decrease in pigmentation was confirmed on histological analysis.

Topical retinoids are an important agent in treating ethnic skin. Retinoids are extremely useful for improving the appearance of hyperpigmentation, as well as improving photodamage. It is important to bear in mind that an excessive use of topical retinoids can result in inflammation of ethnic skin, which can potentially be a cause of PIH. When prescribing topical retinoids to ethnic patients, it is important to start with relatively small amounts and to instruct the patients to decrease or stop the use of these agents if they begin to develop significant irritation.

PROCEDURES TO IMPROVE HYPERPIGMENTATION

Chemical Peels

Chemical peels are another treatment option to attempt to improve hyperpigmentation in ethnic skin patients. Depending on the depth of the pigment, chemical peels may be an effective option. Unfortunately, the deeper the chemical peel, the greater is the risk for developing inflammation and HIP. As a result, relatively superficial chemical peels are often the best treatment option for these patients (22). A series of superficial peels is likely to be safer and ultimately more effective than a single deep peel. Most typically, superficial peels such as salicylic acids, glycolic acids, Jessner's solution, and weaker concentrations of trichloroacetic acids are the treatment options of choice in dark skin–type patients (23).

Laser Treatments

Laser technologies are a potential treatment option for hyperpigmentation. However, caution should be exercised, as these laser technologies may worsen the hyperpigmentation or cause other undesirable side effects in darker skin tones. This is particularly true with short wavelength lasers, such as the frequency doubled neodymium: yttrium-aluminum-garnet (Nd:YAG) (532 nm), alexandrite (755 nm), and diode (810 nm) devices. Lasers with longer wavelengths, such as the Nd:YAG (1064 nm) have less risk of causing these side effects, as the long wavelengths penetrate deeply into the dermis with relatively less absorption by epidermal melanocytes (24). These devices may be a therapeutic option for patients who have previously failed topical agents, and should be performed by a physician with experience treating patients with dark skin tones.

Fractional photothermolysis is a relatively new concept in which only a portion of the skin surface is treated with the laser device; the remainder of the skin is left untreated to help facilitate the healing process. The original fractionated device was a 1550-nm erbium doped laser, although several wavelengths are now utilized in similar fractionated devices. Due to the fact that only a portion of the skin surface is treated, higher energy fluences may be delivered to targeted tissue depths to result in greater clinical efficacy, while also reducing the risk of adverse effects. In clinical studies, nonablative fractional devices have been used to successfully treat melasma and other disorders of hyperpigmentation (25). In general, these devices are very safe. However, as per studies, fractional devices have been reported to cause hyperpigmentation and scarring, particularly in darker skin tones (26). By utilizing conservative parameters with lower treatment densities, low energies, and longer intervals between treatments coupled with strict perioperative photoprotection, ethnic skin patients may be able to achieve significant results with little adverse effects (27).

PREVENTION OF REPIGMENTATION

A final important component of effective treatment of hyperpigmentation is preventing the further development of inflammation and hyperpigmentation. If the hyperpigmentation is related to an underlying dermatitis or source of inflammation, this condition should be treated as early as possible; patients should also be educated to avoid the source of the irritation. This may necessitate the use of topical steroids early in the course of the dermatitis to minimize the risk of PIH.

Ultraviolet exposure can also worsen PIH. Patients should be educated that even if they do not sunburn or tan, ultraviolet exposure can exacerbate their PIH. As a result, patients should be counseled on the use of broad spectrum sunscreens, as well as sun protective clothing, in order to minimize this exposure. This can be challenging, as many ethnic patients with an increased epidermal melanin level, may not have previously used sunscreen (28).

CONCLUSIONS

Hyperpigmentation is one of the most frequent complaints in ethnic skin patients. The increased melanin content of dark ethnic skin makes it more susceptible to pigmentation disorders in response to inflammation, injury, and treatment. Unfortunately, while there are many options available for treatment, improving hyperpigmentation is still a challenge. When selecting a skin-lightening agent, it is important to select the optimal agent for the targeted disorder. It is essential to minimize irritation induced by the depigmenting agent, either by a proper selection of an agent or by combining it with a topical steroid. In many cases, a combination of active ingredients is more efficacious than a single agent. With proper selection and patient instruction, it is possible to use these agents to significantly reduce hyperpigmentation in our ethnic patients.

REFERENCES

1. Callender VD. Acne in ethnic skin: special considerations for therapy. Dermatol Ther 2004; 17: 184–95.
2. Sanquer S, Reenstra WR, Eller MS, Gilchrest BA. Keratinocytes and dermal factors activate CRABP-I in melanocytes. Exp Dermatol 1998; 7: 369–79.
3. Jimbow K, Obata H, Pathak MA, Fitzpatrick TB. Mechanism of depigmentation by hydroquinone. J Invest Dermatol 1974; 62: 436–49.
4. Taylor SC, Torok H, Jones T, et al. Efficacy and safety of a new triple-combination agent for the treatment of facial melasma. Cutis 2003; 72: 67–72.
5. Nordlund J, Grimes P, Ortonne JP. The safety of hydroquinone. J Cosmet Dermatol 2006; 5: 168–9.
6. Maeda K, Fukuda M. Arbutin: mechanism of its depigmenting action in human melanocyte culture. J Pharmacol Exp Ther 1996; 276: 765–9.
7. Fitton A, Goa KL. Azelaic acid. A review of its pharmacological properties and therapeutic efficacy in acne and hyperpigmentary skin disorders. Drugs 1991; 41: 780–98.
8. Guevara IL, Pandya AG. Safety and efficacy of 4% hydroquinone combined with 10% glycolic acid, antioxidants, and sunscreen in the treatment of melasma. Int J Dermatol 2003; 42: 966–72.
9. Lim JT. Treatment of melasma using kojic acid in a gel containing hydroquinone and glycolic acid. Dermatol Surg 1999; 25: 282–4.
10. Holloway VL. Ethnic cosmetic products. Dermatol Clin 2003; 21: 743–9.
11. Nair X, Parab P, Suhr L, Tramposch KM. Combination of 4-hydroxyanisole and all-trans retinoic acid produces synergistic skin depigmentation in swine. J Invest Dermatol 1993; 101: 145–9.
12. Jang D-II. Melanogenesis inhibitor from paper mulberry. Cosmet Toilet 1997; 112: 59–62.
13. Kollias N, Pote J, Wallo W, et al. Improvements in mottled hyperpigmentation with a soy-based moisturizer. Poster presented at: 61st Annual Meeting of the American Academy of Dermatology, San Francisco, CA, March 21–26, 2003.
14. Jarratt M. Mequinol 2%/tretinoin 0.01% solution: an effective and safe alternative to hydroquinone 3% in the treatment of solar lentigines. Cutis 2004; 74: 319–22.
15. Fitzpatrick RE, Rostan EF. Double-blind, half-face study comparing topical vitamin C and vehicle for rejuvenation of photodamage. Dermatol Surg 2002; 28: 231–6.
16. Grimes P, Callender V. Tazarotene cream for postinflammatory hyperpigmentation and acne vulgaris in darker skin: a double-blind, randomized, vehicle-controlled study. Cutis 2006; 77: 45–50.
17. Taylor SC. Skin of color: biology, structure, function, and implications for dermatologic disease. J Am Acad Dermatol 2002; 46(2 Suppl): S41–62.
18. Wolverton S. Comprehensive Dermatologic Drug Therapy, 7th edn. Philadelphia: W.B. Saunders Company, 2001.
19. Bhawan J. Short- and long-term histologic effects of topical tretinoin on photodamaged skin. Int J Dermatol 1998; 37: 286–92.
20. Takahashi S, Iwasaki J. Topical retinoids in Ethnic Skin. In: Grimes P, ed. Aesthetics and Cosmetic Surgery for Darker Skin Types. Philadelphia: Lippincott Williams & Wilkins, 2008: 86.
21. Griffiths CE, Goldfarb MT, Finkel LJ, et al. Topical tretinoin (retinoic acid) treatment of hyperpigmented lesions associated with photoaging in Chinese and Japanese patients: a vehicle-controlled trial. J Am Acad Dermatol 1994; 30: 76–84.
22. Grimes PE. Managment of hyperpigmentation in darker racial ethnic groups. Semin Cutan Med Surg 2009; 28: 77–85.
23. Davis EC, Callender VD. Postinflammatory hyperpigmentation: a review of the epidemiology, clinical features, and treatment options in skin of color. J Clin Aesthetic Dermatol 2010; 3: 20–31.
24. Battle EF Jr, Soden CE Jr. The use of lasers in darker skin types. Semin Cutan Med Surg 2009; 28: 130–40.
25. Katz TM, Glaich AS, Goldberg LH, et al. Treatment of melasma using fractional photothermolysis: a report of eight cases with long-term follow-up. Dermatol Surg 2010; 36: 1273–80.
26. Graber EM, Tanzi EL, Alster TS. Side effects and complications of fractional laser photothermolysis: experience with 961 treatments. Dermatol Surg 2008; 34: 301–5; discussion 305–7.
27. Kono T, Chan HH, Groff WF, et al. Prospective direct comparison study of fractional resurfacing using different fluences and densities for skin rejuvenation in Asians. Lasers Surg Med 2007; 39: 311–14.
28. Hall HI, Rogers JD. Sun protection behaviors among African Americans. Ethn Dis 1999; 9: 126–31.

5.3 Aesthetic treatments
Quyn S. Rahman and Stefani Takahashi

KEY POINTS

- It is important to be aware of the differences in the aging process in ethnic skin, as well as to fully discuss the patients' ultimate treatment goal for their cosmetic procedure
- Botulinum toxin can be used to soften the glabella, reshape eyebrows in ethnic patients, create a more rounded and youthful appearance to the eyes, as well as reshape the lower face of patients
- Dermal filler products can be utilized to improve nasolabial folds, reshape the malar cheeks, improve the appearance of lips, as well as perform rhinoplasty in ethnic patients
- Numerous laser technologies exist to offer photorejuvenation to ethnic patients. Initially, these technologies may have resulted in pigmentary changes and the potential for scarring. With current technologies, low energies and long pulse durations, ethnic patients can be effectively treated with lasers and light sources.

Facial aesthetic enhancement has grown with the development of numerous minimally invasive cosmetic procedures in ethnic groups. Non-Caucasians are slightly less likely to obtain cosmetic procedures compared with their Caucasian counterparts. Nonetheless, ethnic minorities account for a significant population interested in cosmetics procedures and will likely comprise a higher percentage of cosmetic procedures in the future (1). Our ethnic patients have slightly different ideals of beauty and tend to age differently from Caucasians, so it is important that their aesthetic treatments take into account these differences.

BOTULINUM TOXIN

Botulinum toxin is the most common cosmetic procedure performed in the United States. The reasons are simple: patients achieve excellent results to soften dynamic wrinkles through a quick, safe, minimal downtime procedure (2). While the initial studies of botulinum toxins were performed on Caucasian patients, new research is ongoing in the use of botulinum toxin for ethnic groups. These studies attempt to determine the ideal dosage of botulinum toxin, as well as the necessary placement of the botulinum toxin to help ethnic patients achieve their ideals of beauty.

Botulinum Toxin for Glabellar Rejuvenation

Dark skinned patients typically have fewer facial wrinkles compared with their age-matched fair skinned counterparts. Dynamic wrinkles in these individuals are predominantly in the upper face, notably the glabella region. Upper face aging is characterized by rhytides in the glabellar, periorbital, and nasal regions. Periorbital wrinkles are an early sign of facial aging and are caused by photodamage and muscle hyperactivity

(Fig. 5.3.1). Glabellar botulinum toxin injections result in diminished lines and wrinkles as well as enhanced brow position and shape (Fig. 5.3.2). In one study, Grimes et al. treated women of Fitzpatrick's skin types V and VI with botulinum toxin, which resulted in a reduced severity of glabellar lines with a high level of patient satisfaction (3). The effect was safe and lasted for the four-month duration of the study.

A recent study comparing the treatment of glabellar lines in Japanese patients with botulinum toxin in 2 doses of 10U or 20U divided equally across five injection sites, confirmed the safety and efficacy of both doses. Greater efficacy and longer duration of effect were seen with the 20U dose, although the difference was not statistically significant at all time points (4). The ideal dose in Japanese patients remains to be determined, but has been estimated by others to range between 15 and 17.5U total (5).

Botulinum Toxin for Eyelid Rejuvenation

A common complaint among Asian patients is aging eyelids, producing a tired appearance. While absolute redundancy of periorbital tissue is best treated with blepharoplasty, periorbital fat redistribution, and the classic brow lift, subtle yet significant improvement can be gained by the use of botulinum toxin alone. In regards to treating the upper eyelid and brow, Huang et al. examined the use of botulinum toxin as a means to temporarily lift the eyebrow (6). Each brow received 5U of botulinum toxin into the glabellar region, and 10U (in four equally spaced injections) along the lateral orbital rim below the brow. Significant elevations were noted in the brow, leading the authors to conclude that botulinum toxin is a safe and effective treatment for temporary brow lift. Placing the injections below the brow, yet lateral to the orbital rim minimized the incidence of brow ptosis.

(A) (B)

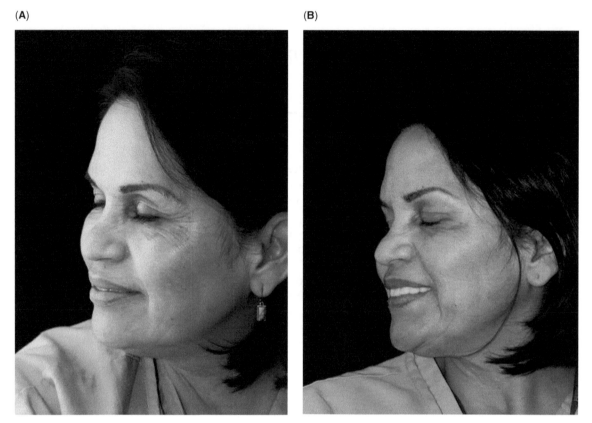

Figure 5.3.1 Periorbital rhytides at baseline (**A**); 1 week after treatment with botulinum toxin A (**B**).

(A) (B)

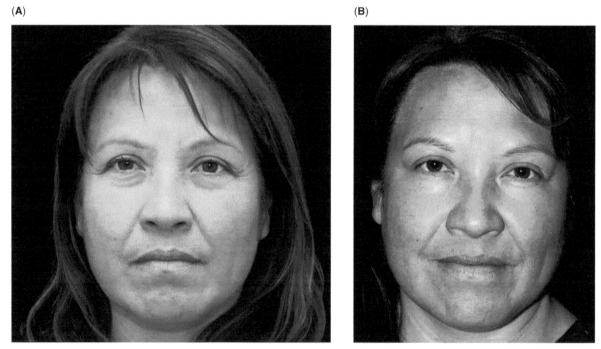

Figure 5.3.2 Before (**A**) and after (**B**) treatment in the glabellar area with 21 units of botulinum toxin A.

Addressing the lower eyelid, Asian patients may seek treatment of bulging in the lower periorbital area. These patients often benefit from injection of small amounts (2U) of botulinum toxin in the midpupillary line just below (3 mm) the inferior ciliary margin (7). This tends to provide a rounder, more youthful look to the eyes.

Treatment of crow's feet and the lateral brow can also help to widen the appearance of the eye, which is often a desired result in African-American, Hispanic, and Asian patients.

Botulinum Toxin for Lower Face Rejuvenation

Botulinum toxin is often used to reverse signs of lower face aging, including perioral wrinkles. However, perioral wrinkles are typically less prominent in African-Americans when compared with Caucasians, likely due to the common fullness of the lips in the African-American population. Botulinum toxin can increase the fullness of the lips and cause slight eversion of the upper lip when used for the correction of perioral wrinkles. This may be seen as an undesirable effect in some African-American patients, so conservative treatment should be undertaken (8). Often, combination treatments with botulinum toxin and hyaluronic acid fillers provide better results than botulinum toxin monotherapy.

A prominent mandibular angle, resulting in the appearance of a square face, is a common reason for aesthetic treatment in Asian women. This feature is thought to be secondary to hypertrophic masseteric muscles in addition to a wider mandibular angle. In a clinical study, 25–30 U of botulinum toxin were injected into each side of the face, spread across 5–6 injection points into the masseter muscle. Ultrasounds and CT scans performed one month after the injection revealed an approximately 20% reduction in the mean masseter thickness. Additionally, 80% of the patients were satisfied with the contouring effects of the treatment (9). Another clinical study demonstrated similar results with another formulation of botulinum toxin (10).

INJECTABLE FILLERS

Dermal fillers are the third most common nonsurgical cosmetic procedure performed, after botulinum toxin and laser hair removal. Fillers are used in the treatment of fine lines, deeper folds, lip augmentation, and volume depletion of the cheeks. Collagen was once the most commonly used dermal filler and has been used with great success for more than 20 years. More recently, hyaluronic acid fillers have become the most popular dermal filler injectable products because of their long duration and excellent safety profile (1).

Photoaging is minimal in dark skin types, partly due to the inherent sun protection factor provided by an increase in melanin and melanosome distribution. Fine and deep rhytides that are characteristic of Caucasian skin are less prevalent in dark skin types. Therefore, younger patients with dark skin tend to need fillers less frequently than their Caucasian counterparts (11).

Dermal Fillers in Ethnic Populations

Dermal fillers in ethnic skin types, particularly African-Americans, have a predominant role in the treatment of midface aging. Loss of volume in the midface and heavier cheeks is a common finding in the aging population, particularly in African-American patients. Treating the nasolabial folds combined with malar augmentation results in a significant improvement for patients. Depending on the specific patient, and their cosmetic goals, the amount of volume necessary as well as the ratio between malar augmentation and nasolabial fold correction will vary.

Lip augmentation is also a common presenting issue in ethnic populations. In Asian populations, lips project more than the nose and chin, whereas in Caucasians, the projection of the nose and chin are more prominent. With aging, the lips of Asian patients tend to deflate and flatten. By contrast, African-American patients often have fuller lips with less loss of volume over time. As a result, these patients may be less likely to seek treatment for lip augmentation. The treatment goal in ethnic patients seeking lip rejuvenation is to restore the volume with filler substances without causing excess protrusion (6). These changes can be readily accomplished with filler products. Historically, fine collagen products were often used for restoring volume to the lips. More recently, hyaluronic acid products have been most commonly used for lip rejuvenation.

Rejuvenation around the perioral area, as well as the chin, is another common reason for patients to seek treatment. Marionette lines, as well as prejowl sulci, often develop in ethnic populations as they age. These areas are easily amenable to treatment with dermal filler products (12). More robust hyaluronic acid filler products may result in greater improvement. It is important to bear in mind that depending on the ethnicity of the patient, injecting fillers into the lower face may lead to a rounder appearance, which may or may not be cosmetically desirable to the patient.

Dermal fillers can also be utilized to reshape eyebrows (13). As we age, the eyebrows may become heavy and develop ptosis. While surgical brow lift remains the most definitive treatment, many patients are increasingly turning to minimally invasive filler injections. Ethnic patients may elect to have these injections performed to reshape their eyebrows, either creating or reducing an angular arched appearance. Dermal fillers should be injected deeply, even periosteally, when rejuvenating these areas.

Filler rhinoplasty, or augmentation rhinoplasty, is an evolving field, and may be suitable for nasal rejuvenation in patients with ethnic skin. With aging, a nasal tip drop is observed, along with a loss of subcutaneous tissue. De Lacerda and Zancanaro reported on the use of dermal fillers (hyaluronic acid and porcine collagen) to obtain changes in the frontonasal angle, nasal dorsum, and columella–philtrum junction (14). Filler injections resulted in an elevated nasal tip, smooth nasal dorsum, and an overall more youthful appearance with the illusion of a smaller nose. Long lasting results can be seen up to one year after the procedure.

It is important that the patients' ultimate goals for rejuvenation be borne in mind. Ethnic populations may have slightly different baseline features and ideals of beauty compared with Caucasian patients. As a result, the exact product and volume necessary to achieve the patient's cosmetic goals will need to be individualized.

Dermal Filler Safety Profile in Ethnic Skin

Studies have shown that hyaluronic acid fillers are effective and well tolerated in persons of color. Grimes et al. compared Juvederm® (hyaluronic acid product manufactured by Allergan Inc, Irvine, California, USA) with bovine collagen for the treatment of nasolabial folds in African-American and Caucasian patients (15). No difference in efficacy based on skin type was observed throughout the 24-week duration of the study. Moreover, there was no increased incidence of hyperpigmentation or hypertrophic scarring in the African-American group.

Currently, there is no evidence that darker racial groups experience a greater complication rate than Caucasians. Since dark skin types are more prone to dyschromic conditions, including ephelides, melasma, and postinflammatory hyperpigmentation, as well as keloid formation and hypertrophic scarring, all injections should proceed gingerly to avoid prolonged trauma to the skin. It appears that any individual demonstrating an inflammatory response is at risk of postinflammatory hyperpigmentation regardless of the color of their skin. Even Caucasians showing prolonged erythema after procedures have the potential to develop dyspigmentation. In all patient populations, especially those with dark racial ethnic skin, an injection technique using fewer injections with a threading pattern rather than multiple injections per treatment area should be considered (9). Any hyperpigmentation that results can be treated with standard therapeutic options such as bleaching agents, retinoids, and exfoliating agents.

LASERS AND LIGHT SOURCES FOR PHOTOREJUVENATION

Photorejuvenation is defined as the use of visible or infrared light energy source to reverse the process of sun-induced or environmental skin damage (16). This may be accomplished in a nondestructive, or nonablative, fashion, where visible disruption of the overlying epidermis does not occur. This is the preferred laser treatment of choice to minimize the risk of postinflammatory hyperpigmentation or hypopigmenation in ethnic populations. Nonablative skin rejuvenation involves the use of a laser or light source together with a cooling device to improve signs of photoaging, namely dyspigmentation, fine wrinkles, textural alterations, prominent pores, telangiectasias, and skin laxity (17).

Patients with a dark skin tone present a greater challenge to laser treatment. Mechanistically, melanin has a wide absorption spectrum, ranging from 250 to 1200 nm, and can be targeted by all visible light and near-infrared dermatologic lasers. Laser energy intended for dermal chromophores such as hemoglobin, follicles, water, and even fat can be easily absorbed by melanin in the basal layer of the epidermis. If sufficient absorption occurs, unintended epidermal damage may result in blistering, permanent hyper- or hypopigmentation, textural changes, atrophy, and scarring (18). In addition, competitive absorption by epidermal melanin substantially decreases the total amount of energy reaching the intended dermal chromophores, resulting in less clinical effects.

While nonablative techniques are the preferred option in dark skinned patients due to the lower association with postprocedure adverse events (19), ablative techniques abound in an attempt to "push the envelope." These ablative technologies have a higher incidence of adverse effects, particularly potentially permanent hyper- and hypopigmentation, as well as scarring. For this reason, we do not advocate performing fully ablative resurfacing on dark skinned ethnic patients. These patients should be referred to a physician specializing in skin resurfacing with significant experience in treating dark skinned ethnic patients.

Nonablative Technologies

A wide range of lasers or light sources are available for nonablative skin rejuvenation, including visible green-yellow (the frequency doubled neodymium: yttrium-aluminum-garnet (Nd:YAG) 532-nm laser; 585-nm or 595-nm pulsed dye laser), near infrared and infrared lasers (1064-nm Nd:YAG, 1320-nm Nd:YAG, 1450-nm diode, 1540-nm erbium glass), and intense pulsed light (IPL) sources. Patients typically experience a mild degree of erythema lasting 24 hours, as well as darkening of the lentigines immediately after the procedure. Repeated monthly treatments, usually for six months, may be necessary to achieve the desired clinical effect (14). Strict perioperative use of topical bleaching agents and sun protective measures is valuable in optimizing outcomes, while performing a small test spot on a representative lesion four weeks before treating the entire area is prudent.

The 532-nm Nd:YAG Laser

Besides being utilized in its ablative Q-switched mode classically, the 532-nm Nd:YAG laser has also been reported for use in treating pigmented and telangiectatic components of photoaging in patients of dark skin phototypes. Rashid et al. reported a 50% improvement rate with the use of the 532-nm quasi-continuous laser in the treatment of lentigines in Fitzpatrick skin type IV patients (20). A 10% incidence of hyperpigmentation and a 25% incidence of hypopigmentation were reported after multiple treatments. The adverse events abated after two to six months. In comparing the long pulsed 532-nm laser with the conventional Q-switched laser for the treatment of lentigines, Chan et al. revealed no significant difference in the degree of clearing (21).

Pulsed Dye Laser (585–595 nm)

Pulsed dye lasers (PDL) target the epidermal pigment and papillary dermal vessels through hemoglobin absorption. Injury to dermal vessels allows an effective treatment of facial telangiectasias and also results in new collagen formation. The microvascular supply of sebaceous glands is affected, reducing sebum production and improving the pore size (14). The pulsed dye laser can be used to safely and effectively treat telangiectasias and vascular lesions in ethnic populations, though pigmentary alterations can result.

Skin cooling is essential when treating ethnic skin with visible and near infrared lasers, including pulsed dye lasers, to decrease the likelihood of pigmentary alterations. Skin cooling allows the thermal energy to penetrate deeper, treating the underlying vessels, dermis, and sebaceous glands. Without efficient cooling, light absorbed by melanin is converted to heat, creating epidermal thermal injury (22). This effect can be utilized by experienced physicians to create controlled epidermal injury. A glass slide can be used to compress the skin, and in the process, block the cryogen spray from cooling the skin. The laser energy is then absorbed by the epidermis. Glass slide compression is sometimes used in Asian patients to treat lentigines, though temporary hyperpigmentation is commonly seen (23,24).

Intense Pulsed Light

Another device for photorejuvenation of ethnic skin is IPL. Negishi et al. investigated the use of IPL in Asians for skin rejuvenation in 97 patients (25). A cutoff filter of 550 nm was used. Investigators found that 90% of patients experienced a reduction in pigmentation, 83% experienced an improvement in telangiectasias, and 65% experienced an improvement in texture after three treatment sessions. The group observed no cases of PIH. However, a lower efficacy of IPL compared with other nonablative laser modalities is generally cited. A split-face study comparing IPL versus PDL in 10 Asian patients revealed a 62% versus 81% improvement in lentigines, respectively, and no difference in wrinkle improvement (26).

The 1064-nm Nd:YAG Laser

Long-pulsed 1064-nm lasers target melanin, hemoglobin, and water, with less preference for melanin compared to their 532-nm counterparts. Nevertheless, epidermal cooling is critical when using this infrared wavelength for rejuvenation in dark skin types (19). Most commonly, the long-pulsed 1064-nm laser is used for laser hair removal in dark skinned patients. Previously, ethnic patients could not undergo laser hair removal without significant risk of hyperpigmentation or scarring. The development of the long-pulsed 1064-nm laser revolutionized the field of laser hair removal in dark skinned patients. The increased wavelength allows for decreased epidermal melanin absorption and increased penetration depth. The long pulse duration causes slower heating, and results in a lower incidence of dyspigmentation (27,28).

In addition to its use in laser hair removal, the long-pulsed 1064-nm laser can be used for photorejuvenation. Lee et al. treated 150 patients with the long-pulsed potassium titanyl phosphate (KTP) 532-nm laser and long-pulsed Nd:YAG 1064-nm laser separately and in combination (29). Patients were treated monthly, three to six times, and followed up to 18 months after the last treatment. All 150 patients were found to have a mild to moderate degree of improvement in wrinkling, a moderate degree of improvement in skin tone and texture, and a significant degree of improvement in redness and pigmentation. The KTP and Nd:YAG laser combination was superior to either laser used alone.

The 1320-nm Nd:YAG Laser

Infrared lasers that strictly target water as a chromophore are important for avoiding melanin in ethnic skin. The wavelengths used in ethnic skin for treatment of wrinkles and acne scars are 1320 nm, 1450 nm, and 1540 nm (19).

Several studies have been conducted using the 1320-nm Nd:YAG on ethnic skin. Trelles et al. evaluated rejuvenation in patients with type IV skin and found histologic improvement and fair to significant clinical improvement four to six months after twice-weekly treatments for four weeks (30). However, there was ultimately low patient satisfaction, as the laser did not result in significant efficacy particularly with the treatment of dynamic rhytides.

Fractional Photothermolysis

Fractional photothermolysis utilizes a nonablative erbium-doped (1540 nm) laser treatment for facial rejuvenation; however, instead of treating the entire skin surface, its laser output is broken up into small columns of light known as microthermal zones (31). It is thought that by breaking up the laser energy into these microthermal zones, the risk of adverse events would be decreased with no significant change in the treatment efficacy. Fractionated technologies are an attempt to balance the increased clinical efficacy of aggressive or ablative technologies with the reduced downtime and decreased risk of nonablative technologies.

Fractional photothermolysis has been reported to be efficacious in the treatment of many conditions, including facial tone and texture, rhytides, photodamage, dyspigmentation, melasma, lentigines, acne, striae, and scarring (32). In general, these fractional technologies are very safe and effective, both in fair skinned and ethnic populations. Chan et al. reported a successful use of fractional resurfacing in Asian patients with Fitzpatrick's type IV skin (33). The investigators found that patients treated with high energy but low density of microthermal zones [16 mJ, 1000 microscopic treatment zone (MTZ)] had a lower prevalence of PIH than those treated with a low energy but high density of microthermal zones (8 mJ, 2000 MTZ). Numerous other erbium and carbon dioxide lasers touting similar pixilated patterns of treatment are being used to successfully treat patients with dark skin phototypes.

When using fractionated technologies to treat patients with dark skin tones, caution should be used as these patients are likely to have increased risk of post-treatment hyperpigmentation and/or scarring. In general, conservative parameters stressing lower treatment densities, low energies, and longer intervals between treatments coupled with strict perioperative photoprotection may bring significant results with little adverse effects.

CONCLUSIONS

The growth of cosmetic procedures is increasing rapidly in dark skinned racial ethnic groups. While many aesthetic treatments have shown to be effective and well tolerated in ethnic skin, a consideration of skin type and pigmentation is crucial in selecting optimal treatment approaches for these patients. Botulinum toxin, dermal fillers, and laser technologies can all be safely utilized to help our ethnic patients achieve their ideals of beauty. The approach to aesthetic treatment of ethnic skin, like that of all patients, must take into account personal and cultural concepts, as well as the bone structure and musculature of their face. When treating this population, the physician should view each individual's presentation uniquely in order to provide a balanced aesthetic outcome. Sensitivity and consideration of cultural and ethnic aesthetic ideals should play a major role in the treatment plan. Individual and ethnic identification must be maintained to provide a natural and enhanced cosmetic outcome (6).

REFERENCES

1. Beddingfield F, Kim J. Fillers in ethnic skin. In: Grimes P, ed. Aesthetics and Cosmetic Surgery for Darker Skin Types. Philadelphia: Lippincott Williams & Wilkins, 2008: 225.
2. Carruthers J, Carruthers A. BOTOX use in the mid and lower face and neck. Semin Cutan Med Surg 2001; 20: 85–92.
3. Grimes P. A four-month randomized, double masked evaluation of the efficacy of botulinum toxin type A for the treatment of glabellar lines in women with skin types V and VI. In American Academy of Dermatology 62nd Annual Meeting. Washington DC, 2004.

4. Harii K, Kawashima M. A double-blind, randomized, placebo-controlled, two-dose comparative study of botulinum toxin type A for treating glabellar lines in Japanese subjects. Aesthetic Plast Surg 2008; 32: 724–30.

5. Kane MA. A double-blind, randomized, placebo-controlled, two-dose comparative study of botulinum toxin type A for treating glabellar lines in Japanese subjects. Aesthetic Plast Surg 2008; 32: 933–5.

6. Huang W, Rogachefsky AS, Foster JA. Browlift with botulinum toxin. Dermatol Surg 2000; 26: 55–60.

7. Carruthers JD, Glogau RG, Blitzer A. Advances in facial rejuvenation: botulinum toxin type a, hyaluronic acid dermal fillers, and combination therapies–consensus recommendations. Plast Reconstr Surg 2008; 121 (5 Suppl): 5S–30.

8. Semchyshyn N, Sengelmann RD. Botulinum toxin A treatment of perioral rhytides. Dermatol Surg 2003; 29: 490–5.

9. Park MY, Ahn KY, Jung DS. Botulinum toxin type A treatment for contouring of the lower face. Dermatol Surg 2003; 29: 477–83.

10. Yu CC, Chen PK, Chen YR. Botulinum toxin a for lower facial contouring: a prospective study. Aesthetic Plast Surg 2007; 31: 445–51.

11. Beddingfield F, Kim J. Fillers in Ethnic Skin. In: Grimes P, ed. Aesthetics and Cosmetic Surgery for Darker Skin Types. Philadelphia: Lippincott Williams & Wilkins, 2008: 236–7.

12. Weinkle S. Injection techniques for revolumization of the perioral region with hyaluronic acid. J Drugs Dermatol 2010; 9: 367–71.

13. Andre P. New trends in face rejuvenation by hyaluronic acid injections. J Cosmet Dermatol 2008; 7: 251–8.

14. DeLacerda DA, Zancanaro P. Filler rhinoplasty. Dermatol Surg 2007; 33(Suppl 2): S207–12.

15. Grimes P, Thomas J, Carruthers J. Efficacy and safety of novel hyaluronic acid-based fillers and crosslinked bovine collagen in Caucasians and persons of color. In American Academy of Dermatology's 2006 Summer Meeting. San Diego, CA, 2006.

16. Weiss RA, McDaniel DH, Geronemus RG, Weiss MA. Clinical trial of a novel non-thermal LED array for reversal of photoaging: clinical, histologic, and surface profilometric results. Lasers Surg Med 2005; 36: 85–91.

17. Chan HH. Ablative and Nonablative Resurfacing in Darker Skin. In: Grimes P, ed. Aesthetics and Cosmetic Surgery for Darker Skin Types. Philadelphia: Lippincott Williams & Wilkins, 2008: 179–82.

18. Tanzi EL, Williams CM, Alster TS. Treatment of facial rhytides with a nonablative 1,450-nm diode laser: a controlled clinical and histologic study. Dermatol Surg 2003; 29: 124–8.

19. Ruiz-Esparza J, Barba Gomez JM, Gomez de la Torre OL, Huerta Franco B, Parga Vazquez EG. UltraPulse laser skin resurfacing in Hispanic patients. A prospective study of 36 individuals. Dermatol Surg 1998; 24: 59–62.

20. Rashid T, Hussain I, Haider M, Haroon TS. Laser therapy of freckles and lentigines with quasi-continuous, frequency-doubled, Nd:YAG (532 nm) laser in Fitzpatrick skin type IV: a 24-month follow-up. J Cosmet Laser Ther 2002; 4: 81–5.

21. Chan HH, Fung WK, Ying SY, Kono T. An in vivo trial comparing the use of different types of 532 nm Nd:YAG lasers in the treatment of facial lentigines in oriental patients. Dermatol Surg 2000; 26: 743–9.

22. Munavalli GS, Weiss RA, Halder RM. Photoaging and nonablative photorejuvenation in ethnic skin. Dermatol Surg 2005; 31(9 Pt 2): 1250–60.

23. Kono T, Chan HH, Groff WF, et al. Long-pulse pulsed dye laser delivered with compression for treatment of facial lentigines. Dermatol Surg 2007; 33: 945–50.

24. Kono T, Manstein D, Chan HH, Nozaki M, Anderson RR. Q-switched ruby versus long-pulsed dye laser delivered with compression for treatment of facial lentigines in Asians. Lasers Surg Med 2006; 38: 94–7.

25. Negishi K, Tezuka Y, Kushikata N, Wakamatsu S. Photorejuvenation for Asian skin by intense pulsed light. Dermatol Surg 2001; 27: 627–31.

26. Kono T, Groff WF, Sakurai H, et al. Comparison study of intense pulsed light versus a long-pulse pulsed dye laser in the treatment of facial skin rejuvenation. Ann Plast Surg 2007; 59: 479–83.

27. Greppi I. Diode laser hair removal of the black patient. Lasers Surg Med 2001; 28: 150–5.

28. Alster TS, Bryan H, Williams CM. Long-pulsed Nd:YAG laser-assisted hair removal in pigmented skin: a clinical and histological evaluation. Arch Dermatol 2001; 137: 885–9.

29. Lee MW. Combination visible and infrared lasers for skin rejuvenation. Semin Cutan Med Surg 2002; 21: 288–300.

30. Trelles MA, Allones I, Luna R. Facial rejuvenation with a nonablative 1320 nm Nd:YAG laser: a preliminary clinical and histologic evaluation. Dermatol Surg 2001; 27: 111–16.

31. Manstein D, Herron GS, Sink RK, Tanner H, Anderson RR. Fractional photothermolysis: a new concept for cutaneous remodeling using microscopic patterns of thermal injury. Lasers Surg Med 2004; 34: 426–38.

32. Sherling M, Friedman PM, Adrian R, et al. Consensus recommendations on the use of an erbium-doped 1,550-nm fractionated laser and its applications in dermatologic laser surgery. Dermatol Surg 2010; 36: 461–9.

33. Chan HH. Effective and safe use of lasers, light sources, and radiofrequency devices in the clinical management of Asian patients with selected dermatoses. Lasers Surg Med 2005; 37: 179–85.

Index